Alternative Uses of Dermatoscopy

Editors

GIUSEPPE MICALI

FRANCESCO LACARRUBBA

DERMATOLOGIC CLINICS

www.derm.theclinics.com

Consulting Editor

BRUCE H. THIERS

October 2018 • Volume 36 • Number 4

ELSEVIER

1600 John F. Kennedy Boulevard • Suite 1800 • Philadelphia, Pennsylvania, 19103-2899

http://www.theclinics.com

DERMATOLOGIC CLINICS Volume 36, Number 4
October 2018 ISSN 0733-8635, ISBN-13: 978-0-323-64123-4

Editor: Jessica McCool
Developmental Editor: Sara Watkins

Dermatologic Clinics (ISSN 0733-8635) is published quarterly by Elsevier Inc., 360 Park Avenue South, New York, NY 10010-1710. Months of publication are January, April, July, and October. Business and editorial offices: 1600 John F. Kennedy Blvd., Suite 1800, Philadelphia, PA 19103-2899. Customer service office: 11830 Westline Drive, St. Louis, MO 63146. Periodicals postage paid at New York, NY, and additional mailing offices. Subscription prices are USD 392.00 per year for US individuals, USD 701.00 per year for US institutions, USD 451.00 per year for Canadian individuals, USD 855.00 per year for Canadian institutions, USD 505.00 per year for international individuals, USD 855.00 per year for international institutions, USD 100.00 per year for US students/residents, and USD 240.00 per year for Canadian and international students/residents. International air speed delivery is included in all *Clinics* subscription prices. All prices are subject to change without notice. **POSTMASTER:** Send address changes to *Dermatologic Clinics*, Elsevier Health Sciences Division, Subscription Customer Service, 3251 Riverport Lane, Maryland Heights, MO 63043. **Customer Service: 1-800-654-2452 (U.S. and Canada); 314-447-8871 (outside U.S. and Canada). Fax: 314-447-8029. E-mail: journalscustomerservice-usa@elsevier.com (for print support); journalsonlinesupport-usa@elsevier.com (for online support).**

Reprints. For copies of 100 or more, of articles in this publication, please contact the Commercial Reprints Department, Elsevier Inc., 360 Park Avenue South, New York, New York 10010-1710. Tel.: 212-633-3874; Fax: 212-633-3820; Email: reprints@elsevier.com.

The *Dermatologic Clinics* is covered in *MEDLINE/PubMed (Index Medicus), Current Contents/Clinical Medicine, Excerpta Medica, Chemical Abstracts,* and *ISI/BIOMED*.

Contributors

CONSULTING EDITOR

BRUCE H. THIERS, MD
Professor and Chairman Emeritus, Department of Dermatology and Dermatologic Surgery, Medical University of South Carolina, Charleston, South Carolina, USA

EDITORS

GIUSEPPE MICALI, MD
Full Professor, Chair, Dermatology Clinic, University of Catania, Catania, Italy

FRANCESCO LACARRUBBA, MD
Assistant Professor, Dermatology Clinic, University of Catania, Catania, Italy

AUTHORS

AURORA ALESSANDRINI, MD
Specialist, Department of Specialised Experimental and Diagnostic Medicine, Dermatology, Alma Mater Studiorum, Università di Bologna, Bologna, Italy

ROBERTO ALFANO, MD
Department of Anesthesiology, Surgery and Emergency, Second University of Naples, Naples, Italy

ZOE APALLA, MD, PhD
1st Department of Dermatology – Venereology, State Clinic of Dermatology, Aristotle University of Thessaloniki, Hospital of Skin and Venereal Diseases, Thessaloniki, Greece

MARCO ARDIGÒ, MD
Department of Clinical Dermatology, San Gallicano Dermatological Institute, Rome, Italy

GIUSEPPE ARGENZIANO, MD, PhD
Dermatology Unit, University of Campania Luigi Vanvitelli, Naples, Italy

JOSÉ BAÑULS, MD, PhD
Dermatology Department, Hospital General Universitario de Alicante, ISABIAL, Alicante, Spain

CATERINA BOMBONATO, MD
Centro Oncologico ad Alta Tecnologia Diagnostica, Azienda Unità Sanitaria Locale – IRCCS di Reggio Emilia, Italy

ALESSANDRO BORGHI, MD
Professor, Department of Medical Sciences, Section of Dermatology and Infectious Diseases, University of Ferrara, Ferrara, Italy

GABRIELLA BRANCACCIO, MD
Dermatology Unit, University of Campania Luigi Vanvitelli, Naples, Italy

MANAS CHATTERJEE, MD, DNB
Senior Adviser, Professor, HOD, Department of Dermatology, INHS Asvini, Mumbai, India

ELISA CINOTTI, MD, PhD
Department of Medical, Surgical and Neurological Science, Dermatology Section, University of Siena, S. Maria alle Scotte Hospital, Siena, Italy

MONICA CORAZZA, MD
Professor, Department of Medical Sciences, Section of Dermatology and Infectious Diseases, University of Ferrara, Ferrara, Italy

ALESSANDRO DI STEFANI, MD
Institute of Dermatology, Catholic University of the Sacred Heart, Rome, Italy

FRANCO DINOTTA, MD
Dermatology Clinic, University of Catania, Catania, Italy

ENZO ERRICHETTI, MD, MSc, DVD
Department of Medical Area, Institute of Dermatology, University of Udine, Udine, Italy

MICHELE FIMIANI, MD
Department of Medical, Surgical and Neurological Science, Dermatology Section, University of Siena, S. Maria alle Scotte Hospital, Siena, Italy

IGNACIO GÓMEZ-MARTÍN, MD
Dermatology Department, Hospital Sant Pau i Santa Tecla, Tarragona, Spain

PELLACANI GIOVANNI, MD
Dermatology Department, University of Modena and Reggio Emilia, Italy

DAMIEN GRIVET, MD
Department of Ophthalmology, University Hospital of Saint-Etienne, Laboratory Biology, Engineering and Imaging of Corneal Graft, Jean Monnet University, Saint-Etienne, France

DIMITRIOS IOANNIDES, MD, PhD
1st Department of Dermatology – Venereology, State Clinic of Dermatology, Aristotle University of Thessaloniki, Hospital of Skin and Venereal Diseases, Thessaloniki, Greece

MATHILDE KASPI, MD
Department of Ophthalmology, University Hospital of Saint-Etienne, Laboratory Biology, Engineering and Imaging of Corneal Graft, Jean Monnet University, Saint-Etienne, France

ALEXANDER KATOULIS, MD, PhD
2nd Department of Dermatology – Venereology, National Kapodistrian University of Athens, ATTIKON University Hospital, Athens, Greece

ANNA LA ROCCA, MD
Department of Medical, Surgical and Neurological Science, Dermatology Section, University of Siena, S. Maria alle Scotte Hospital, Siena, Italy

BRUNO LABEILLE, MD
Department of Dermatology, University Hospital of Saint-Etienne, Saint-Etienne, France

FRANCESCO LACARRUBBA, MD
Assistant Professor, Dermatology Clinic, University of Catania, Catania, Italy

AIMILIOS LALLAS, MD, MSc, PhD
1st Department of Dermatology – Venereology, State Clinic of Dermatology, Aristotle University of Thessaloniki, Hospital of Skin and Venereal Diseases, Thessaloniki, Greece

VICTOR LAMBERT, MD
Department of Ophthalmology, University Hospital of Saint-Etienne, Laboratory Biology, Engineering and Imaging of Corneal Graft, Jean Monnet University, Saint-Etienne, France

CATERINA LONGO, MD, PhD
Centro Oncologico ad Alta Tecnologia Diagnostica, Azienda Unità Sanitaria Locale – IRCCS di Reggio Emilia, Dermatology Department, University of Modena and Reggio Emilia, Italy

JOSÉ MARÍA MARTIN, MD, PhD
Dermatology Department, Hospital Clínico Universitario, Valencia, Spain

GIUSEPPE MICALI, MD
Full Professor, Chair, Dermatology Clinic, University of Catania, Catania, Italy

ELVIRA MOSCARELLA, MD
Dermatology Unit, University of Campania Luigi Vanvitelli, Naples, Italy

NICCOLÒ NAMI, MD
Department of Medical, Surgical and Neurological Science, Dermatology Section, University of Siena, S. Maria Alle Scotte Hospital, Siena, Italy

SHEKHAR NEEMA, MD
Assistant Professor, Department of Dermatology, Command Hospital, Kolkata, West Bengal, India

CHAU YEE NG, MD
Department of Dermatology, College of Medicine, Chang Gung Memorial Hospital, Taoyuan, Taiwan

MAŁGORZATA OLSZEWSKA, MD, PhD
Professor, Department of Dermatology, Medical University of Warsaw, Warsaw, Poland

RICCARDO PAMPENA, MD
Centro Oncologico ad Alta Tecnologia Diagnostica, Azienda Unità Sanitaria Locale – IRCCS di Reggio Emilia, Italy

JEAN LUC PERROT, MD, PhD
Department of Dermatology, University Hospital of Saint-Etienne, Saint-Etienne, France

VINCENZO PICCOLO, MD
Dermatology Unit, University of Campania Luigi Vanvitelli, Naples, Italy

BIANCA MARIA PIRACCINI, MD, PhD
Professor, Associate Professor, Department of Specialised Experimental and Diagnostic Medicine, Dermatology, Alma Mater Studiorum, Università di Bologna, Bologna, Italy

RODRIGO PIRMEZ, MD
Dermatologist, Dermatology Department, Instituto de Dermatologia Professor Rubem David Azulay, Santa Casa de Misericórdia do Rio de Janeiro, Rio de Janeiro, Rio de Janeiro, Brazil

ENRICA QUATTROCCHI, MD
Dermatology Clinic, University of Catania, Catania, Italy

ADRIANA RAKOWSKA, MD, PhD
Associate Professor, Department of Dermatology, Medical University of Warsaw, Warsaw, Poland

DIMITRIOS RIGOPOULOS, MD, PhD
1st Department of Dermatology – Venereology, National Kapodistrian University of Athens, A. Syggros Hospital, Athens, Greece

PIETRO RUBEGNI, MD, PhD
Department of Medical, Surgical and Neurological Science, Dermatology Section, University of Siena, S. Maria alle Scotte Hospital, Siena, Italy

LIDIA RUDNICKA, MD, PhD
Professor, Department of Neuropeptides, Mossakowski Medical Research Centre Polish Academy of Sciences, Warsaw, Poland

TERESA RUSSO, MD
Dermatology Unit, University of Campania Luigi Vanvitelli, Naples, Italy

DIMITRIOS SGOUROS, MD
2nd Department of Dermatology – Venereology, National Kapodistrian University of Athens, ATTIKON University Hospital, Athens, Greece

ELENA SOTIRIOU, MD, PhD
1st Department of Dermatology – Venereology, State Clinic of Dermatology, Aristotle University of Thessaloniki, Hospital of Skin and Venereal Diseases, Thessaloniki, Greece

MICHELA STARACE, MD, PhD
Fellow Researcher, Department of Specialised Experimental and Diagnostic Medicine, Dermatology, Alma Mater Studiorum, Università di Bologna, Bologna, Italy

GIUSEPPE STINCO, MD, MSc, DVD
Department of Medical Area, Institute of Dermatology, University of Udine, Udine, Italy

ALEXANDER STRATIGOS, MD, PhD
1st Department of Dermatology – Venereology, National Kapodistrian University of Athens, A. Syggros Hospital, Athens, Greece

LINDA TOGNETTI, MD
Department of Medical, Surgical and Neurological Science, Dermatology Section, University of Siena, S. Maria alle Scotte Hospital, Siena, Italy

ANTONELLA TOSTI, MD
Professor, Department of Dermatology and Cutaneous Surgery, University of Miami Miller School of Medicine, University of Miami, Miami, Florida, USA

EFSTRATIOS VAKIRLIS, MD, PhD
1st Department of Dermatology – Venereology, State Clinic of Dermatology, Aristotle University of Thessaloniki, Hospital of Skin and Venereal Diseases, Thessaloniki, Greece

ANNA ELISA VERZÌ, MD
Dermatology Clinic, University of Catania, Catania, Italy

ANNAROSA VIRGILI, MD
Professor, Department of Medical Sciences, Section of Dermatology and Infectious Diseases, University of Ferrara

ANNA WAŚKIEL, MD
Research Assistant, Department of Dermatology, Medical University of Warsaw, Warsaw, Poland

PEDRO ZABALLOS, MD, PhD
Dermatology Department, Hospital Sant Pau i Santa Tecla, Tarragona, Spain

Contents

Erratum xiii

Preface: The Expanding Use of Dermatoscopy xv

Giuseppe Micali and Francesco Lacarrubba

Dermatoscopy: Instrumental Update 345

Giuseppe Micali and Francesco Lacarrubba

Dermatoscopy is a noninvasive technique that allows in vivo magnified observation of skin details and structures not visible to the naked eye. It may be performed using handheld devices or computer-assisted digital systems or videodermatoscopes. The handheld dermatoscope is the most used device because it is user-friendly and relatively inexpensive. It is not a mere magnifying glass but a more complex instrument that allows the visualization of the cutaneous microstructures of the different skin layers. Videodermatoscopes are more expensive systems that allow higher magnifications and simplify the process of image viewing, storage, organization, analysis, and retrieval.

Dermatoscopy of Parasitic and Infectious Disorders 349

Anna Elisa Verzì, Francesco Lacarrubba, Franco Dinotta, and Giuseppe Micali

The use of dermatoscopy in the diagnosis and management of parasitic and infectious skin disorders has been defined as entodermoscopy, and several studies have confirmed its advantages in dermatology. Dermatoscopic patterns of several parasitic, viral, and fungal skin infections have been identified and herein described. A noninvasive, fast, and accurate diagnosis plays an important role in containing the spread of contagious skin disorders.

Dermoscopy of Common Inflammatory Disorders 359

Dimitrios Sgouros, Zoe Apalla, Dimitrios Ioannides, Alexander Katoulis, Dimitrios Rigopoulos, Elena Sotiriou, Alexander Stratigos, Efstratios Vakirlis, and Aimilios Lallas

In addition to its “traditional” application for the early diagnosis of melanoma and nonmelanoma skin cancers, dermoscopy gains appreciation in fields beyond dermatooncology. Nowadays, dermoscopy has been established as a reliable adjunctive tool to the everyday clinical practice of general dermatology. Morphology and distribution of vascular structures, background colors, follicular abnormalities, and the presence of scales are important features that should be evaluated. Clinical examination remains the undoubted mainstay of diagnosis in inflammatory and infectious diseases.

Dermatoscopy of Granulomatous Disorders 369

Enzo Errichetti and Giuseppe Stinco

Although diagnosis of cutaneous granulomatous disorders (CGDs) is usually suspected based on morphologic findings, localization, and anamnestic data, clinical differentiation from each other and from similar dermatoses may be challenging.

Recently, dermatoscopy has been demonstrated to be a useful tool for assisting the recognition of several CGDs. This article provides a current overview of the dermatoscopic features of the main noninfectious and infectious CGDs, including sarcoidosis, necrobiosis lipoidica, granuloma annulare, rheumatoid nodules, and leishmaniasis. Other, less common, CGDs are briefly addressed, including granulomatous rosacea, acne agminata, and leprosy.

Dermoscopy of Lymphomas and Pseudolymphomas **377**

Caterina Bombonato, Riccardo Pampena, Aimillios Lallas, Pellacani Giovanni, and Caterina Longo

Primary cutaneous lymphomas are a heterogeneous group that includes 2 main groups of primary T- and B-cell lymphomas, which can involve the skin with distinct variability in clinical presentation, histopathology, immunophenotypes, molecular signature, and prognosis. We sought to describe the clinical and dermoscopic features of the most frequent clinical forms of cutaneous lymphomas. The diagnosis of these entities is still based on a cellular level and there are very few reports in literature about dermoscopy of cutaneous lymphomas. Nevertheless, we think that their dermoscopic features can be useful for helping in clinical diagnosis.

Dermatoscopy of Vascular Lesions **389**

Vincenzo Piccolo, Teresa Russo, Elvira Moscarella, Gabriella Brancaccio, Roberto Alfano, and Giuseppe Argenziano

Cutaneous vascular lesions (VLs) represent a very common reason for dermatologic consultation for patients. In most cases, VLs are benign and self-limiting. However, because they often mimic malignant skin tumors, their correct and prompt identification is very important in daily practice. Dermoscopy may play a key role in achieving that purpose. This article reviews current knowledge of dermoscopic features of the most frequent VLs.

Dermoscopy of Adnexal Tumors **397**

Pedro Zaballos, Ignacio Gómez-Martín, José María Martin, and José Bañuls

Cutaneous adnexal tumors include lesions with apocrine, eccrine, follicular, sebaceous, and mixed differentiation. Most are benign and sporadic, although malignant forms are occasionally observed and some cases develop in the setting of inherited syndromes. These tumors often cause immense diagnostic difficulty. Dermoscopy is a noninvasive technique that has greatly improved the diagnostic accuracy of different skin lesions, including these tumors. The authors provide a review of the literature on the dermoscopic structures and patterns associated with adnexal tumors. Most patterns associated with this kind of tumor are nonspecific and are observed in other nonadnexal tumors, especially in basal cell carcinomas.

Trichoscopy Tips **413**

Rodrigo Pirmez and Antonella Tosti

Although trichoscopy has only recently been introduced in the assessment of hair and scalp disorders, it is already considered an essential diagnostic tool by many experts in the field. This article discusses topics that are often a source of doubt among clinicians and tips that may help dermatologists better perform trichoscopy. Subjects include fundamental concepts needed to start performing the method, basic trichoscopic structures, tips to identify a scarring condition and to approach a patient with a receding hairline, features that are unique to children, those that are typically seen in the dark scalp, and pitfalls of the technique.

Trichoscopy in Hair Shaft Disorders 421

Lidia Rudnicka, Małgorzata Olszewska, Anna Waśkiel, and Adriana Rakowska

Trichoscopy allows analyzing the structure and size of growing hair shafts in their natural environment in children and adults. The method replaces light microscopy, which requires pulling of multiple hairs for investigation. In monilethrix, trichoscopy shows uniform elliptical nodosities with intermittent constrictions. In trichorrhexis nodosa nodular thickenings along hair shafts are visible (low magnification) or splitting into numerous small fibers along the hair shaft may be observed (high magnification). In trichorrhexis invaginata (bamboo hair) the hair shaft telescopes into itself at several points along the shaft. Trichoscopy shows small nodules along the shaft. Hairs bend and break in these diseases. Trichoscopy of pili torti shows twists of hair shafts along their long axis. In pili annulati hair shafts with alternating white and dark bands are visible. In woolly hair the examination demonstrates hair shafts with waves at very short intervals. For trichothiodystrophy polarized trichoscopy should be used. In ectodermal dysplasias, trichoscopy shows a variety of hair abnormalities, but the most characteristic finding is hair shaft pigmentation heterogeneity.

Onychoscopy: Dermoscopy of the Nails 431

Bianca Maria Piraccini, Aurora Alessandrini, and Michela Starace

Onychoscopy is the examination of the nail unit using a dermoscope. The dermoscopic criteria for a valid diagnosis have been developed and assessed in numerous papers. However, in all nail alterations that are suspicious or potentially malignant, a surgical intervention with subsequent histopathologic evaluation should be performed. A simple visualization may not be helpful in diagnosing many nail conditions nor is a nail biopsy diagnostic in all cases. Onychoscopy is a valuable aid in enhancing visible nail features and in revealing cryptic features of diagnostic value.

Dermoscopy for the Diagnosis of Conjunctival Lesions 439

Elisa Cinotti, Anna La Rocca, Bruno Labeille, Damien Grivet, Linda Tognetti, Victor Lambert, Mathilde Kaspi, Niccolò Nami, Michele Fimiani, Jean Luc Perrot, and Pietro Rubegni

This article describes the present literature on dermoscopy of conjunctiva and shows the results of a dermoscopy study of 147 conjunctival tumors. Melanomas were characterized by a heavy pigmentation, irregular dots, and a higher prevalence of gray color compared with nevi. Squamous cell carcinomas had peculiar hairpin and glomerular vessels. Primary acquired melanoses were characterized by regularly distributed light brown dots. A large part of nevi had small cysts.

Dermoscopy of Inflammatory Genital Diseases: Practical Insights 451

Alessandro Borghi, Annarosa Virgili, and Monica Corazza

Diagnosis of genital inflammatory disorders may be difficult for several reasons, such as their similar appearance, possible misdiagnosis with infectious and malignant conditions, and peculiar anatomic conditions that may lead to modification of clinical features. Dermoscopy could be included as a part of the clinical inspection of genital diseases to support diagnosis, as well as to ideally avoid unnecessary invasive investigation. Practical guidance for the use of dermoscopy in the assessment of the main inflammatory genital diseases is provided, namely, for lichen sclerosus, lichen planus, psoriasis, lichen simplex chronicus, and plasma cell mucositis.

Dermatoscopy of Common Lesions in Pediatric Dermatology **463**

Giuseppe Micali, Anna Elisa Verzì, Enrica Quattrocchi, Chau Yee Ng, and Francesco Lacarrubba

The use of dermatoscopy to assist in the diagnosis of a variety of proliferative, pigmentary, inflammatory, infectious, congenital, and genetic cutaneous and skin appendage disorders is constantly increasing, as it is effective, affordable, noninvasive, and quick to perform.

Dermoscopy of Pigmentary Disorders in Brown Skin **473**

Manas Chatterjee and Shekhar Neema

Dermoscopy is a noninvasive technique for the diagnosis, prognosis, and monitoring of pigmentary disorders in brown skin. It can be used for the diagnosis of various facial melanoses, which can avoid the need for biopsy in many cases. It can also help in early identification of the adverse effect of topical steroids and hydroquinone when they are used for the treatment of these disorders. Dermoscopy can also reliably differentiate vitiligo from other disorders of hypopigmentation. It can also help in assessing the stability of vitiligo before surgery.

Dermatoscopy and Reflectance Confocal Microscopy Correlations in Nonmelanocytic Disorders **487**

Francesco Lacarrubba, Marco Ardigò, Alessandro Di Stefani, Anna Elisa Verzì, and Giuseppe Micali

Dermatoscopy and in vivo reflectance confocal microscopy are noninvasive techniques that provide a horizontal approach, with an en face view of the skin structures. Both techniques assist in the clinical diagnosis of a variety of inflammatory and infectious cutaneous disorders. In many cases, they have shown concordance. Their combined use represents, in several instances, a promising option to reach the final diagnosis without the need for invasive procedures.

DERMATOLOGIC CLINICS

FORTHCOMING ISSUES

January 2019
Hot Topics in Dermatology
Kenneth J. Tomecki, *Editor*

April 2019
Therapeutic Hotline: New Developments in Dermatology
Seemal R. Desai, *Editor*

July 2019
Cutaneous Oncology and Dermatologic Surgery
Rajiv Nijhawan and Divya Srivastava, *Editors*

RECENT ISSUES

July 2018
Pruritis
Gil Yosipovitch, *Editors*

April 2018
Rosacea
Steven R. Feldman, Leah A. Cardwell, and Sarah L. Taylor, *Editors*

January 2018
Cosmetic Dermatology for Men
Neil S. Sadick, *Editor*

ISSUE OF RELATED INTEREST

Clinics in Laboratory Medicine, September 2017 (Vol. 37, No. 3)
Dermatopathology
Steven D. Billings, *Editor*
Available at: https://www.labmed.theclinics.com/

Erratum

In the July 2018 issue of *Dermatologic Clinics* (Volume 36, Issue 3) devoted to Pruritus, the Guest Editor's affiliation was listed incorrectly on the Contributors page. The correct affiliation for Gil Yosipovitch, MD is "Department of Dermatology and Cutaneous Surgery, Miami Itch Center, University of Miami Miller School of Medicine, University of Miami Hospital, Miami, Florida, USA."

Dermatol Clin 36 (2018) xiii
https://doi.org/10.1016/j.det.2018.07.010
0733-8635/18/© 2018 Published by Elsevier Inc.

Preface
The Expanding Use of Dermatoscopy

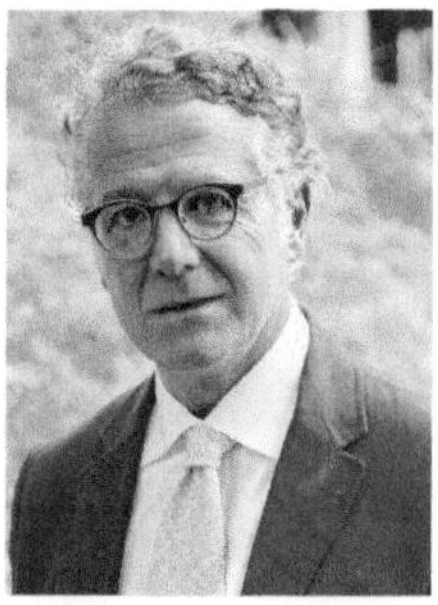
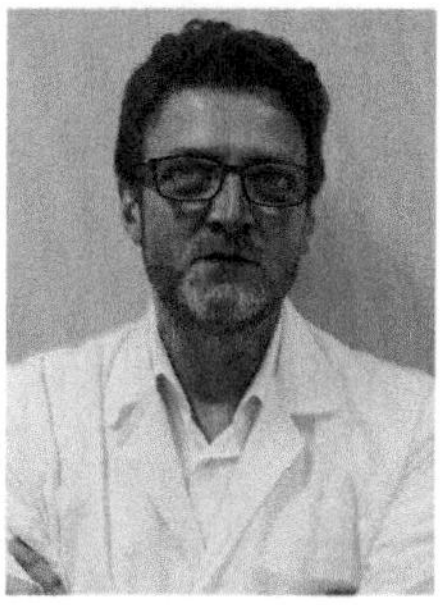

Giuseppe Micali, MD   Francesco Lacarrubba, MD
Editors

We are pleased to introduce this issue of *Dermatologic Clinics* that deals with the "Alternative Uses of Dermatoscopy" beyond the classical use on the diagnosis of pigmented lesions. As known, dermatoscopy (or dermoscopy; the two terms are synonyms and they will be used interchangeably in this issue) is a noninvasive technique that has greatly enhanced the diagnostic accuracy of nevi, melanoma, and other benign and malignant skin tumors. Throughout the years, the use of dermatoscopy has been extended to a variety of skin disorders for diagnosis enhancement, follow-up, and therapeutic monitoring. Its current applications include several inflammatory, infectious, and appendage disorders, along with other skin conditions. The introduction of new terms in the literature, such as *inflammoscopy*, *entodermoscopy*, *trichoscopy*, and *onychoscopy*, confirms the scientific community's interest in these novel dermatoscopy indications. Although the simple handheld dermatoscope, allowing $\times 10$ magnification, is adequate for the evaluation of most of these disorders, in some cases, the use of videodermatoscope, allowing higher magnifications up to $\times 500$, is preferable.

The purpose of this issue of *Dermatologic Clinics*, which hosts contributions from renowned international experts in the field, is to advance the knowledge of the "alternative" uses of dermatoscopy by providing an overview of the existing data. The issue also includes articles focusing on "special" body areas (genital and conjunctival mucosae) and populations (pediatric age and brown skin individuals), dermatoscopy tips to use in daily practice, and interesting correlations with reflectance confocal microscopy.

Dermatoscopy may represent an important and relatively simple aid in daily clinical practice, and dermatologists should be encouraged to use this technique beyond pigmented lesions, so as to enhance the clinical diagnosis and to reduce the need for semi-invasive or invasive procedures such as skin scrapings and/or biopsy.

Giuseppe Micali, MD
Dermatology Clinic
University of Catania
Via Santa Sofia, 78
Catania 95123, Italy

Francesco Lacarrubba, MD
Dermatology Clinic
University of Catania
Via Santa Sofia, 78
Catania 95123, Italy

E-mail addresses:
gimicali1@hotmail.it (G. Micali)
franclacarrubba@gmail.com (F. Lacarrubba)

Dermatol Clin 36 (2018) xv
https://doi.org/10.1016/j.det.2018.06.001
0733-8635/18/© 2018 Published by Elsevier Inc.

Dermatoscopy
Instrumental Update

Giuseppe Micali, MD*, Francesco Lacarrubba, MD

KEYWORDS

• Dermatoscopy • Dermoscopy • Videodermatoscopy • Videomicroscopy • Instrumentation

KEY POINTS

- Dermatoscopy is a non-invasive technique used for the evaluation of pigmented (melanocytic and nonmelanocytic) skin lesions and in several dermatology fields, including inflammatory disorders, infectious diseases, and hair and nails abnormalities.
- The handheld dermatoscope is the most used device because it is user-friendly and relatively inexpensive. It allows 10 times magnification and may be connected to digital cameras and/or smartphones.
- Videodermatoscopes are more expensive devices that allow higher magnifications (up to 1000 times) and simplify the process of image storage, analysis, and retrieval.

INTRODUCTION

Dermatoscopy (or dermoscopy) is a noninvasive technique that allows in vivo, magnified observation of skin details and structures not visible to the naked eye. It was first used for the evaluation of pigmented (melanocytic and non-melanocytic) skin lesions but currently its use has been extended to several dermatology fields, including inflammatory disorders, infectious diseases, and hair and nails abnormalities.[1] Dermatoscopy may be performed using handheld devices or computer-assisted digital systems or videodermatoscopes.

HANDHELD DERMATOSCOPY

The handheld dermatoscope represents the most used device because it is user-friendly and relatively inexpensive. It is not a mere magnifying glass but a more complex instrument that allows the visualization of the cutaneous microstructures of the different skin layers, from the surface to the mid-dermis.[2,3] These microstructures appear of different colors, depending on their composition and depth. Because they are observed from the top, they appear superimposed.

A wide variety of handheld dermatoscopes are commercially available with an approximate cost of 1000 Euros (**Table 1**).

The classic handheld dermatoscope includes a high-quality lens that generally allows 10 times magnification and a transilluminating lighting system that uses an incident light source (at an angle of ~30°–45°). To overcome the light scattering on the skin surface, a medium (eg. oil, alcohol, glycerin, water) at the interface between the skin and the device's glass slide is required (epiluminescence technique). This immersion technique makes the skin surface optically homogeneous and translucent, and allows the observation of the deeper structures.[2,3] Because the epiluminescence technique requires contact between the device and the skin, it has the disadvantage of compressing the microvasculature. Moreover, the instrument needs to be cleaned after the observation of each patient, especially in case of evaluation of contagious disorders (eg, warts, molluscum contagiosum, scabies). In some cases, the use of dermatoscopy without the immersion fluid (dry dermatoscopy) is recommended, including the evaluation of scaling, follicular hyperkeratosis, hair shaft disorders, and nail plate surface.[4,5]

Other handheld devices are provided with polarized light that absorbs all the scattered waves. These instruments do not require the use of a liquid medium and offer the capability of viewing the skin while avoiding the surface contact

Disclosures: None.
Dermatology Clinic, University of Catania, Via S. Sofia 78, Catania 95123, Italy
* Corresponding author. Dermatology Clinic, University of Catania, Via S. Sofia 78, Catania 95123, Italy.
E-mail address: cldermct@gmail.com

Dermatol Clin 36 (2018) 345–348
https://doi.org/10.1016/j.det.2018.05.001

Table 1
Main available handheld dermatoscopes

Name	Company
Handheld Dermatoscopes (×10)	
Dermatoscope Holtex	Holtex (Aix en Provence, France)
Dermatoscope compact	ProximaMedTech (Cokot, Serbia)
DermLite	3Gen (San Juan Capistrano, USA)
DermoGenius ultra	Dermoscan (Regensburg, Germany)
Heine Delta	Heine (Dover, USA)
Horus	Miis (Hsinchu, Taiwan)
IDS-1100	Illuco (Gunpo-si, South Korea)
Kawe	Kirchner & Wilhelm GmbH + Co. KG (Asperg, Germany)
MicroDERM	Visiomed AG (Bielefeld, Germany)
Orion Dermatoscope	Sklar Surgical Instruments (West Chester, USA)
Proscope	American Diagnostic Corporation (Hauppauge, USA)
Ri-derma	Riester (Jungingen, Germany)
Sigma 1000	Medical devices Ltd (Ugoki, Pakistan)
Veos	Canfield (Parsippany, USA)
Dermatoscopes with an integrated camera	
Dermaview	3Tmedical (Camposano, Italy)
DermLite Foto	3Gen (San Juan Capistrano, USA)
LiteScope kit	Quantificare (Valbonne, France)
Photomax pro	Derma Medical (Vienna, Austria)
Veos SLR	Canfield (Parsippany, USA)
Dermatoscopes with camera/smartphone adapter	
DermLite connection kit	3Gen (San Juan Capistrano, USA)
DermoGenius pro	Dermoscan (Regensburg, Germany)
Handyscope	FotoFinder (Bad Birnbach, Germany)
Heine iC1	Heine (Dover, USA)
IDS-1100 adapter	Illuco (Gunpo-si, South Korea)
MoleScope	MetaOptima (Vancouver, Canada)
Veos DS3	Canfield (Parsippany, USA)

(noncontact dermatoscopy). This modality is especially useful in cases of infectious disorders.

A study comparing nonpolarized and polarized devices concluded that there are similarities, as well as differences, in the visualization of skin lesions.[6] The investigators observed that, in general, nonpolarized dermatoscopy revealed superficial features and polarized dermatoscopy revealed deeper structures. They concluded that the use of both methods can provide complementary information.[6] The same conclusions were reported in another study comparing polarized and nonpolarized dermatoscopy for hair and scalp disorders. Certain features, such as vascular patterns, scaling, and reticular pigmentation, were better appreciated in a polarized mode, whereas others, such as black dots and tapered hair, were better documented in a nonpolarized mode.[7]

Some handheld dermatoscope devices are equipped with both nonpolarized and polarized light, providing the capability of viewing the skin both with and without a liquid interface and direct skin contact.

Although handheld devices do not allow image storage, this may be obtained by connecting the dermatoscope to a digital camera or a smartphone. Some manufacturing companies provide specially designed adapters for this purpose (**Figs. 1** and **2**; **Table 1**).

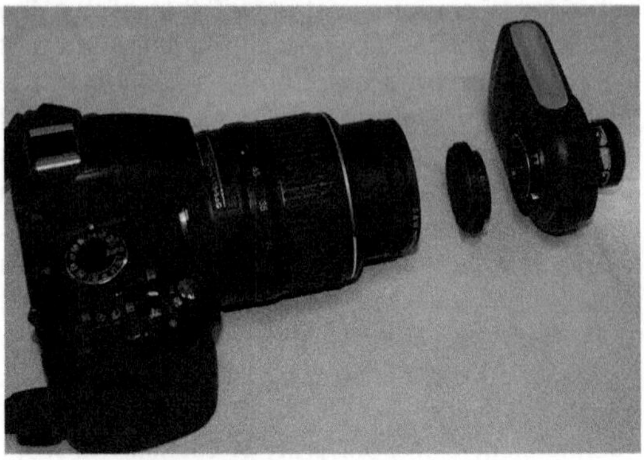

Fig. 1. Handheld dermatoscope and adapter for connection to a digital camera.

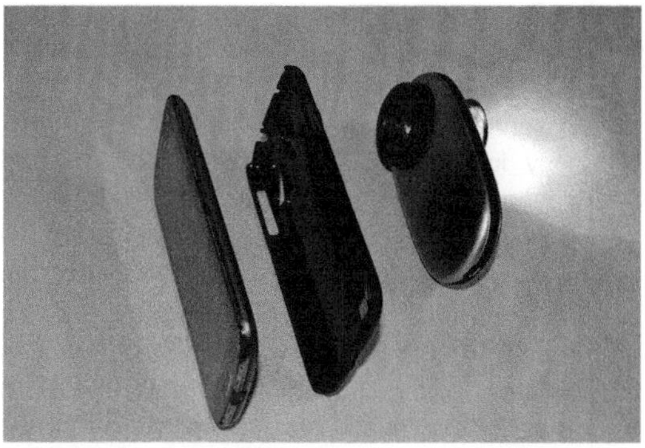

Fig. 2. Handheld dermatoscope and adapter for connection to a smartphone.

VIDEODERMATOSCOPY

Videodermatoscopes are more expensive systems (~15,000–25,000 Euros), that simplify image viewing and the process of image acquisition, storage, organization, analysis, and retrieval.[8] These systems are equipped with high-resolution color videocameras that reveal. In a monitor, images obtained using nonpolarized or polarized light (**Fig. 3**, **Table 2**). The image quality of these systems is generally not superior to handheld devices but they are equipped with lenses that ensure real-time zooming up to 1000 times magnification. This is a great advantage for the evaluation of some conditions such as scabies, psoriasis, and hair shafts disorders as well as for the study of the vascular pattern that is crucial in most cases.

Low-cost videomicroscopes (~30–100 Euros) are available on the Web for nonmedical use in entomology, botany, and microelectronics. These consist of low-resolution, digital devices able to provide magnification ranging from 10 to 1000 times; they must be connected to a personal computer via a universal serial bus (USB) to visualize and store the images. These low-cost devices are not recommended for the evaluation of pigmented lesions and hair or scalp disorders because of the low color quality and/or resolution.[9,10] However, they have been demonstrated to be useful for the diagnosis of scabies, being able to identify its typical signs similarly to a standard videodermatoscope.[9] Their use should be limited to those skin disorders (eg, entomodermatoses and hair shaft disorders) in which image color quality and resolution are not crucial for the diagnosis.[9,10]

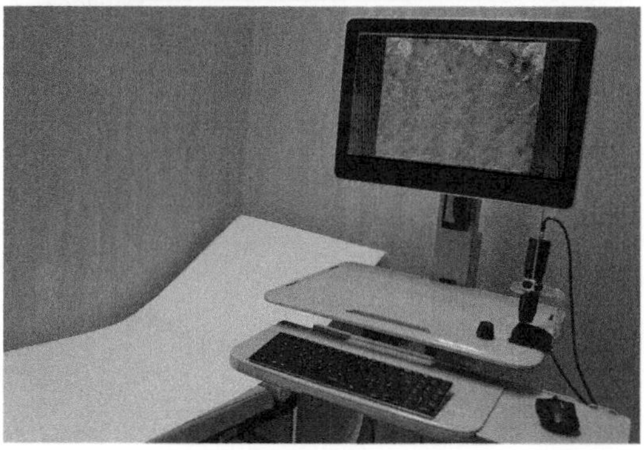

Fig. 3. Videodermatoscope.

Table 2
Main available videodermatoscopes

Name	Company	Magnification
DermoGenius ultra	Dermoscan (Regensburg, Germany)	×10
Dino-lite	AnMo Electronics Corporation (New Taipey City, Taiwan)	×10–×200
FotoFinder dermoscope	FotoFinder (Bad Birnbach, Germany)	×20–×70
Hi-scope	Hirox (Tokyo, Japan)	×4–×1000
Horus	Adamo s.r.l. (Trapani, Italy)	×30–×150
IRSkin	CA-MI (Langhirano, Italy)	×10–×100
Molemax HD	Derma Medical (Vienna, Austria)	×20–×100
Optilia	Optilia Instruments (Sollentuna, Sweden)	×20–×50
Skin Cam	Medicam (Mumbai, India)	×10–×200
Videocap 3.0	D.S. Medica (Milano, Italy)	×20–×200
Vidix	Medicimedical (Piumazzo di Castelfranco Emilia, Italy)	×7–×100

SOFTWARE FOR IMAGE ANALYSIS

In the evaluation of pigmented skin lesions, different types of software have been developed for computer-assisted diagnosis based on the analysis of variables such as diameter, symmetry, and colors of the acquired dermatoscopic images. On the other hand, digital image analysis currently has few applications regarding alternative uses of dermatoscopy.[11] A software (Trichoscan,Tricholog

GmbH & Datinf GmbH, Freiburg, Germany) has been developed to monitor hair loss and treatment response, although its reliability remains to be confirmed.[11,12]

NEW TECHNIQUES

Polarized transilluminating dermoscopy (PTD) is a new interesting technique that has recently been proposed for the diagnosis of trichothiodystrophy.[12] With the use of the handheld dermatoscope, it mimics a polarizing microscope, an instrument used by dermatopathologists that allows the examination of skin sections or hair shafts with polarized light.[13,14] In trichothiodystrophy, polarizing microscopy shows characteristic alternate dark and white bands of the hair shaft with a tiger-tail appearance that is not visualized on standard light microscopy and is highly suggestive of the disorder.

PTD can be performed using 2 dermatoscopes and a light source or 1 dermatoscope and a mirror. In both cases, the hair shaft is transilluminated by the polarized light, allowing the visualization of the typical tiger-tail pattern of trichothiodystrophy.[14]

If PTD will be validated by further studies, its use could be extended to other disorders in which polarizing microscopy is used for the evaluation of hair abnormalities, such as gray hair syndromes, argininosuccinase deficiency, acrodermatitis enteropathica, keratitis ichthyosis deafness syndrome, and steroid sulfatase deficiency, thus avoiding the use of more complex tools and/or time-consuming consultation with the pathologist.[14]

REFERENCES

1. Micali G, Lacarrubba F, Massimino D, et al. Dermatoscopy: alternative uses in daily clinical practice. J Am Acad Dermatol 2011;64:1135–46.
2. Tanaka M. Dermoscopy. J Dermatol 2006;33(8): 513–7.
3. Campos-do-Carmo G, Ramos-e-Silva M. Dermoscopy: basic concepts. Int J Dermatol 2008;47(7):712–9.
4. Inui S, Nakajima T, Itami S. Dry dermoscopy in clinical treatment of alopecia areata. J Dermatol 2007; 34(9):635–9.
5. Alessandrini A, Starace M, Piraccini BM. Dermoscopy in the evaluation of nail disorders. Skin Appendage Disord 2017;3(2):70–82.
6. Lake A, Jones B. Dermoscopy: to cross-polarize, or not to cross-polarize, that is the question. J Vis Commun Med 2015;38(1–2):36–50.
7. Nikam VV, Mehta HH. A nonrandomized study of trichoscopy patterns using nonpolarized (contact) and polarized (noncontact) dermatoscopy in hair and shaft disorders. Int J Trichology 2014;6(2): 54–62.
8. Fleming MG. Digital dermoscopy. Dermatol Clin 2001;19(2):359–67.
9. Verzì AE, Lacarrubba F, Micali G. Use of low-cost videomicroscopy versus standard videodermatoscopy in trichoscopy: a controlled, blinded noninferiority trial. Skin Appendage Disord 2016;1(4): 172–4.
10. Micali G, Lacarrubba F, Verzì AE, et al. Low-cost equipment for diagnosis and management of endemic scabies outbreaks in underserved populations. Clin Infect Dis 2015;60(2):327–9.
11. Micali G, Verzì AE, Lacarrubba F. Alternative uses of dermatoscopy in daily clinical practice: an update. J Am Acad Dermatol 2018 Jun 16. pii: S0190-9622(18)32143-1. [Epub ahead of print].
12. Bilgiç Temel A, Gülkesen KH, Dicle Ö. Automated digital image analysis (TrichoScan) in male patients with androgenetic alopecia; comparison with manual marking of hairs on trichoscopic images. Skin Res Technol 2018. https://doi.org/10.1111/srt.12449.
13. Yang YW, Yarbrough K, Mitkov M, et al. Polarized transilluminating dermoscopy: bedside trichoscopic diagnosis of trichothiodystrophy. Pediatr Dermatol 2018;35(1):147–9.
14. Lacarrubba F, Tosti A. Polarized transilluminating dermoscopy. Pediatr Dermatol 2018;35(1):150–1.

Dermatoscopy of Parasitic and Infectious Disorders

Anna Elisa Verzì, MD, Francesco Lacarrubba, MD, Franco Dinotta, MD, Giuseppe Micali, MD*

KEYWORDS

• Dermatoscopy • Dermoscopy • Entomodermoscopy • Videodermatoscopy • Skin infection • Skin infestation • Ectoparasites

KEY POINTS

- The increasing reports of several diverse dermatoscopic patterns confirm the important role of dermatoscopy in many dermatologic fields.
- Dermatoscopy has proved to be a helpful auxiliary tool in the diagnosis of parasitic and infectious disorders.
- Among different skin infestations and infections, characteristic dermoscopic patterns have been described for scabies, pediculosis, tungiasis, leishmaniasis, larva migrans, trombiculiasis, viral warts, molluscum contagiosum, tinea capitis, and tinea nigra.

INTRODUCTION

Dermatoscopy is traditionally used for the evaluation of pigmented skin lesions, improving the diagnostic accuracy of malignant lesions significantly above that of a naked eye examination. In the past years, its use has been extended to other dermatology fields, including parasitic and infectious disorders; the term entodermoscopy has been introduced.[1] Several studies have reported the usefulness of dermatoscopy in assisting the clinical diagnosis of these conditions and in reducing the need of semi-invasive or invasive procedures, such as skin scrapings and/or biopsies. This article provides a review of the main dermatoscopic patterns seen in selected parasitic, viral, and fungal skin disorders.

PARASITIC DISORDERS

Scabies

Scabies is caused by infestation by the host-specific mite *Sarcoptes scabiei var hominis*, which lives its entire life within the epidermis. It is a worldwide problem that may involve all ages, races, and socioeconomic groups, although higher incidences occur in overcrowded environments, including schools, hospitals, prisons, and refugee camps. Scabies may be transmitted directly by close contact or indirectly via fomites. Clinical diagnosis is based on the presence of intense itching accentuated at nighttime, typical distribution (wrists, axillae, waist, umbilicus, ankles, buttocks, genitalia, areolae, and nipples), and types of lesions (small erythematous papules, excoriations, secondary bacterial infections) along with a positive history for similar symptoms in household members or close personal contacts. The pathognomonic sign is the burrow, appearing as a small (3–10 mm long), wavy, thread-like, grayish-whitish trait. However, at clinical observation intact burrows may be hard to detect because of intense scratching. Confirmation of the diagnosis can be achieved by light microscopic examination of skin scrapings that reveals the presence of adult mites, eggs, and/or fecal pellets. However, the results of this method are limited to the tested areas and false-negative results are common.

Disclosures: None declared.
Dermatology Clinic, University of Catania, Via Santa Sofia 78, Catania 95123, Italy
* Corresponding author.
E-mail address: cldermct@gmail.com

Dermatol Clin 36 (2018) 349–358
https://doi.org/10.1016/j.det.2018.05.002

Dermatoscopy has been proved to be an effective tool for the diagnosis of scabies, allowing a rapid, noninvasive, in vivo examination of the entire skin surface in a few minutes.[2–6]

At low magnifications (×10), dermatoscopy enables the visualization of a small, dark-brown triangular structure "circumflex accent" located at the end of a subtle linear segment (**Fig. 1**A); both structures resemble a jet with contrail whereby the triangular structure corresponds to the pigmented anterior part of the mite (mouth and 2 anterior pairs of legs), whereas the contrail-shaped segment correlates with the burrow.[1,2] The use of low magnification, however, requires good experience, as these features may be confused with excoriations and/or splinters that may frequently occur because of repeated scratching. Higher magnifications (up to ×600) reveal unequivocal images of burrows and mites; they also allow the recognition of eggs or feces (invisible at low magnifications) that also represent diagnostic signs[7,8] (**Fig. 1**B). Using higher magnifications, anatomic details of *Sarcoptes scabiei* may be revealed, including the roundish translucent body, the head, the anterior and posterior legs, and the dorsal spiculae. In some cases, the mite moving inside the burrows may be highlighted.[9] A double-blinded study has demonstrated that high-magnification dermatoscopy is equivalent to scraping in terms of diagnostic accuracy.[7] Another study in children has confirmed a better acceptance in the pediatric population, as it is not painful and does not require blades for skin scraping.[8] Dermatoscopy is also particularly useful to screen asymptomatic contacts and family members and for post-therapeutic follow-up, ruling out the persistence of viable mites, thus, reducing the risk of infestation spread.[9–13] Recently, low-cost videomicroscopes (about $30), which permit high magnifications (up to ×500) and are available for nonmedical use in entomology, botany, and/or microelectronics, have been demonstrated to be able to allow for a definitive scabies diagnosis, showing the typical signs of the infestation as did the medically marketed videodermatoscope.[14] The impact of these inexpensive videomicroscopes, whose usefulness has not been confirmed in other dermatologic conditions,[15] seems to be significant and cost-effective in scabies, both in institutional settings (hospitals, nursing homes, long-term care facilities, and prisons) as well as in underdeveloped countries experiencing endemic outbreaks, where the availability of affordable, noninvasive techniques is crucial.[14]

Pediculosis

Dermatoscopy has demonstrated to be useful for the diagnosis and therapeutic monitoring of 2 common, highly contagious, cutaneous infestations due to human obligate, blood-sucking arthropods: pediculosis capitis and phthiriasis pubis.[16]

Pediculosis capitis is caused by *Pediculus humanus var capitis* (head louse). It is dorsoventrally elongated (2–3 mm), flattened, and wingless, with 3 pairs of clawed legs. The oval eggs (nits) are cemented to hair shafts close to the scalp with a chitinous material secreted by the female louse. Pediculosis capitis is worldwide and usually occurs in school-aged children causing small epidemics in classmates and in members of the same household. Girls seem to be more frequently affected, probably because of long hair and common sharing of brushes and hair accessories. Patients typically complain of intense pruritus of the scalp, mainly involving the occipital and retroauricular regions. The itching induces scratching, which can lead to excoriations, secondary bacterial infection, and lymphadenopathy.

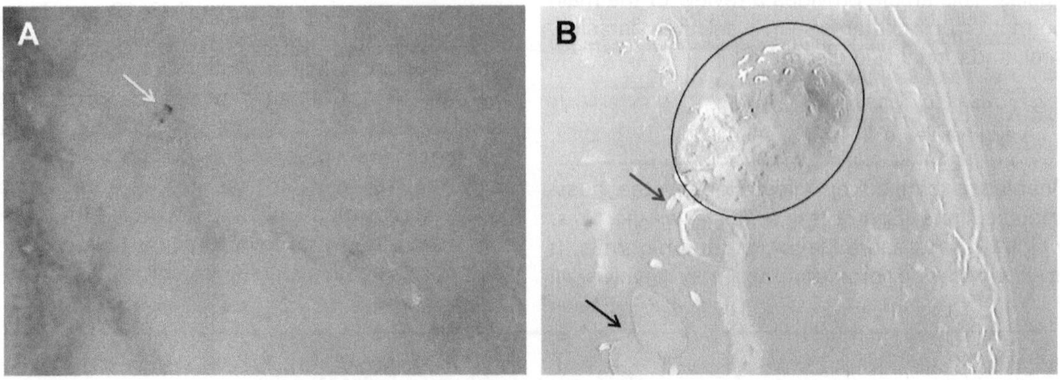

Fig. 1. Scabies. (*A*) Low-magnification dermatoscopy of a burrow shows a small dark brown triangular structure (*yellow arrow*) located at the end of a wavy, whitish segment (original magnification ×10). (*B*) High-magnification videodermatoscopy reveals unequivocal images of *Sarcoptes scabiei* body (*circle*) along with eggs (*black arrow*) and feces (*red arrow*) (original magnification ×400).

The diagnosis of pediculosis capitis is usually made by closely examining the scalp hair for the presence of lice or nits. Dermatoscopy allows the unequivocal identification of the nits,[17–20] which appear as ovoid, brownish structures firmly attached to the hair shafts, and a clear and real-time differentiation from pseudonits. The latter, clinically resembling nits, may be represented by scales of seborrheic dermatitis (whitish, amorphous masses),[21] hair casts (whitish, elongated, tubular structures encircling the hair shaft),[22–24] white piedra (whitish, ovular masses along the shafts),[25–27] or trichorrhexis nodosa (broken hair shafts with a brushed tip).[25] Moreover, dermatoscopy can be used for a detailed identification of full versus empty nits: the first, which contain nymphs and indicate a potential active infestation, present a convex extremity, whereas empty nits, which may persist after the healing, are translucent and typically show a plane and fissured free ending. This differentiation provides crucial information about the therapeutic approach.[21,28] Dermatoscopy has also been used to study the pediculicidal activity of different topical products by ex vivo evaluation of the movements and physiology of the mite.[29]

Interestingly, a case report described a patient with recalcitrant pruritus of the scalp and unresponsive to repeated pediculicidal treatments, who exhibited self-collected specimens of presumed head lice claimed to be recovered after combing the hair. Ex vivo high-magnification videodermatoscopy of the samples unequivocally excluded pediculosis capitis, and an entomologic consultation identified the arthropods as *collembola* (springtails). The latter may be confused with nymph-stage head lice, being quite similar in size and shape at a naked-eye observation or using magnification lenses/handheld dermatoscopy.[30]

Phthiriasis pubis is caused by *Pthirus pubis* (crab louse). It is classified as a sexually transmitted disease, as lice are typically found in pubic hair spreading from direct contact. However, it can affect any hair-bearing region, including the scalp, eyebrows, and eyelashes (phthiriasis palpebrarum). The roundish body of a pubic louse is 1 to 2 mm long and resembles a microscopic crab. As in pediculosis capitis, patients typically present with pruritus, sometimes associated with the presence of slate-gray to blue macules (maculae ceruleae) on the thighs or trunk.

In phthiriasis pubis, dermatoscopy clearly shows the presence of lice firmly attached to the pubic hairs and allows a more detailed identification of full versus empty nits.[31,32] In case of phthiriasis palpebrarum, lice are sometimes clinically difficult to identify, so the infestation may be misdiagnosed with scaling of atopic or seborrheic dermatitis. In these cases, dermatoscopy can rapidly reveal the presence of lice and/or nits.[33,34]

Tungiasis

Tungiasis is an infestation caused by the flea *Tunga penetrans*, which is endemic in Central and South America, Africa, Pakistan, and India. The typical lesion of tungiasis is caused by the female flea that burrows into the skin. In the early stage it appears as a small black dot surrounded by a halo of erythema. With time, it evolves into a pearl-like whitish papule and then into a larger nodule with a clearly demarcated white halo surrounding a black central punctum. The most common site of infestation is the periungual area of the toes, toe webs, and soles.

The use of dermatoscopy has been reported to be a valuable diagnostic tool, especially in nonendemic areas.[35–42] Dermatoscopy shows a whitish homogeneous lesion with a central brown-pigmented ring around a pore, corresponding to the pigmented chitin that surrounds the posterior opening of the flea exoskeleton.[35,39] Within the papule, eggs have been described as gray-blue blotches[39] or as whitish oval structures linked together to form chain-like structures.[36] Clusters of eggs can also be detected as jelly-like bags after a careful superficial shaving of the lesion and compression of its edges.[36] Finally, after extraction of the intact parasite, ex vivo dermatoscopy can be used for diagnosis confirmation by revealing the flea with a distended jelly sac abdomen full of eggs.[40]

Cutaneous Leishmaniasis

Leishmaniases are a group of tropical and subtropical diseases that are endemic in Asia, Africa, the Americas, and the Mediterranean region. They are caused by *Leishmania spp*, obligate intracellular parasites of macrophages. In cutaneous leishmaniasis, the protozoa are transmitted by dogs to humans through the bites of phlebotomine sandflies,[43] so it generally occurs in unclothed body areas including the ears, nose, lips, cheeks, legs, hands, forearms, and ankles. The typical onset is an erythematous papule that enlarges in a few weeks to form an infiltrated nodule with central ulceration and crust (**Fig. 2**A). The diagnosis of cutaneous leishmaniasis may be suggested by history and clinical examination, but laboratory confirmation with microscopic identification of the protozoa (Leishman-Donovan bodies) in Giemsa-stained lesion smears is mandatory.

In the last few years, dermatoscopy has been reported to enhance the clinical diagnosis.[44–47] The

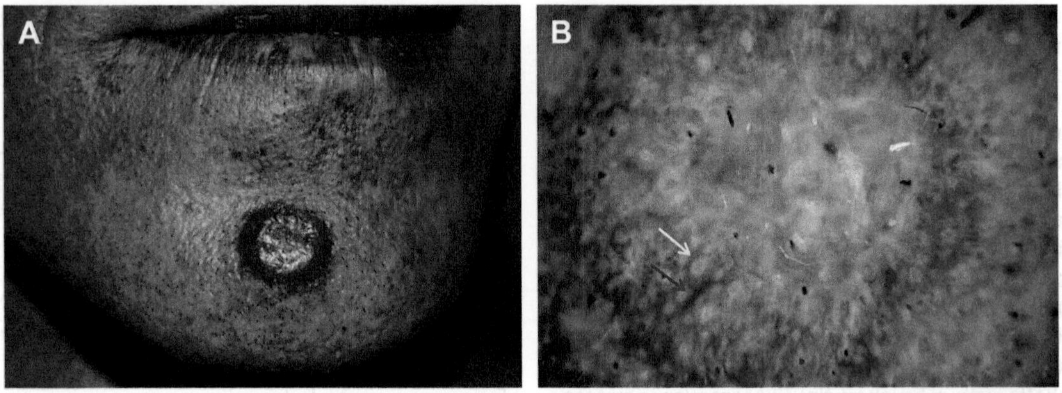

Fig. 2. Cutaneous leishmaniasis. (*A*) Infiltrated nodule on the chin. (*B*) Dermatoscopy shows diffuse erythema, central erosion, yellow tear-like structures (*yellow arrow*), and linear vessels (*red arrow*) (original magnification ×10).

most typical dermatoscopic findings are the yellow tear-like structures (**Fig. 2**B), corresponding to keratin plugs, and the peripheral white starburst-like pattern, histologically correlated to the parakeratotic hyperkeratosis.[47] Diffuse erythema and yellow to salmon-colored areas are frequently observed; but their diagnostic value is low, as they are visible in other granulomatous disorders (sarcoidosis, foreign body reaction, lupus vulgaris). Other dermatoscopic features are represented by vessels of various shape (dotted, linear-irregular, comma-shaped, polymorphous atypical, hairpin, arborizing, telangiectatic, glomerular-like, corkscrew-like), central hyperkeratosis/scales and erosions/ulcers, milia-like cysts, and a perilesional hypopigmented halo.[45,46] In a study, the different dermatoscopic patterns have been correlated with the evolution of the lesions: a predominance of yellow tear-like structures and vessels were found in early papular lesions, whereas chronic and/or advanced lesions were characterized by central erosion/ulcerations combined with scales, a white starburst-like pattern, and vascular structures at the periphery.[44]

Cutaneous Larva Migrans

Cutaneous larva migrans is a common infestation in tropical and subtropical geographic areas that is caused by different nematodes, mainly *Ancylostoma braziliense*. Humans are accidentally infested by contact with the larvae present in a soil contaminated with feces of dogs, cats, and wild animals. The larvae penetrate into the skin where they migrate and burrow intraepidermal, linear/serpentine cutaneous trails. The lesions are generally erythematous and itchy and typically involve the feet but also buttocks, hands, and knees. A creeping eruption associated with recent exposure to sand or soil is the basis for the diagnosis.

Few studies evaluated the usefulness of dermatoscopy in the diagnosis of cutaneous larva migrans, showing a low sensitivity of the technique.[48,49] When detected, the body of the larva appears as translucent brownish structureless areas in a segmental arrangement.[1] In a report using polarized dermatoscopy, the serpiginous tract showed oval structures with a yellow periphery and a brown center.[50]

Trombiculiasis

Trombiculiasis is an epi-zoonosis that occurs worldwide and is caused by various types of chiggers that usually inhabit heated and humid environments. *Neotrombicula autumnalis* has been reported as the most frequent causative agent of human infestation in Europe.[51] Larvae feed on their hosts by using chelicerae to inject lytic enzymes into the upper layers of the skin. As cutaneous findings are unspecific, consisting of multiple, erythematous, and/or excoriated papules associated with intense itching, the infestation is often misdiagnosed leading to inadequate treatments.[52] For this reason, although the infestation is self-limiting, a correct identification of the parasite is advisable.

The usefulness of dermatoscopy in diagnosing trombiculiasis has been described in 2 reports, in which the mite has been detected on the skin presenting a strong fluorescent orange-reddish color.[52,53]

VIRAL DISORDERS

Cutaneous and Anogenital Warts

Warts are common, cutaneous, benign proliferations caused by *Human papillomaviruses* (HPV).[54,55] According to anatomic or morphologic grounds, they are classified into common warts (verrucae vulgares), palmoplantar warts, flat warts (verrucae planae), and anogenital warts (condylomata acuminata). Cutaneous HPV infection may occur via direct skin-to-skin contact or indirectly through contaminated surfaces and objects, whereas anogenital infection most commonly results from intimate contact. Common warts present as single or multiple exophytic papules with a rough surface that may involve any area of the body, especially hands and fingers. Pedunculated and filiform warts can also develop, especially in periorificial areas of the face and neck. Palmoplantar warts usually appear as endophytic, hyperkeratotic, often painful papules. Superficial lesions coalescing into large plaques are referred to as mosaic warts or myrmecia. Flat warts are skin colored or slightly pigmented, roundish, flat-topped papules with smooth surface usually occurring on the dorsal hands, arms, or face, often in a linear distribution. Anogenital warts involve the external genitalia, the perineum, the perianal areas, and the inguinal folds. They may appear as sessile, exophytic, skin-colored, brown, or whitish (especially when macerated in moist areas) papules or as pedunculated, broad-based papillomas (cauliflower-like genital warts) (**Fig. 3**A).

The diagnosis of cutaneous and anogenital warts is generally based on their typical clinical appearance even though dermatoscopy may be useful for a more accurate examination.

At dermatoscopy, common warts appear as well-demarcated lesions composed of multiple papillae containing hemorrhagic red to black dots and globules and surrounded by a whitish halo. Exophytic lesions display multiple, finger-like whitish projections containing elongated and dilated vessels.[1,56–59] Palmoplantar warts reveal yellowish structureless areas associated with multiple irregularly distributed red to brown to black dots or linear streaks.[60] Typically, the disruption of dermatoglyphics can be easily noted, enhancing the differential diagnosis with traumatic thickening.[61,62] Flat warts display regularly distributed, tiny, red dots (histopathologically corresponding to the top of dilated capillaries in the papillary dermis) on a whitish or light-brown background.[63,64] Dermatoscopy allows an easy differential diagnosis from acne comedones, which typically reveal a central white to yellow pore corresponding to hair follicle opening.

Papular anogenital warts are dermatoscopically characterized by the presence of a whitish network associated with regularly distributed dotted vessels (mosaic pattern).[11,65–68] These features correlate with hyperkeratosis and acanthosis and tortuous/dilated capillaries in the papillary dermis, respectively.[68] In papillomatous lesions, multiple, whitish, finger-like projections arising from a common base and comprising elongated and dilated vessels (**Fig. 3**B) are observed.[11] Dermatoscopy may help to differentiate anogenital warts from other anogenital growths, such as molluscum contagiosum, pearly penile papules, vestibular papillae, Fordyce spots, lymphangiomas, and lichen nitidus.[11,66,68]

Molluscum Contagiosum

Molluscum contagiosum is a highly contagious infection caused by a *Molluscipox* virus, whose transmission occurs directly by skin-to-skin contact. It is common in children and in sexually active adults. Lesions typically appear as dome-shaped, flesh-colored, or pearly papules with an umbilicated center (**Fig. 4**A) and may occur anywhere on the body. The clinical diagnosis is usually easy, especially in pediatric patients, as lesions are characteristic in appearance. However, it may be occasionally misdiagnosed with other disorders, particularly in adulthood.

Dermatoscopy is very useful to enhance the clinical diagnosis of molluscum contagiosum.[69–73] It is characterized by the presence of single or multiple,

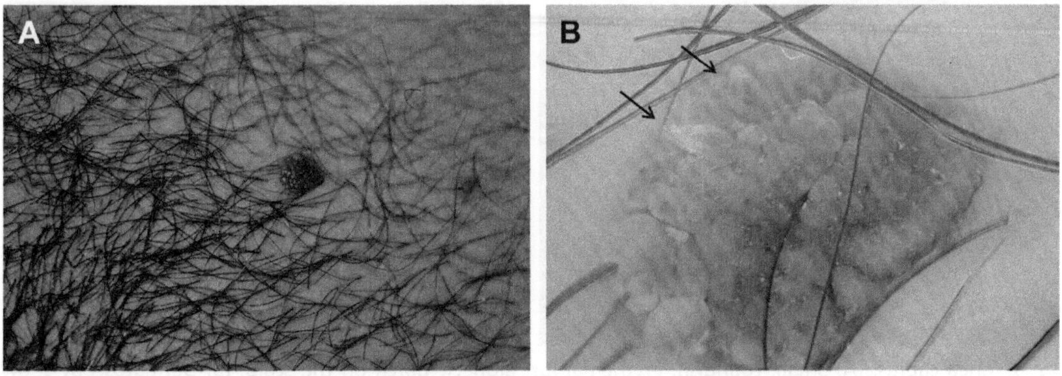

Fig. 3. Genital warts. (*A*) Papillomatous lesion on the pubic area. (*B*) Dermatoscopy shows multiple, whitish, finger-like projections comprising elongated vessels (*arrows*) (original magnification ×10).

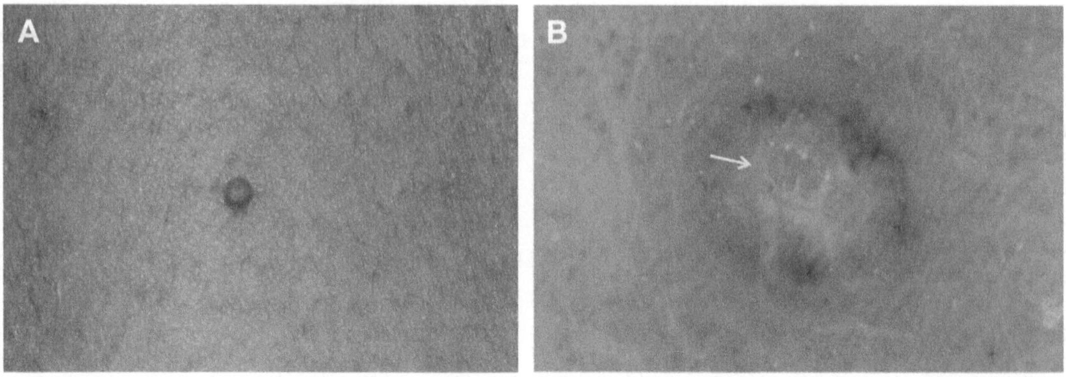

Fig. 4. Molluscum contagiosum. (*A*) Dome-shaped, flesh-colored papule on the trunk. (*B*) Dermatoscopy shows an amorphous central structure (*arrow*) surrounded by fine, linear vessels (original magnification ×10).

yellowish-white, lobulated, amorphous structures in the center of the lesion associated with a surrounding crown of linear, fine, or branching vessels (Fig. 4B). Histopathologically, these features correlate with the lobulated, endophytic epidermal hyperplasia with intracytoplasmic inclusion bodies (Henderson-Paterson bodies) and with the dilated vessels in the dermis, respectively. Dermatoscopy allows an easy differential diagnosis with acne, cysts, and other genital growth.[11,72]

FUNGAL DISORDERS

Tinea Capitis

Tinea capitis is a superficial dermatophyte infection quite common in children. Although several different species of fungi may be responsible, the main causative pathogens are members of 2 genera, *Microsporum* (zoophilic dermatophytes) and *Trichophyton* (anthropophilic dermatophytes). Risk factors include promiscuity, poor hygiene, and direct contact with pets. Based on the mechanism of hair shaft invasion, 2 main types of parasitism can be identified. In ectothrix infection, fungi (eg, *Microsporum canis*) spread around and into the hair shaft before descending into the follicles to penetrate the cortex, whereas in endothrix infection (eg, *Trichophyton tonsurans* and *soudanense*) only the inside of the hair shaft is filled with hyphae and spores replacing the intrapilary keratin.[74]

The clinical presentation of tinea capitis is quite variable, depending on the type of hair invasion, the level of host resistance, and the degree of the inflammatory host response. The typical lesions of ectothrix-type infection vary from patches of partial alopecia, revealing several broken hairs with fine scaling and slight inflammatory changes (Fig. 5A) to painful inflammatory masses sometimes discharging pus (kerion). In endothrix infections, noninflammatory grayish alopecic patches with several black dots, corresponding to swollen hair shafts, are usually seen.

The diagnosis of tinea capitis is established based on microscopic direct examination of skin scraping for hyphae and mycological cultures that allow the identification of the causative agent.

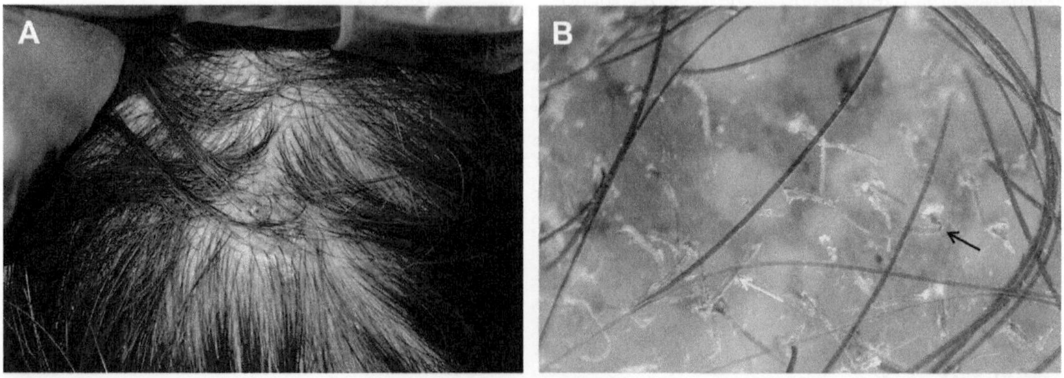

Fig. 5. Tinea capitis. (*A*) Small, roundish, erythematous, alopecic patch on the scalp. (*B*) Dermatoscopy shows diffuse scaling, broken hairs, comma hairs (*black arrow*), and interrupted hairs (*yellow arrow*) (original magnification ×10).

Several recent studies have reported the usefulness of dermatoscopy in the diagnosis of tinea capitis, characterized by the presence of diffuse scaling, broken hairs, bent hairs, and black dots[75–93] (**Fig. 5**B). A typical finding is the presence of comma hairs, appearing as short, C-shaped, homogeneously thickened and sharp slating ended hairs that are related to the bending and breakage of hair shafts filled with hyphae. In black patients and in patients with curly hair, the so-called corkscrew hairs (short hairs with multiple twists) are usually observed.[78–80] Another typical finding is represented by the interrupted hairs (also known as Morse code-like or bar-code hairs) characterized by horizontal, irregularly alternating, whitish and dark bands.[75,91,92] At high magnification (150), the whitish bands appear as empty areas of the shaft likely related to fungal invasion and representing loci minoris resistentiae causing bending and breakage.[89] The interrupted hairs have also been observed in tinea of the eyebrows.[79] Another dermatoscopic finding is represented by zigzag hairs, consisting of hairs with consecutive bending. Finally, inflammatory tinea capitis (kerion) is characterized by blotchy pigmentation, erythema, scaling, pustules, and follicular scale-crust formation.[94]

Dermatoscopy is useful to easily rule out other forms of patchy alopecia, in particular alopecia areata and trichotillomania.

Tinea Nigra

Tinea nigra is a superficial phaeohyphomycosis, a cutaneous infection usually caused by Hortaea werneckii, a fungus that produces distinct brown to black hyphae. Clinically it appears as a single, sharply marginated, brown, nonscaly patch usually occurring on the palms and soles. Because the lesions grossly resemble acquired acral melanocytic lesions, biopsy is often considered. At dermatoscopy, tinea nigra is characterized by fine, brownish spicules and dots in a reticular-like or filamentous arrangement that do not follow the furrows and ridges.[95–106] They correspond to pigmented hyphae in the stratum corneum. This dermatoscopic pattern is quite characteristic, allowing the differentiation from malignant melanoma, junctional melanocytic nevi, or other nonmalignant disorders and avoiding unnecessary biopsies.[95,102,107] However, few cases of tinea nigra showing a parallel ridge pattern (generally observed in melanoma) have been described.[98,99]

SUMMARY

Dermatoscopy has been demonstrated to enhance the diagnostic accuracy of several common parasitic and infectious skin disorders.[108] The main advantages of this technique are that it is noninvasive, quick to perform, and relatively inexpensive. Moreover, training for the dermatoscopic recognition of these disorders is simple compared with that required for pigmented skin lesions. The routine use of dermatoscopy in dermatology in daily clinical practice may play an important role to contain the spreading of skin contagious disorders.

REFERENCES

1. Zalaudek I, Giacomel J, Cabo H, et al. Entodermoscopy: a new tool for diagnosing skin infections and infestations. Dermatology 2008;216:14–23.
2. Argenziano G, Fabbrocini G, Delfino M. Epiluminescence microscopy. A new approach to in vivo detection of Sarcoptes scabiei. Arch Dermatol 1997;133:751–3.
3. Prins C, Stucki L, French L, et al. Dermoscopy for the in vivo detection of sarcoptes scabiei. Dermatology 2004;208:241–3.
4. Dupuy A, Dehen L, Bourrat E, et al. Accuracy of standard dermoscopy for diagnosing scabies. J Am Acad Dermatol 2007;56:53–62.
5. Lacarrubba F, Micali G. Videodermatoscopy and scabies. J Pediatr 2013;163:1227–1227.e1.
6. Micali G, Lacarrubba F, Verzì AE, et al. Scabies: advances in noninvasive diagnosis. PLoS Negl Trop Dis 2016;10(6):e0004691.
7. Micali G, Lacarrubba F, Lo Guzzo G. Scraping versus videodermatoscopy for the diagnosis of scabies: a comparative study [letter]. Acta Derm Venereol 2000;79:396.
8. Lacarrubba F, Musumeci ML, Caltabiano R, et al. High-magnification videodermatoscopy: a new noninvasive diagnostic tool for scabies in children. Pediatr Dermatol 2001;18:439–41.
9. Park JH, Kim CW, Kim SS. The diagnostic accuracy of dermoscopy for scabies. Ann Dermatol 2012; 24(2):194–9.
10. Lacarrubba F, Micali G. Videodermatoscopy enhances the diagnostic capability in a case of scabies of the scalp. G Ital Dermatol Venereol 2008;143:351–2.
11. Micali G, Lacarrubba F, Massimino D, et al. Dermatoscopy: alternative uses in daily clinical practice. J Am Acad Dermatol 2011;64:1135–46.
12. Micali G, Lacarrubba F, Tedeschi A. Videodermatoscopy enhances the ability to monitor efficacy of scabies treatment and allows optimal timing of drug application. J Eur Acad Dermatol Venereol 2004;18:153–4.
13. Lacarrubba F, D'Amico V, Nasca MR, et al. Use of dermatoscopy and videodermatoscopy in therapeutic follow-up: a review. Int J Dermatol 2010; 49(8):866–73.
14. Micali G, Lacarrubba F, Verzì AE, et al. Low-cost equipment for diagnosis and management of

endemic scabies outbreaks in underserved populations. Clin Infect Dis 2015;60:327–9.
15. Verzì AE, Lacarrubba F, Micali G. Use of low-cost videomicroscopy versus standard videodermatoscopy in trichoscopy: a controlled, blinded noninferiority trial. Skin Appendage Disord 2016;1(4): 172–4.
16. Devore CD, Schutze GE, Council on School Health and Committee on Infectious Diseases, American Academy of Pediatrics. Head lice. Pediatrics 2015;135(5):e1355–65.
17. Criado PR. Entodermoscopy: dermoscopy for the diagnosis of pediculosis. An Bras Dermatol 2011; 86:370–1.
18. Di Stefani A, Hofmann-Wellenhof R, Zalaudek I. Dermoscopy for diagnosis and treatment monitoring of pediculosis capitis. J Am Acad Dermatol 2006;54:909–11.
19. Martins LG, Bernardes Filho F, Quaresma MV, et al. Dermoscopy applied to pediculosis corporis diagnosis. An Bras Dermatol 2014;89(3):513–4.
20. Nikam VV, Mehta HH. A nonrandomized study of trichoscopy patterns using nonpolarized (contact) and polarized (noncontact) dermatoscopy in hair and shaft disorders. Int J Trichology 2014;6:54–62.
21. Zalaudek I, Argenziano G. Images in clinical medicine. Dermoscopy of nits and pseudonits. N Engl J Med 2012;367(18):1741.
22. Doche I, Vincenzi C, Tosti A. Casts and pseudocasts. J Am Acad Dermatol 2016;75(4):e147–8.
23. Albayrak H, Yanik ME. Dermoscopic appearance of hair casts. J Dermatol 2017;44(8):e182–3.
24. Tang JQ, You ZM, Yang Q, et al. Image gallery: dermoscopy for hair casts due to traction. Br J Dermatol 2017;176(4):e37.
25. Miteva M, Tosti A. Dermatoscopy of hair shaft disorders. J Am Acad Dermatol 2013;68(3):473–81.
26. Zhuang K, Ran X, Dai Y, et al. An unusual case of white piedra due to Trichosporon inkin mimicking trichobacteriosis. Mycopathologia 2016;181(11–12):909–14.
27. Sandoval-Tress C, Arenas-Guzmán R, Guzmán-Sánchez DA. Hair shaft yellow nodules in a pediatric female patient. Skin Appendage Disord 2015; 1(2):62–4.
28. Micali G, Tedeschi A, West DP, et al. The use of videodermatoscopy to monitor treatment of scabies and pediculosis. J Dermatolog Treat 2011;22(3):133–7.
29. Lacarrubba F, Nardone B, Milani M, et al. Head lice: ex vivo videodermatoscopy evaluation of the pediculocidal activity of two different topical products. G Ital Dermatol Venereol 2006;141:233–5.
30. Nasca MR, Lacarrubba F, Micali G. Collembola vs head lice: a puzzling case solved by videodermoscopy. J Am Acad Dermatol 2015;72:S76–7.
31. Chuh A, Lee A, Wong W, et al. Diagnosis of Pediculosis pubis: a novel application of digital epiluminescence dermatoscopy. J Eur Acad Dermatol Venereol 2007;21:837–8.
32. Budimcić D, Lipozencić J, Pastar Z, et al. Pediculosis pubis and dermoscopy. Acta Dermatovenerol Croat 2009;17:77–8.
33. Lacarrubba F, Micali G. The not-so-naked eye: phthiriasis palpebrarum. Am J Med 2013;126: 960–1.
34. Micali G, Lacarrubba F. Images in clinical medicine. Phthiriasis Palpebrarum in a child. N Engl J Med 2015;373(27):e35.
35. Bauer J, Forschner A, Garbe C, et al. Dermoscopy of tungiasis. Arch Dermatol 2004;140(6):761–3.
36. Cabrera R, Daza F. Tungiasis: eggs seen with dermoscopy. Br J Dermatol 2008;158:635–6.
37. Bakos RM, Bakos L. "Whitish chains": a remarkable in vivo dermoscopic finding of tungiasis. Br J Dermatol 2008;159:991–2.
38. Cabrera R, Daza F. Dermoscopy in the diagnosis of tungiasis. Br J Dermatol 2009;160:1136–7.
39. Di Stefani A, Rudolph CM, Hofmann-Wellenhof R, et al. An additional dermoscopic feature of tungiasis. Arch Dermatol 2005;141:1045–6.
40. Dunn R, Asher R, Bowling J. Dermoscopy: ex vivo visualization of fleas head and bag of eggs confirms the diagnosis of Tungiasis. Australas J Dermatol 2012;53:120–2.
41. Criado PR, Landman G, Reis VM, et al. Tungiasis under dermoscopy: in vivo and ex vivo examination of the cutaneous infestation due to Tunga penetrans. An Bras Dermatol 2013;88:649–51.
42. Abarzua A, Cataldo K, Alvarez S. Dermoscopy in tungiasis. Indian J Dermatol Venereol Leprol 2014;80:371–3.
43. Torres-Guerrero E, Quintanilla-Cedillo MR, Ruiz-Esmenjaud J, et al. Leishmaniasis: a review. F1000Res 2017;6:750.
44. Llambrich A, Zaballos P, Terrasa F, et al. Dermoscopy of cutaneous leishmaniasis. Br J Dermatol 2009;160:756–61.
45. Taheri AR, Pishgooei N, Maleki M, et al. Dermoscopic features of cutaneous leishmaniasis. Int J Dermatol 2013;52:1361–6.
46. Yücel A, Günaşti S, Denli Y, et al. Cutaneous leishmaniasis: new dermoscopic findings. Int J Dermatol 2013;52:831–7.
47. Ayhan E, Ucmak D, Baykara SN, et al. Clinical and dermoscopic evaluation of cutaneous leishmaniasis. Int J Dermatol 2015;54:193–201.
48. Elsner E, Thewes M, Worret WI. Cutaneous larva migrans detected by epiluminescence microscopy. Acta Derm Venereol 1997;77:487–8.
49. Veraldi S, Schianchi R, Carrera C. Epiluminescence microscopy in cutaneous larva migrans. Acta Derm Venereol 2000;80:233.
50. Aljasser MI, Lui H, Zeng H, et al. Dermoscopy and near-infrared fluorescence imaging of cutaneous

larva migrans. Photodermatol Photoimmunol Photomed 2013;29:337–8.
51. Guarneri C, Lanteri G, Tchernev G, et al. Trombiculiasis: the uninvited trekker. IDCases 2017;9:4–5.
52. Nasca MR, Lacarrubba F, Micali G. Diagnosis of trombiculosis by videodermatoscopy. Emerg Infect Dis 2014;20:1059–60.
53. di Meo N, Fadel M, Trevisan G. Pushing the edge of dermoscopy in new directions: entomodermoscopy of Trombicula autumnalis. Acta Dermatovenerol Alp Pannonica Adriat 2017;26(2):45–6.
54. Al Aboud AM, Nigam PK. Wart (plantar, verruca vulgaris, verrucae). StatPearls. Treasure Island (FL): StatPearls Publishing; 2017.
55. Forcier M, Musacchio N. An overview of human papillomavirus infection for the dermatologist: disease, diagnosis, management, and prevention. Dermatol Ther 2010;23(5):458–76.
56. Micali G, Lacarrubba F. Possible applications of videodermatoscopy beyond pigmented lesions. Int J Dermatol 2003;42:430–3.
57. Micali G, Lacarrubba F. Augmented diagnostic capability using videodermatoscopy on selected infectious and non-infectious penile growths. Int J Dermatol 2011;50:1501–5.
58. Yoong C, Di Stefani A, Hofmann-Wellenhof R, et al. Unusual clinical and dermoscopic presentation of a wart. Australas J Dermatol 2009;50:228–9.
59. Lacarrubba F, Verzì AE, Dinotta F, et al. Dermatoscopy in inflammatory and infectious skin disorders. G Ital Dermatol Venereol 2015;150(5):521–31.
60. Lee DY, Park JH, Lee JH, et al. The use of dermoscopy for the diagnosis of plantar wart. J Eur Acad Dermatol Venereol 2009;23:726–7.
61. Kim HO, Bae JM, Kim YY, et al. Differential diagnosis of wart from callus and healed wart with aid of dermoscopy. Abstract Proceedings First Congress of the International Dermoscopy Society (IDS). Dermatology 2006;212:307.
62. Bae JM, Kang H, Kim HO, et al. Differential diagnosis of plantar wart from corn, callus and healed wart with the aid of dermoscopy. Br J Dermatol 2009;160:220–2.
63. Vázquez-López F, Kreusch J, Marghoob AA. Dermoscopic semiology: further insights into vascular features by screening a large spectrum of nontumoral skin lesions. Br J Dermatol 2004;150:226–31.
64. Kim WJ, Lee WK, Song M, et al. Clinical clues for differential diagnosis between verruca plana and verruca plana-like seborrheic keratosis. J Dermatol 2015;42(4):373–7.
65. Kim SH, Seo SH, Ko HC, et al. The use of dermatoscopy to differentiate vestibular papillae, a normal variant of the female external genitalia, from condyloma acuminata. J Am Acad Dermatol 2009;60:353–5.
66. Watanabe T, Yoshida Y, Yamamoto O. Differential diagnosis of pearly penile papules and penile condyloma acuminatum by dermoscopy. Eur J Dermatol 2010;20:414–5.
67. Dong H, Shu D, Campbell TM, et al. Dermatoscopy of genital warts. J Am Acad Dermatol 2011;64:859–64.
68. Lacarrubba F, Dinotta F, Nasca MR, et al. Enhanced diagnosis of genital warts with videodermatoscopy: histopatologic correlation. G Ital Dermatol Venereol 2012;147:215–6.
69. Zaballos P, Ara M, Puig S, et al. Dermoscopy of molluscum contagiosum: a useful tool for clinical diagnosis in adulthood. J Eur Acad Dermatol Venereol 2006;20:482–3.
70. Morales A, Puig S, Malvehy J, et al. Dermoscopy of molluscum contagiosum. Arch Dermatol 2005;141:1644.
71. Ianhez M, Cestari Sda C, Enokihara MY, et al. Dermoscopic patterns of molluscum contagiosum: a study of 211 lesions confirmed by histopathology. An Bras Dermatol 2011;86:74–9.
72. Alfaro-Castellón P, Mejía-Rodríguez SA, Valencia-Herrera A, et al. Dermoscopy distinction of eruptive vellus hair cysts with molluscum contagiosum and acne lesions. Pediatr Dermatol 2012;29:772–3.
73. Lacarrubba F, Verzì AE, Ardigò M, et al. Handheld reflectance confocal microscopy for the diagnosis of molluscum contagiosum: histopathology and dermoscopy correlation. Australas J Dermatol 2017;58(3):e123–5.
74. Verna S, Heffernan MP. Superficial fungal infection: dermatophytosis, onychomycosis, tinea nigra, piedra. In: Wolff K, Goldsmith LA, Katz SI, et al, editors. Fitzpatrick's dermatology in general medicine. 7th edition. New York: McGraw-Hill; 2008. p. 1811–2.
75. Mapelli ET, Gualandri L, Cerri A, et al. Comma hairs in tinea capitis: a useful dermatoscopic sign for diagnosis of tinea capitis. Pediatr Dermatol 2012;29:223–4.
76. Slowinska M, Rudnicka L, Schwartz RA, et al. Comma hairs: a dermatoscopic marker for tinea capitis: a rapid diagnostic method. J Am Acad Dermatol 2008;59:S77–9.
77. Rudnicka L, Olszewska M, Rakowska A, et al. Trichoscopy update 2011. J Dermatol Case Rep 2011;5:82–8.
78. Schechtman RC, Silva ND, Quaresma MV, et al. Dermatoscopic findings as a complementary tool in the differential diagnosis of the etiological agent of tinea capitis. An Bras Dermatol 2015;90(3 Suppl 1):13–5.
79. Neri I, Starace M, Patrizi A, et al. Corkscrew hair: a trichoscopy marker of tinea capitis in an adult white patient. JAMA Dermatol 2013;149:990–1.
80. Hughes R, Chiaverini C, Bahadoran P, et al. Corkscrew hair: a new dermoscopic sign for diagnosis of tinea capitis in black children. Arch Dermatol 2011;147:355–6.

81. Pinheiro AM, Lobato LA, Varella TC. Dermoscopy findings in tinea capitis: case report and literature review. An Bras Dermatol 2012;87:313–4.
82. Hernández-Bel P, Malvehy J, Crocker A, et al. Comma hairs: a new dermoscopic marker for tinea capitis. Actas Dermosifiliogr 2012;103:836–7.
83. Ekiz O, Sen BB, Rifaioğlu EN, et al. Trichoscopy in paediatric patients with tinea capitis: a useful method to differentiate from alopecia areata. J Eur Acad Dermatol Venereol 2014;28:1255–8.
84. Brasileiro A, Campos S, Cabete J, et al. Trichoscopy as an additional tool for the differential diagnosis of tinea capitis: a prospective clinical study. Br J Dermatol 2016;175(1):208–9.
85. Amer M, Helmy A, Amer A. Trichoscopy as a useful method to differentiate tinea capitis from alopecia areata in children at Zagazig University Hospitals. Int J Dermatol 2017;56(1):116–20.
86. Bourezane Y, Bourezane Y. Analysis of trichoscopic signs observed in 24 patients presenting tinea capitis: hypotheses based on physiopathology and proposed new classification. Ann Dermatol Venereol 2017;144(8–9):490–6.
87. Elghblawi E. Idiosyncratic findings in trichoscopy of tinea capitis: comma, zigzag hairs, corkscrew, and morse code-like hair. Int J Trichology 2016; 8(4):180–3.
88. Gómez Moyano E, Crespo Erchiga V, Martínez Pilar L, et al. Correlation between dermoscopy and direct microscopy of morse code hairs in tinea incognito. J Am Acad Dermatol 2016;74(1):e7–8.
89. Lacarrubba F, Verzì AE, Micali G. Newly described features resulting from high-magnification dermoscopy of tinea capitis. JAMA Dermatol 2015;151:308–10.
90. Errichetti E, Stinco G. Dermoscopy as a useful supportive tool for the diagnosis of pityriasis amiantacea-like tinea capitis. Dermatol Pract Concept 2016;6(3):63–5.
91. Lu M, Ran Y, Dai Y, et al. An ultrastructural study on corkscrew hairs and cigarette-ash-shaped hairs observed by dermoscopy of tinea capitis. Scanning 2016;38(2):128–32.
92. Lekkas D, Ioannides D, Apalla Z, et al. Dermoscopy for discriminating between trichophyton and microsporum infections in tinea capitis. J Eur Acad Dermatol Venereol 2017. https://doi.org/10.1111/jdv.14755.
93. Wang HH, Lin YT. Bar code-like hair: dermoscopic marker of tinea capitis and tinea of the eyebrow. J Am Acad Dermatol 2015;72:S41–2.
94. Jain N, Doshi B, Khopkar U. Trichoscopy in alopecias: diagnosis simplified. Int J Trichology 2013;5: 170–8.
95. Criado PR, Delgado L, Pereira GA. Dermoscopy revealing a case of Tinea Nigra. An Bras Dermatol 2013;88:128–9.
96. Gupta G, Burden AD, Shankland GS, et al. Tinea nigra secondary to Exophiala werneckii responding to Itraconazole. Br J Dermatol 1997;137:483–4.
97. Maia Abinader MV, Carvalho Maron SM, Araújo LO, et al. Tinea nigra dermoscopy: a useful assessment. J Am Acad Dermatol 2016;74(6):e121–2.
98. Nazzaro G, Ponziani A, Cavicchini S. Tinea nigra: a diagnostic pitfall. J Am Acad Dermatol 2016;75(6): e219–20.
99. Noguchi H, Hiruma M, Inoue Y, et al. Tinea nigra showing a parallel ridge pattern on dermoscopy. J Dermatol 2015;42:518–20.
100. Paschoal FM, de Barros JA, de Barros DP, et al. Study of the dermatoscopic pattern of tinea nigra: report of 6 cases. Skinmed 2010;8:319–21.
101. Piliouras P, Allison S, Rosendahl C, et al. Dermoscopy improves diagnosis of tinea nigra: a study of 50 cases. Australas J Dermatol 2011; 52:191–4.
102. Rossetto AL, Corrêa PR, Cruz RC, et al. A case of Tinea nigra associated to a bite from a European rabbit (Oryctolagus cuniculus, Leporidae): the role of dermoscopy in diagnosis. An Bras Dermatol 2014;89(1):165–6.
103. Smith SB, Beals SL, Elston DM, et al. Dermoscopy in the diagnosis of tinea nigra plantaris. Cutis 2001; 68:377–80.
104. Thomas CL, Samarasinghe V, Natkunarajah J, et al. Entodermoscopy: a spotlight on tinea nigra. Int J Dermatol 2016;55(2):e117–8.
105. Veasey JV, Avila RB, Ferreira MAMO, et al. Reflectance confocal microscopy of tinea nigra: comparing images with dermoscopy and mycological examination results. An Bras Dermatol 2017; 92(4):568–9.
106. Xavier MH, Ribeiro LH, Duarte H, et al. Dermatoscopy in the diagnosis of tinea nigra. Dermatol Online J 2008;14:15.
107. Lacarrubba F, Dall'Oglio F, Dinotta F, et al. Photoletter to the editor: exogenous pigmentation of the sole mimicking in situ acral melanoma on dermoscopy. J Dermatol Case Rep 2012;6(3): 100–1.
108. Micali G, Verzì AE, Lacarrubba F. Alternative uses of dermatoscopy in daily clinical practice: an update. J Am Acad Dermatol 2018 Jun 16. pii: S0190-9622(18)32143-1. [Epub ahead of print].

Dermoscopy of Common Inflammatory Disorders

Dimitrios Sgouros, MD[a], Zoe Apalla, MD, PhD[b], Dimitrios Ioannides, MD, PhD[b], Alexander Katoulis, MD, PhD[a], Dimitrios Rigopoulos, MD, PhD[c], Elena Sotiriou, MD, PhD[b], Alexander Stratigos, MD, PhD[c], Efstratios Vakirlis, MD, PhD[b], Aimilios Lallas, MD, MSc, PhD[b,*]

KEYWORDS

• Dermoscopy • General dermatology • Inflammoscopy • Inflammatory dermatoses • Dermatoscopy • Vessels

KEY POINTS

- Dermoscopy gains appreciation in fields beyond dermato-oncology, in addition to its "traditional" application for the early diagnosis of melanoma and nonmelanoma skin cancers.
- Nowadays, dermoscopy serves as an additional tool for the assessment of skin lesions in general dermatology, following the well-known clinical diagnostic steps.
- A stepwise approach scheme for the dermoscopic evaluation of skin lesions in general dermatology should be stratified.
- The main parameters that should be evaluated are morphology and distribution of vessels, color and distribution of scales, background colors, follicular abnormalities, and specific clues.
- Dermoscopic findings should be always viewed within patient's clinical context and interpreted in conjunction with all relevant information from patients' history, symptomatology, and macroscopic morphology.

INTRODUCTION

Dermoscopy has been established as the dermatologist's key tool for the evaluation of pigmented and nonpigmented skin tumors.[1–3] In addition to its "traditional" application for the early diagnosis of melanoma and nonmelanoma skin cancers, dermoscopy gains appreciation in fields beyond dermato-oncology. This is because dermoscopy reveals clues and patterns that cannot be seen with the naked eye. Therefore, it adds morphologic information in any type of skin lesion or eruption. Indeed, the dermoscopic patterns of several inflammatory skin diseases have been described. Dermoscopy is nowadays considered as an additional valuable method for the assessment of skin lesions in general dermatology, which follows and completes the well-known clinical diagnostic steps, such as medical history and clinical examination. Clinical examination remains the undoubted mainstay of diagnosis in inflammatory and infectious diseases, representing a synthesis of several components to which dermoscopy contributes additional morphologic information in a submacroscopic level, thus completing the puzzle of clinical diagnosis.[4–8]

An issue of great importance is the definition of a stepwise approach for the dermoscopic evaluation

Disclosure: None.

[a] 2nd Department of Dermatology – Venereology, National Kapodistrian University of Athens, ATTIKON University Hospital, 1 Rimini Street, Chaidari, Athens 12462, Greece; [b] 1st Department of Dermatology – Venereology, State Clinic of Dermatology, Aristotle University of Thessaloniki, Hospital of Skin and Venereal Diseases, 124 Delfon Street, Thessaloniki 54643, Greece; [c] 1st Department of Dermatology – Venereology, National Kapodistrian University of Athens, A. Syggros Hospital, 5 I.Dragoumi Street, Athens 16121, Greece
* Corresponding author.
E-mail address: emlallas@gmail.com

Dermatol Clin 36 (2018) 359–368
https://doi.org/10.1016/j.det.2018.05.003

of skin lesions in general dermatology. Taking into account all the existing knowledge of the dermoscopic characteristics of inflammatory and infectious skin diseases, the main categories of criteria that should be evaluated are the following: (1) morphology of the vascular structures (eg, dotted, linear); (2) arrangement of vascular structures; (3) color and distribution of scales; (4) background colors; (5) follicular abnormalities; and (6) other specific features (clues).[5] Obviously, the observed (described) dermatoscopic features of a given lesion should always be considered within the overall clinical context.

Regarding the selection of the optimal dermoscopic equipment, the introduction of the new-generation devices in everyday clinical practice, combining noncontact, polarized light dermoscopy with the classic contact dermoscopy, has resolved the issue of altering or even obscuring the vascular structures of inflammatory lesions. This is critical for the accurate dermoscopic examination of skin disorders in general dermatology, because the pattern of vessels (morphology, distribution etc) often represents the predominant dermoscopic characteristic.[4]

For more than a decade from the first publications on the use of dermoscopy in inflammatory dermatoses, the authors' knowledge was based on a few case reports and case series studies. However, in the last years, several case series and case-control studies have been published, some of them including well-documented data and large numbers of patients.[9–14] In addition, nowadays dermoscopy is not only used for strictly diagnostic purposes but also to evaluate the physical course of diseases and the response to treatments.[15–17]

This article aims to provide an up-to-date overview of existing data on dermoscopic findings in common inflammatory skin diseases. This field is often described under the term "inflammoscopy." For structural purposes, the review is subdivided into 5 categories of dermatologic disorders: (1) erythemato-squamous skin diseases, (2) autoimmune cutaneous diseases (3) intolerance reactions and vasculitides, (4) rosacea and demodecidosis, and (5) disorders of keratinization and porokeratosis.

ERYTHEMATO-SQUAMOUS SKIN DISEASES

Psoriasis

Psoriasis is the most typical representative of the category of erythemato-squamous skin diseases, clinically manifesting with red plaques with prominent white scales. The dermoscopic pattern of psoriasis was firstly described in the early 2000s.[18,19] The most striking dermoscopic features of psoriasis are the evenly distributed red dots or globules over a pale red erythematous background along with white scaling of the lesion.[11,18–20] These red roundish structures appear under higher magnification (×100 to ×400) as convoluted loops, mirroring the underlying histopathologic finding of spiraled capillaries within the dermal papillae, associated with the psoriasiform epidermal hyperplasia.[5,20,21] Moreover, clinical experience has clarified that the differentiation between the descriptive terms of dots (smaller diameter of 0.1 mm) and globules (larger diameter than dots) is insignificant in the dermoscopic classification of psoriatic lesions despite their importance in the dermoscopy of melanocytic lesions. Red dots or globules in psoriasis are typically monomorphic, of similar diameter and shape, and symmetrically distributed in a given plaque. However, vascular structures of different diameters might occasionally coexist in the same lesion.[4]

An additional dermoscopic finding of high relevance for psoriasis is the white scaling, which can be a very helpful clue for the differential diagnosis between psoriasis and other inflammatory skin diseases as well as neoplastic disorders. Specifically, the white color of psoriatic scales is of particular value for the diagnosis of psoriasis compared with the yellow scales or crusts that are usually suggestive of dermatitis.[12] Even in hyperkeratotic psoriatic plaques, the removal of scales can reveal the characteristic vascular pattern of psoriasis, possibly together with tiny red blood drops, representing the dermoscopic "Auspitz sign."[4] In addition, the color and distribution of scales along with the dermoscopic vascular pattern contribute in the differentiation of psoriasis from Bowen disease. As mentioned earlier, typically, in psoriasis there are red globules regularly distributed throughout the lesion, accompanied with fine white scales (**Fig. 1**). In contrast, glomerular vessels, commonly similar to globules, scattered in clusters along with yellowish crusts or unevenly distributed "islands" of whitish scales compose the dermoscopic pattern of Bowen disease.[22,23] Finally, the pattern of dotted vessels versus short, fine telangiectasias is helpful in the differentiation of similarly appearing patches of psoriasis and superficial basal cell carcinoma, respectively.[24]

The dermoscopic variability of psoriatic lesions according to the anatomic site has also been investigated. It was shown that the typical vascular findings of psoriasis (regularly distributed red globules) prevails even on special anatomic locations such as the scalp, face, palms, soles, folds, and

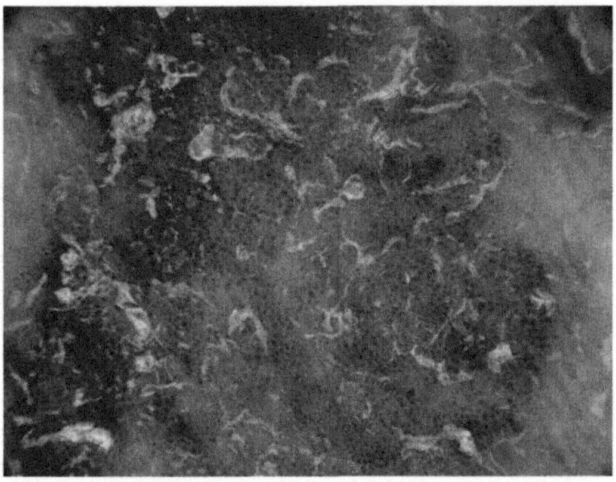

Fig. 1. Dermoscopy of psoriasis: regularly distributed dotted vessels and white scales (original magnification ×10).

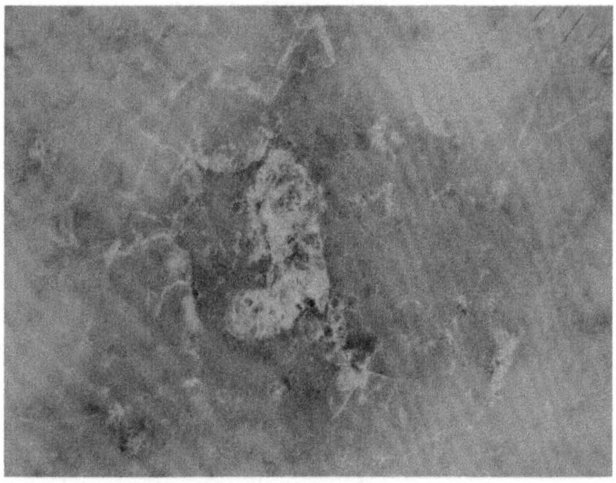

Fig. 2. Dermoscopy of dermatitis: yellow serocrusts (original magnification ×10).

genitalia.[25,26] In contrast, scaling reasonably varies according to the anatomic site. Specifically, scales appear diffuse on the scalp and palmoplantar psoriasis while there is lack of scaling, and thus better visualization of the vessels, in the genitalia and the folds.[13]

Apart from diagnosis, dermoscopy is also used as a tool for the evaluation of treatment of psoriasis. It helps monitor patients on systemic therapies for psoriasis and it is also a predictor of early response to treatment or recurrence.[15,21,27] Hemorrhagic dots in a given psoriatic plaque have been suggested to represent a positive predictive sign, suggesting a favorable clinical outcome in psoriasis treated with biological agents. Special attention should be given in the differentiation of the typical red globular vessels of psoriasis from these recently described hemorrhagic dots.[15] Furthermore, dermoscopy can reveal an otherwise not clinically evident, skin atrophy with telangiectatic vessels in cases of psoriasis following treatment with potent topical steroids.[28]

Dermatitis-Eczema-Seborrheic Dermatitis

The term "dermatitis" comprises several distinct clinical entities sharing common histopathologic features, such as contact/allergic dermatitis, atopic dermatitis, and seborrheic dermatitis. Beyond their clinical presentation and epidemiologic characteristics, dermoscopy is useful for their distinction and the differential diagnosis from similarly looking diseases such as psoriasis or even mycosis fungoides.[4,9,12,29–31] Dotted vessels in a patchy distribution and yellow serocrusts represent the most common dermoscopic findings in all subtypes of dermatitis (**Fig. 2**).[5] The dermoscopic pattern varies according to the evolution stage of dermatitis. Specifically, the acute phase of blistering and exudative dermatitis is dermoscopically typified by yellow serocrusts, corresponding to the spongiotic reaction, and dotted vessels irregularly distributed within the lesion.[29,32] The term "yellow clod sign" was described for nummular eczema and refers to these yellowish serum crusts.[32] In chronic types of dermatitis the most prevalent dermoscopic features are the dotted vessels in a patchy distribution, often surrounded by white halos that histopathologically correspond to the epidermal hyperplasia of the lichenoid reaction.[29]

Recent studies report the use of dermoscopy in the differential diagnosis of several types of dermatitis (ie, atopic dermatitis, palmar eczema etc.) from psoriasis. Lacarrubba and colleagues[8,9] described the difference between intensely dilated "bushy vessels" in psoriasis and slightly dilated capillary loops in atopic and contact dermatitis by the use of videodermoscopy, which offers higher magnifications (×150). Errichetti and Stinco studied the dermoscopic patterns in chronic hand eczema and palmar psoriasis confirming the above-described characteristic findings in both skin disorders.[30]

Dermoscopy has also been suggested to improve the clinical differential diagnosis between chronic, resistant-to-treatment or relapsing eczema and early stage mycosis fungoides. Specifically, dermoscopy of the patches of mycosis fungoides reveals thin linear vessels alone or in combination with red dots, forming the peculiar "spermatozoon-like" structures (**Fig. 3**), whereas dermatitis usually lacks linear vessels, unless overtreated with topical steroids.[5,31]

Finally, seborrheic dermatitis is a type of chronic erythemato-squamous disease with a tendency to affect scalp and face. In terms of dermoscopy, seborrheic dermatitis exhibits the typical findings of other types of dermatitis, that is, dotted vessels

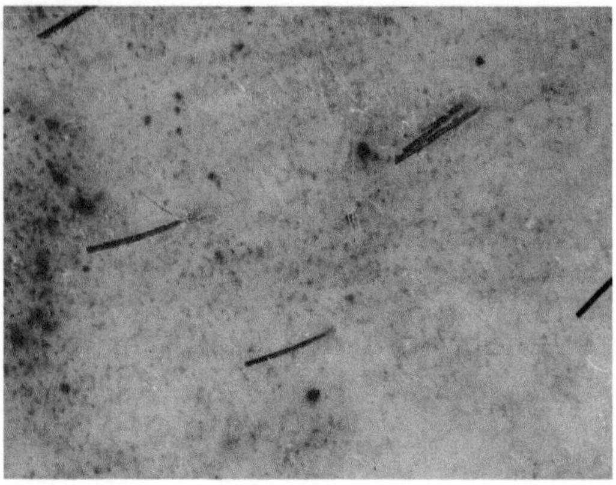

Fig. 3. Dermoscopy of mycosis fungoides: short linear vessels (original magnification ×10).

with a patchy distribution and yellow scales.[33] However, several other vascular forms have been reported especially for seborrheic dermatitis of the scalp, such as arborizing, looped, and comma-like vessels.[11,34]

Lichen Planus

Lichen planus is a papulosquamous disease involving skin, scalp, nails, and mucosal membranes. The so-called "Wickham striae," previously known as a clinical sign of mucosal lichen planus, is considered the dermoscopic hallmark of the disease. In detail, the typical dermoscopic pattern of lichen planus consists of white crossing or annular lines surrounded by red pinpoint or globular vessels at their periphery distributed in lines or rings, respectively, over a dull erythematous background (**Fig. 4**).[4,12,29,35] This feature is also of value for the differentiation of genital lichen planus from other dermatoses of the genital area such as condylomata, balanitis etc.[5] Of note, yellowish scales have been described in variants of lichen planus.[36] Pigmented types of the disease reveal a brownish structureless background admixed with blue, gray, and brown dots.[5,35]

Pityriasis Rosea

Peripheral white scaling, clinically described as "collarette scale," over a pale red to light yellowish background are the striking features in the dermoscopy of pityriasis rosea.[5,12,37,38] Dotted vessels can also be seen within a lesion; however, they do not follow the regular distribution of psoriasis.[4] Any of the aforementioned dermatoscopic features can be observed in either the herald patch or the secondary lesions (**Fig. 5**).

Pityriasis Rubra Pilaris

Pityriasis rubra pilaris is an uncommon erythemato-squamous dermatosis, often clinically resembling psoriasis. Limited data exist on the dermoscopic differentiation between the 2 entities. In a few published cases of pityriasis rubra pilaris, dermoscopy was reported to reveal linear or both linear and dotted vessels, distributed either peripherally or diffusely, whereas psoriasis is known to display regularly distributed dotted vessels. In pityriasis rubra pilaris the scales are characterized by a characteristic yellow coloration and a clustered or diffuse distribution, in contrast to the white scales of psoriasis.[39,40]

Pityriasis Lichenoides Chronica

Pityriasis lichenoides chronica is dermoscopically characterized by a combination of nondotted vessels (ie, linear irregular, branching, milky-red areas), focally distributed dotted vessels, and structureless orange areas. These findings can be of help for the differential diagnosis of pityriasis lichenoides chronica from guttate psoriasis that is

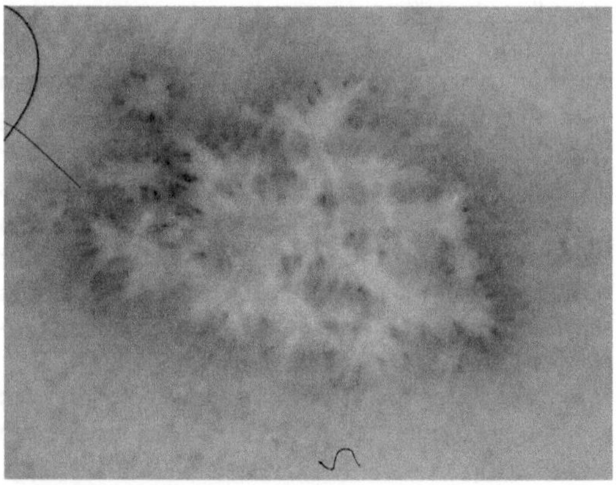

Fig. 4. Dermoscopy of lichen planus: Wickham striae (original magnification ×10).

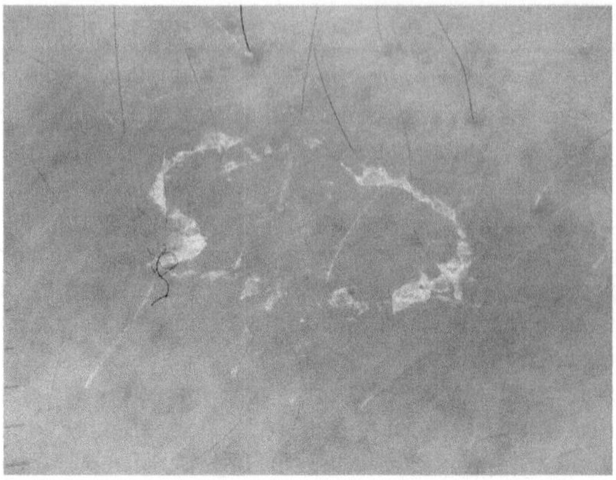

Fig. 5. Dermoscopy of pityriasis rosea: peripheral white scales (original magnification ×10).

typified by a regular distribution of dotted vessels.[6,10]

Erythroderma

Erythroderma is an urgent dermatologic condition that can be secondary to several underlying dermatoses such as psoriasis, atopic dermatitis, cutaneous lymphoma, drugs, and other uncommon diseases (ie, pityriasis rubra pilaris). Dermoscopy can play the role of an auxiliary tool for the investigation of the etiologic factor causing the diffuse erythroderma by revealing features that are not visible to the naked eye.[41]

AUTOIMMUNE CUTANEOUS DISEASES

Discoid Lupus Erythematosus

Dermoscopic manifestations of discoid lupus erythematosus (DLE) vary according to the evolution stage of the disease. Early lesions, especially on the face (extrascalp locations), exhibit intense follicular plugging (yellow clods), perifollicular whitish halo, and white scales (**Fig. 6**). As DLE progresses, signs of fibrosis and scarring become prominent, represented in dermoscopy by blurred, telangiectatic, arborizing vessels; white structureless areas; and hyperpigmentation.[42,43] DLE typically lacks the orange-yellowish pigmentation that prevails in granulomatous cutaneous diseases such as sarcoidosis and lupus vulgaris, which can be simulators of DLE.[5] It is also important to differentiate between DLE and actinic keratosis (AK) that may look quite similar especially on facial skin. Specifically, the dermoscopic pattern of DLE, which consists of red follicular plugs over a white background, can be considered as the negative or inverse pattern of the white-to-yellow targetoid follicles and red pseudonetwork of AK.[44] However, recent reports demonstrate that white, shiny rosettes, a sign formerly attributed to actinic keratosis and squamous cell carcinoma, can also be seen in the spectrum of DLE.[45]

Subacute Lupus Erythematosus

Subacute cutaneous lupus erythematosus is characterized by 2 constant dermoscopic findings, namely whitish scales (diffusely or peripherally distributed) and a mixed vascular pattern (at least 2 types of vessels among dotted, linear-irregular, linear, and branching vessels) over a pinkish-reddish background.[6,42] Focally distributed orange-yellowish structureless areas may also be seen less commonly.[6,46]

Lichen Sclerosus and Morphea

Several studies have been conducted so far investigating the dermoscopic findings in genital and extragenital lichen sclerosus (LS) and morphea according to their clinical stage.[47–52] Regardless the anatomic location and the progression of the disease, the most prevalent dermatoscopic feature of morphea are the bright white or white-yellowish patches, whereas the hallmark of cutaneous LS are the white-yellowish keratotic follicular plugs (**Fig. 7**).[4] A recent study of Errichetti and colleagues[51] correlated the inflammatory, erythematous phase of LS with diffuse erythema and pronounced red focused vessels mostly of the dotted type and the fibrotic clinical stage with white-yellowish plaques admixed with crystalline structures. In the same study the researchers also investigated the dermoscopic pattern of morphea according to the clinical stage. The most characteristic sign of morphea were the white fibrotic beams metaphorically described as "white clouds" in combination with the typical lilac ring representing disease activity.[51] Linear vessels can also accompany the early progressing stage of morphea,

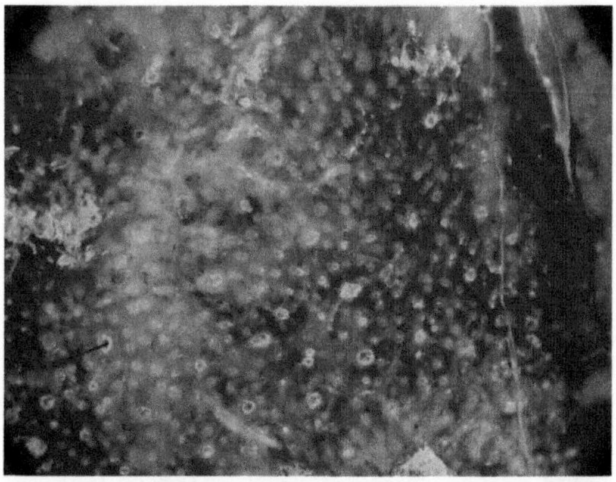

Fig. 6. Dermoscopy of discoid lupus erythematosus (early phase): follicular keratin plugs (original magnification ×10).

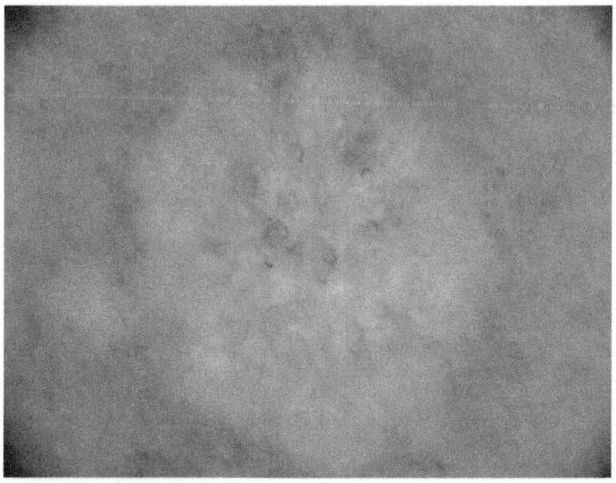

Fig. 7. Dermoscopy of extragenital lichen sclerosus: keratotic plugs over a white background (original magnification ×10).

whereas pigmentary structures are mostly found within postinflammatory plaques.[51,53]

INTOLERANCE REACTIONS AND VASCULITIDES

Urticaria and Urticarial Vasculitis

Very limited data exist about the dermoscopic manifestations of urticaria and urticarial vasculitis. Vázquez-López and colleagues[54] suggested a red network of linear vessels surrounding areas devoid of vascular structures, which correspond to massive dermal edema, as a distinct feature for urticaria. On the other hand urticarial vasculitis typically presents with purpuric dots or globules on an orange-brown background.[55] In ambiguous lesions, these purpuric dots observed through a dermatoscope may be of help in the differential diagnosis between these 2 clinical entities.[56]

Pigmented Purpuric Dermatoses

Pigmented purpuric dermatoses (PPD) represent a category of diseases characterized by extravasation of red blood cells and comprise 5 distinct clinical entities: Schamberg disease, Majocchi purpura, eczematoid purpura of Doucas and Kapetanakis, lichen aureus, and pigmented purpuric lichenoid dermatitis of Gougerot and Blum. Dermoscopically, all PPDs are typified by the presence of purpuric dots or globules within areas of orange-brown pigmentation (**Fig. 8**).[57,58]

Vasculitides

Scarce evidence exists in dermoscopic findings of true vasculitis. Irregularly shaped red patches with blurred borders are described as features of Henoch-Schönlein purpura.[4] Choo JY and colleagues suggested that blue-gray blotches are a typical finding in true vasculitis, resulting from vascular injury with severe inflammation. In contrast, a mottled purpuric pattern with purpuric dots/globules over a brown-orange background can be seen in several vasculopathies.[59]

Granuloma faciale is an uncommon, benign disease located on the face that is included in the group of vasculitides and should be differentiated from several other facial dermatoses such as lupus vulgaris, rosacea, DLE, sarcoidosis etc.[33] Dilated follicular openings, elongated-linear vessels, and surrounding perifollicular whitish halos are the most characteristic findings that might enhance the recognition of granuloma faciale among other types of facial erythema.[33,60,61]

ROSACEA AND DEMODICOSIS

Rosacea is a common skin disease involving the face and characterized by flushing, pronounced telangiectasia, permanent erythema, papulopustules, and facial edema depending on the subtype of the disease. The vascular alterations of erythematotelangiectatic rosacea (ER) are highlighted by dermoscopy.[33,62] Typically, linear vessels are arranged in horizontal and vertical lines forming polygons (polygonal vessels) (**Fig. 9**). The dermoscopic pattern of rosacea is considered as highly specific, because similar findings have not been reported in any other inflammatory disease. These vascular polygons should be differentiated from telangiectatic vessels in sun-exposed, atrophic skin that typically lack this characteristic polygonal arrangement.[4,62] Dermoscopic findings of the papulopustular rosacea include less prominent vascular alterations and more evident follicular disturbances, such as tiny pustules and dilated follicles. Phymatous rosacea displays red-yellowish masses in addition to follicular plugging. Dermoscopy always serves as a tool for the evaluation of treatment in all types of rosacea.[62,63]

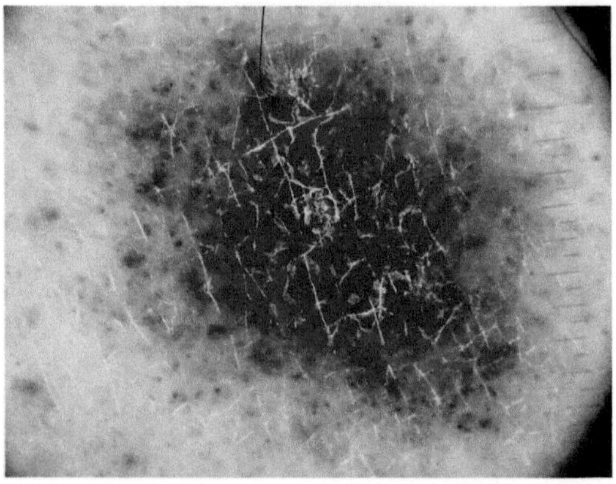

Fig. 8. Dermoscopy of pigmented purpuric dermatosis: purpuric globules on an orange-brown background (original magnification ×10).

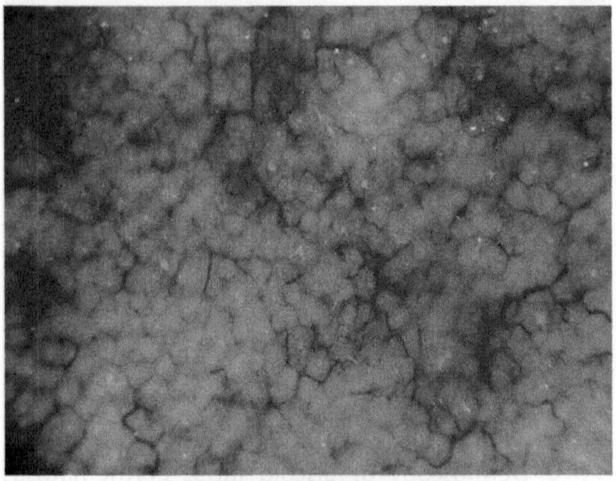

Fig. 9. Dermoscopy of rosacea: characteristic polygonal vessels (original magnification ×10).

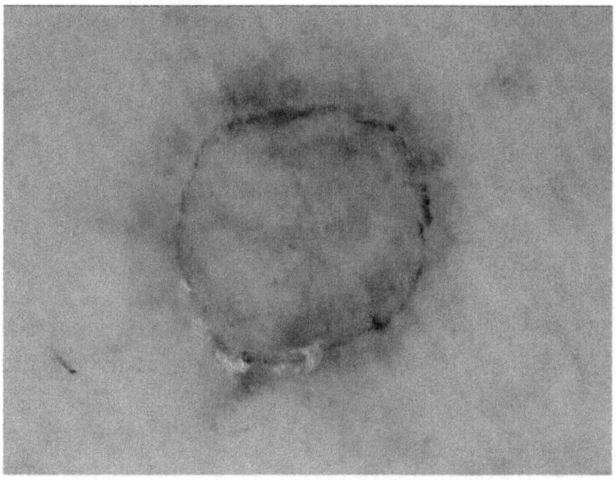

Fig. 10. Dermoscopy of porokeratosis: peripheral keratotic rim (original magnification ×10).

Demodex is a parasite of the hair follicle that might play a role in the pathogenesis of rosacea. Dermoscopy reveals signs of demodicosis such as the so-called "Demodex tails" plus white, amorphic follicular material and erythema.[64,65]

DISORDERS OF KERATINIZATION AND POROKERATOSIS

Darier Disease and Grover Disease

Dermoscopic findings in Darier disease (DD) consist of the characteristic prominent pseudocomedones and other additional nonspecific features.[66] These pseudocomedones are central yellowish or brownish areas surrounded by a whitish halo and histopathologically correspond to dyskeratosis and acantholysis, which is typical of DD. Dotted or linear vessels over a structureless pinkish background are additional features.[66–68]

As a disease sharing similar histopathologic features with DD, Grover disease also displays similar dermoscopic characteristics. There might be a subtle difference between the 2 diseases in the color of the pseudocomedones, which is more brownish in Grover disease and rather yellowish in DD.[69,70]

Porokeratosis

"Cornoid lamella" is the typical histologic finding of porokeratosis. Dermoscopy highlights this feature as a well-defined, thin, white-yellow peripheral annular rim (**Fig. 10**). The feature has also been described as a "white track" that is similar to the outlines of a volcanic crater observed from a height. The rim might be hyperpigmented in disseminated superficial actinic porokeratosis.[71–77] The center of the lesion might display either a brownish pigmentation and dotted or a structureless whitish area.[71–74]

SUMMARY

Dermoscopy has been established as a reliable adjunctive tool to the everyday clinical practice of general dermatology.[4,78] It contributes not only to the diagnosis of inflammatory and infectious skin conditions but also to the monitoring of treatment response. Dermoscopic findings should always be interpreted within the clinical context of a given patient and interpreted in conjunction with all relevant information from patients' history, symptomatology, and macroscopic morphology.

REFERENCES

1. Argenziano G, Albertini G, Castagnetti F, et al. Early diagnosis of melanoma: what is the impact of dermoscopy? Dermatol Ther 2012;25:403–9.
2. Zalaudek I, Kreusch J, Giacomel J, et al. How to diagnose nonpigmented skin tumors: a review of vascular structures seen with dermoscopy: part II. Nonmelanocytic skin tumors. J Am Acad Dermatol 2010;63:377–86 [quiz: 387–8].
3. Lallas A, Argenziano G, Zendri E, et al. Update on non-melanoma skin cancer and the value of dermoscopy in its diagnosis and treatment monitoring. Expert Rev Anticancer Ther 2013;13:541–58.
4. Lallas A, Zalaudek I, Argenziano G, et al. Dermoscopy in general dermatology. Dermatol Clin 2013;13:679–94.
5. Lallas A, Giacomel J, Argenziano G, et al. Dermoscopy in general dermatology: practical tips for the clinician. Br J Dermatol 2014;170(3):514–26.
6. Erichetti E, Stinco G. Dermoscopy in general dermatology: a practical overview. Dermatol Ther 2016;6:471–507.
7. Zalaudek I, Argenziano G, Di Stefani A, et al. Dermoscopy in general dermatology. Dermatology 2006;212:7–18.
8. Lacarrubba F, Verzì AE, Dinotta F, et al. Dermatoscopy in inflammatory and infectious skin disorders. G Ital Dermatol Venereol 2015;150(5):521–31.
9. Lacarrubba F, Musumeci ML, Ferraro S, et al. A three-cohort comparison with videodermatoscopic evidence of the distinct homogeneous bushy capillary microvascular pattern in psoriasis vs atopic dermatitis and contact dermatitis. J Eur Acad Dermatol Venereol 2016;30(4):701–3.
10. Errichetti E, Lacarrubba F, Micali G, et al. Differentiation of pityriasis lichenoides chronica from guttate psoriasis by dermoscopy. Clin Exp Dermatol 2015;40(7):804–6.
11. Kibar M, Aktan Ş, Bilgin M. Dermoscopic findings in scalp psoriasis and seborrheic dermatitis; two new signs; signet ring vessel and hidden hair. Indian J Dermatol 2015;60(1):41–5.
12. Lallas A, Kyrgidis A, Tzellos TG, et al. Accuracy of dermoscopic criteria for the diagnosis of psoriasis,

dermatitis, lichen planus and pityriasis rosea. Br J Dermatol 2012;166(6):1198–205.
13. Lallas A, Apalla Z, Argenziano G, et al. Dermoscopic pattern of psoriatic lesions on specific body sites. Dermatology 2014;228(3):250–4.
14. Haliasos EC, Kerner M, Jaimes-Lopez N, et al. Dermoscopy for the pediatric dermatologist part I: dermoscopy of pediatric infectious and inflammatory skin lesions and hair disorders. Pediatr Dermatol 2013;30(2):163–71.
15. Lallas A, Argenziano G, Zalaudek I, et al. Dermoscopic hemorrhagic dots: an early predictor of response of psoriasis to biologic agents. Dermatol Pract Concept 2016;6(4):7–12. eCollection 2016.
16. Lacarrubba F, D'Amico V, Nasca MR, et al. Use of dermatoscopy and videodermatoscopy in therapeutic follow-up: a review. Int J Dermatol 2010;49(8): 866–73.
17. Rossi A, Prandeta G, Iorio A, et al. Efficacy of Iralfaris shampoo in the treatment of scalp psoriasis: a videodermoscopy evaluation prospective study in 70 patients. G Ital Dermatol Venereol 2012;147(6):625–30.
18. Vázquez-López F, Manjón-Haces JA, Maldonado-Seral C, et al. Dermoscopic features of plaque psoriasis and lichen planus: new observations. Dermatology 2003;207:151–6.
19. De Angelis R, Bugatti L, Del Medico P, et al. Videocapillaroscopic findings in the microcirculation of the psoriatic plaque. Dermatology 2002;204:236–9.
20. Zalaudek I, Argenziano G. Dermoscopy subpatterns of inflammatory skin disorders. Arch Dermatol 2006; 142:808.
21. Lacarrubba F, Pellacani G, Gurgone S, et al. Advances in non-invasive techniques as aids to the diagnosis and monitoring of therapeutic response in plaque psoriasis: a review. Int J Dermatol 2015; 54(6):626–34.
22. Zalaudek I, Argenziano G, Leinweber B, et al. Dermoscopy of Bowen's disease. Br J Dermatol 2004; 150:1112–6.
23. Zalaudek I, Giacomel J, Schmid K, et al. Dermatoscopy of facial actinic keratosis, intraepidermal carcinoma, and invasive squamous cell carcinoma: a progression model. J Am Acad Dermatol 2012;66:589–97.
24. Giacomel J, Zalaudek I. Dermoscopy of superficial basal cell carcinoma. Dermatol Surg 2005;31:1710–3.
25. Micali G, Nardone B, Scuderi A, et al. Videodermatoscopy enhances the diagnostic capability of palmar and/or plantar psoriasis. Am J Clin Dermatol 2008;9(2):119–22.
26. Lacarrubba F, Nasca MR, Micali G. Videodermatoscopy enhances diagnostic capability in psoriatic balanitis. J Am Acad Dermatol 2009;61(6):1084–6.
27. Gniadecki R, Kragballe K, Dam TN, et al. Comparison of drug survival rates for adalimumab, etanercept and infliximab in patients with psoriasis vulgaris. Br J Dermatol 2011;164:1091–6.
28. Vázquez-López F, Marghoob AA. Dermoscopic assessment of long-term topical therapies with potent steroids in chronic psoriasis. J Am Acad Dermatol 2004;51:811–3.
29. Goncharova Y, Attia E, Souid K, et al. Dermoscopic features of clinically inflammatory dermatoses and their correlation with histopathologic reaction patterns. Arch Dermatol Res 2015;307: 23–30.
30. Errichetti E, Stinco G. Dermoscopy in differential diagnosis of palmar psoriasis and chronic hand eczema. J Dermatol 2016;43:423–5.
31. Lallas A, Apalla Z, Lefaki I, et al. Dermoscopy of early stage mycosis fungoides. J Eur Acad Dermatol Venereol 2013;27:617–21.
32. Navarini AA, Feldmeyer L, Töndury B, et al. The yellow clod sign. Arch Dermatol 2011;147:1350.
33. Lallas A, Argenziano G, Apalla Z, et al. Dermoscopic patterns of common facial inflammatory skin diseases. J Eur Acad Dermatol Venereol 2014;28: 609–14.
34. Ross EK, Vincenzi C, Tosti A. Videodermoscopy in the evaluation of hair and scalp disorders. J Am Acad Dermatol 2006;55:799–806.
35. Friedman P, Cohen-Sabban E, Marcucci C, et al. Dermoscopic findings in different clinical variants of lichen planus. Is dermoscopy useful? Dermatol Pract Concept 2015;5:51–5.
36. Papageorgiou C, Apalla Z, Lazaridou E, et al. Atypical case of lichen planus recognized by dermoscopy. Dermatol Pract Concept 2016;6: 39–42.
37. Chuh AA. Collarette scaling in pityriasis rosea demonstrated by digital epiluminescence dermatoscopy. Australas J Dermatol 2001;42:288–90.
38. Chuh AAT. The use of digital epiluminescence dermatoscopy to identify peripheral scaling in pityriasis rosea. Comput Med Imaging Graph 2002;26: 129.
39. Lallas A, Apalla Z, Karteridou A, et al. Photoletter to the editor: dermoscopy for discriminating between pityriasis rubra pilaris and psoriasis. J Dermatol Case Rep 2013;7:20–2.
40. Abdel-Azim NE, Ismail SA, Fathy E. Differentiation of pityriasis rubra pilaris from plaque psoriasis by dermoscopy. Arch Dermatol Res 2017;309(4): 311–4.
41. Errichetti E, Piccirillo A. Dermoscopy as an auxiliary tool in the differentiation of the main types of erythroderma due to dermatological disorders. Int J Dermatol 2016;55(12):e616–8.
42. Lallas A, Apalla Z, Lefaki I, et al. Dermoscopy of discoid lupus erythematosus. Br J Dermatol 2012; 168:284–8.
43. Lopez-Tintos BO, Garcia-Hidalgo L, Orozco-Topete R. Dermoscopy in active discoid lupus. Arch Dermatol 2009;145:358.

44. Lallas A, Apalla Z, Argenziano G, et al. Clues for differentiating discoid lupus erythematosus from actinic keratosis. J Am Acad Dermatol 2013; 69:e5–6.
45. Ankad BS, Shah SD, Adya KA. White rosettes in discoid lupus erythematosus: a new dermoscopic observation. Dermatol Pract Concept 2017;7(4):9–11.
46. Errichetti E, Piccirillo A, Viola L, et al. Dermoscopy of subacute cutaneous lupus erythematosus. Int J Dermatol 2016;55(11):e605–7.
47. Larre Borges A, Tiodorovic-Zivkovic D, Lallas A, et al. Clinical, dermoscopic and histopathologic features of genital and extragenital lichen sclerosus. J Eur Acad Dermatol Venereol 2013;27(11):1433–9.
48. Garrido-Ríos AA, Alvarez-Garrido H, Sanz-Muñoz C, et al. Dermoscopy of extragenital lichen sclerosus. Arch Dermatol 2009;145:1468.
49. Apalla Z, Lallas A. Dermoscopy of atypical lichen sclerosus involving the tongue. J Dermatol Case Rep 2012;6(2):57–8.
50. Shim W-H, Jwa S-W, Song M, et al. Diagnostic usefulness of dermatoscopy in differentiating lichen sclerous et atrophicus from morphea. J Am Acad Dermatol 2012;66:690–1.
51. Errichetti E, Lallas A, Apalla Z, et al. Dermoscopy of morphea and cutaneous lichen sclerosus: clinicopathological correlation study and comparative analysis. Dermatology 2017;233(6):462–70.
52. Lacarrubba F, Pellacani G, Verzì AE, et al. Extragenital lichen sclerosus: clinical, dermoscopic, confocal microscopy and histologic correlations. J Am Acad Dermatol 2015;72(1 Suppl):S50–2.
53. Vazquez-Lopez F, Kreusch J, Marghoob AA. Dermoscopic semiology: further insights into vascular features by screening a large spectrum of nontumoral skin lesions. Br J Dermatol 2004;150:226–31.
54. Vázquez-López F, Fueyo A, Sanchez-Martin J, et al. Dermoscopy for the screening of common urticaria and urticaria vasculitis. Arch Dermatol 2008;144:568.
55. Vázquez-López F, Maldonado-Seral C, Soler-Sánchez T, et al. Surface microscopy for discriminating between common urticaria and urticarial vasculitis. Rheumatology (Oxford) 2003;42:1079–82.
56. Suh KS, Kang DY, Lee KH, et al. Evolution of urticarial vasculitis: a clinical, dermoscopic and histopathological study. J Eur Acad Dermatol Venereol 2014; 28:674–5.
57. Zalaudek I, Ferrara G, Brongo S, et al. Atypical clinical presentation of pigmented purpuric dermatosis. J Dtsch Dermatol Ges 2006;4:138–40.
58. Zaballos P, Puig S, Malvehy J. Dermoscopy of pigmented purpuric dermatoses (lichen aureus): a useful tool for clinical diagnosis. Arch Dermatol 2004; 140:1290–1.
59. Choo JY, Bae JM, Lee JH, et al. Blue-gray blotch: a helpful dermoscopic finding in optimal biopsy site selection for true vasculitis. J Am Acad Dermatol 2016;75:836–8.
60. Lallas A, Sidiropoulos T, Lefaki I, et al. Dermoscopy of granuloma faciale. J Dermatol Case Rep 2012;6:59–60.
61. Caldarola G, Zalaudek I, Argenziano G, et al. Granuloma faciale: a case report on long-term treatment with topical tacrolimus and dermoscopic aspects. Dermatol Ther 2011;24:508–11.
62. Lallas A, Argenziano G, Longo C, et al. Polygonal vessels of rosacea are highlighted by dermoscopy. Int J Dermatol 2014;53:e325–7.
63. Micali G, Dall'Oglio F, Verzì AE, et al. Treatment of erythemato-telangiectatic rosacea with brimonidine alone or combined with vascular laser based on preliminary instrumental evaluation of the vascular component. Lasers Med Sci 2017. https://doi.org/10.1007/s10103-017-2318-3.
64. Segal R, Mimouni D, Feuerman H, et al. Dermoscopy as a diagnostic tool in demodicidosis. Int J Dermatol 2010;49:1018–23.
65. Friedman P, Cohen-Sabban E, Cabo H. Usefulness of dermoscopy in the diagnosis and monitoring treatment of demodicidosis. Dermatol Pract Concept 2017;7:35–8.
66. Vázquez-López F, Lopez-Escobar M, Maldonado-Seral C, et al. The handheld dermoscope improves the recognition of giant pseudocomedones in Darier's disease. J Am Acad Dermatol 2004;50:454–5.
67. Lacarrubba F, Verzì AE, Errichetti E, et al. Darier disease: dermoscopy, confocal microscopy, and histologic correlations. J Am Acad Dermatol 2015;73(3):e97–9.
68. Errichetti E, Stinco G, Lacarrubba F, et al. Dermoscopy of Darier's disease. J Eur Acad Dermatol Venereol 2016;30:1392–4.
69. Errichetti E, De Franzesco V, Pegolo E, et al. Dermoscopy of Grover's disease: variability according to histological subtype. J Dermatol 2016;43:937–9.
70. Lacarrubba F, Boscaglia S, Nasca MR, et al. Grover's disease: dermoscopy, reflectance confocal microscopy and histopathological correlation. Dermatol Pract Concept 2017;7(3):51–4.
71. Delfino M, Argenziano G, Nino M. Dermoscopy for the diagnosis of porokeratosis. J Eur Acad Dermatol Venereol 2004;18:194–5.
72. Zaballos P, Puig S, Malvehy J. Dermoscopy of disseminated superficial actinic porokeratosis. Arch Dermatol 2004;140:1410.
73. Pizzichetta MA, Canzonieri V, Massone C, et al. Clinical and dermoscopic features of porokeratosis of Mibelli. Arch Dermatol 2009;145:91–2.
74. Uhara H, Kamijo F, Okuyama R, et al. Open pores with plugs in porokeratosis clearly visualized with the dermoscopic furrow ink test: report of 3 cases. Arch Dermatol 2011;147:866–8.
75. Oiso N, Kawada A. Dermoscopic features in disseminated superficial actinic porokeratosis. Eur J Dermatol 2011;21:439–40.

76. Panasiti V, Rossi M, Curzio M, et al. Disseminated superficial actinic porokeratosis diagnosed by dermoscopy. Int J Dermatol 2008;47:308–10.
77. Sotoodian B, Mahmood MN, Salopek TG. Clinical and dermoscopic features of pigmented disseminated superficial actinic porokeratosis: case report and literature review. J Cutan Med Surg 2017;22(2):229–31.
78. Micali G, Verzì AE, Lacarrubba F. Alternative uses of dermatoscopy in daily clinical practice: an update. J Am Acad Dermatol 2018 Jun 16 [pii:S0190-9622(18)32143-1]. [Epub ahead of print].

Dermatoscopy of Granulomatous Disorders

Enzo Errichetti, MD, MSc, DVD*, Giuseppe Stinco, MD, MSc, DVD

KEYWORDS

• Dermatoscopy • Dermoscopy • Differential diagnosis • Granulomatous disorders • Inflammoscopy

KEY POINTS

- The main dermatoscopic clue of granulomatous dermatoses is the presence of focal or diffused structureless orangish or yellowish-orange areas histologically corresponding to dermal granulomas.
- Vessels and whitish areas are also frequently seen in granulomatous dermatoses, with the former being more common in early or active phases and the latter being more typical of more long-standing lesions.
- Although most granulomatous dermatoses share several dermatoscopic features, their accurate analysis, along with the detection of peculiar additional dermatoscopic features, may be helpful for distinguishing between the various forms.

INTRODUCTION

Cutaneous granulomatous disorders (CGDs) encompass a heterogeneous group of diseases sharing the common histologic denominator of granuloma formation, namely a focal compact collection of histiocytes with or without other inflammatory cells (eg, plasma cells, eosinophils, neutrophils), necrosis, vasculitis, fibrosis, calcification, or foreign bodies.[1,2] They may be divided into 2 main categories: infectious and noninfectious, with the former mainly including leishmaniasis, mycobacterioses, and fungal infections; and the latter mainly encompassing sarcoidosis, necrobiotic granulomas (ie, granuloma annulare, necrobiosis lipoidica, and rheumatoid nodules), and foreign body granulomas.[1,2]

Diagnosis of CGDs is usually suspected based on morphologic findings, localization, and anamnestic data, though clinical differentiation from each other and from similar dermatoses is often troublesome.[1,2]

Over the last few years, dermatoscopy has been shown to aid in assisting the recognition of several CGDs, including sarcoidosis, necrobiosis lipoidica, granuloma annulare, rheumatoid nodules, cutaneous leishmaniasis, and lupus vulgaris.[3,4]

This article provides an up-to-date overview of the dermatoscopic features of the main noninfectious and infectious CGDs, with a brief mention of other less common CGDs.

The dermatoscopic hallmark of all CGDs is represented by the presence of structureless orangish or yellowish-orange areas, which may be distributed in a focal or diffuse pattern.[3,4] This finding is strictly related to the presence of the dense and compact granulomatous infiltrate in the dermis (mass effect) and is better visualized by applying slight pressure on the skin (because of the reduction of erythema).[3,4]

Of note, orangish or yellowish-orange structureless areas are not absolutely specific for CGDs because they may be also appreciated in other dermatoses characterized by dense or compact

Disclosure: None.

Department of Medical Area, Institute of Dermatology, University of Udine, Udine, Italy
* Corresponding author. Institute of Dermatology, "Santa Maria della Misericordia" University Hospital, Piazzale Santa Maria della Misericordia, 15, Udine 33100, Italy.
E-mail address: enzoerri@yahoo.it

Dermatol Clin 36 (2018) 369–375
https://doi.org/10.1016/j.det.2018.05.004
0733-8635/18/

dermal cellular infiltration (eg, Rosai-Dorfman disease, xanthogranuloma, pseudolymphomas)[3–6] or in skin diseases featuring dermal hemosiderin deposition (eg, pityriasis lichenoides chronica, Zoon balanitis, papular syphiloderm).[7–10] Additionally, the absence of such areas does not rule out the diagnosis of CGDs because they may be difficult to see in early stages (because the inflammatory infiltrate may be initially less compact or organized), when granulomas are located too deep, or there are remarkable epidermal changes (eg, hyperkeratosis, ulceration).[3,4]

Vessels and whitish areas are also frequently seen in CGDs, with the former being more common in early or active phases (when vascular dilation is more marked) and the latter being more typical of long-standing lesions (often characterized by dermal fibrosis).[3,4]

Even though all the aforementioned features are commonly visible in most CGDs, an accurate analysis (eg, shape, color, arrangement) of such findings may be often helpful in assisting their distinction.[3,4] Moreover, CGDs may also display additional dermatoscopic features that may further facilitate the differential diagnosis.[3,4] **Table 1** displays the main dermatoscopic clues of each granulomatous dermatosis.

CUTANEOUS SARCOIDOSIS

The main dermatoscopic clue of the various forms of cutaneous sarcoidosis is the presence of focally distributed or diffuse structureless orange or yellowish-orange areas, with a prevalence rate ranging from 84.2% to 100.0% (**Fig. 1**).[3,4,11–14] As previously mentioned, such areas are less commonly seen in early phases, or when granulomatous infiltrate is deeply located (subcutaneous sarcoidosis) or is associated with significant epidermal changes (eg, ulcerative or hyperkeratotic sarcoidosis).[3,4,11–14]

Vascular structures are another relevant dermatoscopic feature of cutaneous sarcoidosis; they have been reported to be present in 73.7% to 100.0% of patients.[3,4,11–14] Notably, vessels in such a condition may display different morphologies (with linear

Table 1
Main dermatoscopic clues of granulomatous dermatoses

Cutaneous sarcoidosis	• Diffuse or localized, structureless, orangish areas • Well-focused linear or branching vessels
Necrobiosis lipoidica	• Diffuse or localized, structureless, yellowish-orange areas • Well-focused vessels with variable shape (according to the disease phase): dotted, globular, comma-shaped (incipient lesions); network-shaped or hairpin-like (more developed lesions); or branching or serpentine (advanced lesions)
Granuloma annulare	• Unfocused vessels having a variable morphology over a more or less evident pinkish-reddish background • Focal or diffuse yellowish-orange (only palisading granuloma histologic variant) and whitish areas
Rheumatoid nodules	• Pink or mixed (pink and white) homogeneous background, with no or dull orangish areas
Cutaneous leishmaniasis	• Polymorphic vascularization and erythema • Whitish or yellowish follicular plugs having a roundish, oval, or tear-drop shape • White starburst-like pattern (peripheral white halo or radiating striae) • Epidermal changes (hyperkeratosis, yellow or white scaling, central erosion or ulceration and crusts)
Lupus vulgaris	• Diffuse or localized, structureless, orangish areas • Well-focused linear-branching vessels
Granulomatous rosacea	• Diffuse or localized, structureless, orangish areas • Linear reddish or purple vessels arranged in a polygonal network (vascular polygons)
Acne agminata	• Discrete (nonconfluent) focal orangish structureless around follicular openings filled with whitish or yellowish keratotic plugs
Borderline tuberculoid leprosy	• White areas • Decreased density of hairs • Yellowish or orangish globules (facial lesions)

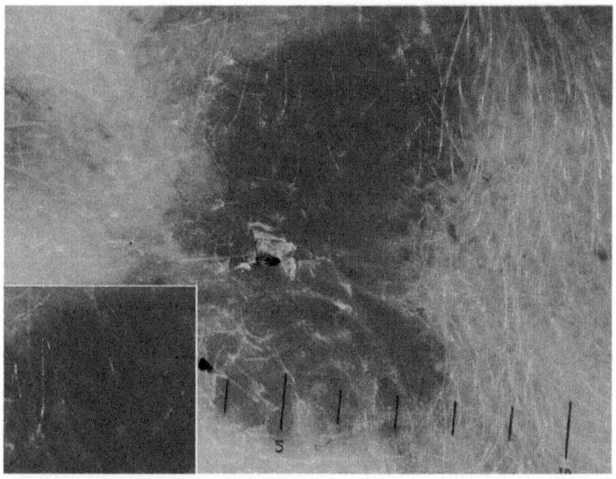

Fig. 1. Dermatoscopy of cutaneous sarcoidosis. Diffuse dull orangish background along with whitish scaling; a well-focused linear-irregular vessel is also visible (*magnified in the box*).

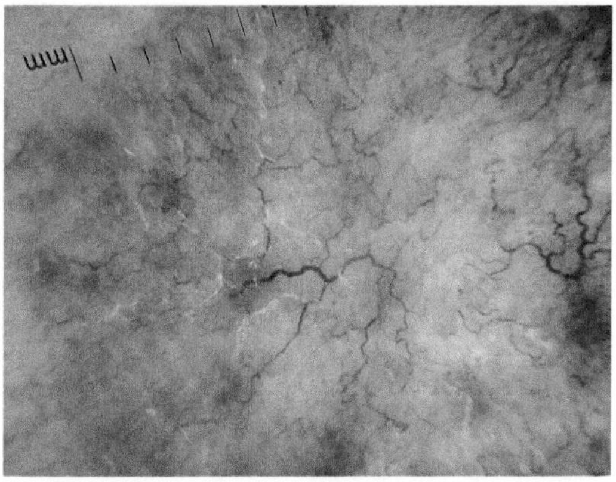

Fig. 2. Dermatoscopy of necrobiosis lipoidica (advanced lesion). Well-focused branching-serpentine vessels. The dimeter decreases from the center to the periphery of the lesion; multifocal yellowish areas and whitish scar-like areas are also present.

or linear-irregular and branching shapes being more common, and dotted or glomerular shapes being rarer) and are usually well-focused (because granulomas push the dermal vessels toward the skin surface, thus looking sharper) (see **Fig. 1**).[3,4,11–14]

Further less frequent or less specific dermatoscopic findings include pigmentation structures (more commonly in darker-skinned patients), follicular plugs, white or yellowish scaling (see **Fig. 1**), dilated follicles, milia-like cysts, whitish structureless areas or scar-like depigmentation, and crystalline structures.[3,4,11–14]

NECROBIOSIS LIPOIDICA

The most peculiar dermatoscopic findings of necrobiosis lipoidica consist of focal or diffuse structureless yellowish-orangish areas (58.3%–100.0% of cases) and well-focused vessels (100.0% of cases) displaying a shape that varies according to the disease phase.[3,12,15–18]

In detail, dotted, comma-shaped, and globular vessels are more frequent in early stages or active border, whereas network-shaped, linear, and hairpin-like vessels are more common in more developed lesions, and branching-serpentine vessels are seen in advanced lesions (**Fig. 2**).[3,12,15–18] Of note, especially in long-standing lesions, vascular structures typically show a sharp appearance and a diameter that decreases from the center to the periphery of the lesion (see **Fig. 2**).[3,12,15–18] This is due to epidermal atrophy, which makes dermal vessels closer to the skin surface, thereby appearing sharper and larger (especially in the center of the lesions because epidermal thinning is more marked in this area).[3,12,15–18]

Additionally, yellowish-orange areas corresponding to dermal granulomatous usually display a yellower hue compared with other granulomatous dermatoses owing to the possible presence of lipid deposits in the dermis (see **Fig. 2**).[3,12,15–18]

Further less common or less specific dermatoscopic findings include ulcerations, whitish or yellowish crusts, whitish scaling, brownish reticular structures, and whitish structureless areas (see **Fig. 2**), with the latter feature being more common in long-standing lesions (characterized by pronounced dermal fibrosis).[3,12,15–18]

GRANULOMA ANNULARE

According to the most recent and large study on dermatoscopy of granuloma annulare, the main dermatoscopic clue (prevalence rate of 88.0%) of this dermatosis is the presence of unfocussed vessels having a variable morphology (dotted in 52.0%, linear-irregular in 44.0%, and/or branching in 28.0% of cases) over a more or less evident pinkish-reddish background (**Figs. 3** and **4**).[19] Notably, earlier studies found lower prevalence rates (41.7%–76.6%), likely because vessels in granuloma annulare are very subtle and may disappear even with minimal pressure on the skin.[12,15,16]

Whitish (irregular or globular) and yellowish-orange (focally or diffusely distributed) areas represent the most common nonvascular findings (see **Figs. 3** and **4**), with the former corresponding to dermal fibrosis and the latter representing dermal granulomas on histology.[19]

Importantly, the dermatoscopic pattern of granuloma annulare significantly varies according to its histologic subtype, with a strict association between yellowish-orange structureless areas

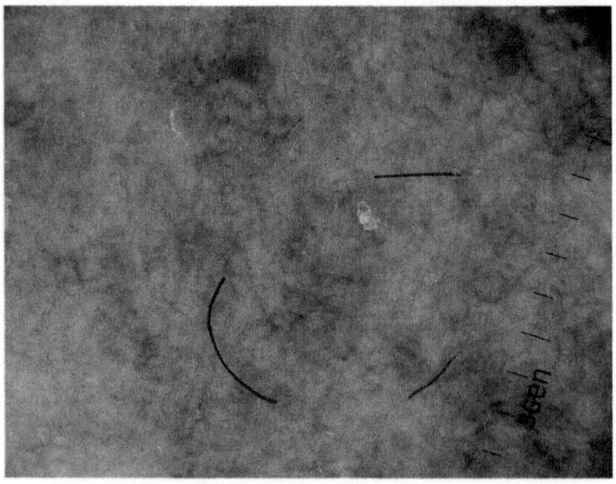

Fig. 3. Dermatoscopy of granuloma annulare (palisading granuloma histologic subtype). Faint linear-irregular vessels over a pinkish background; multifocal yellowish-orange areas and several globular white areas are also evident.

(especially those having diffuse distribution) and palisading granuloma histologic variants (see **Fig. 3**).[19] Indeed, yellowish-orangish areas are usually absent in lesions having an interstitial histologic pattern (see **Fig. 4**).[19] Of note, yellowish-orange areas may be absent or scarcely visible even in lesions with palisading granuloma histology if granulomas are located too deeply.[19]

Rosettes, crystalline structures and whitish scaling may also be seen less commonly in granuloma annulare.[19]

RHEUMATOID NODULES

Albeit rheumatoid nodules are histologically characterized by a granulomatous infiltrate,[12] the typical structureless orange or yellowish-orange areas are usually absent[12] or subtle (duller) because granulomas are located too deeply (authors' personal observations). On the other hand, the most common dermatoscopic findings is pink or mixed (pink and white) homogeneous background and reticulate pigmentation; arborizing or short linear vessels may be seen less frequently.[12]

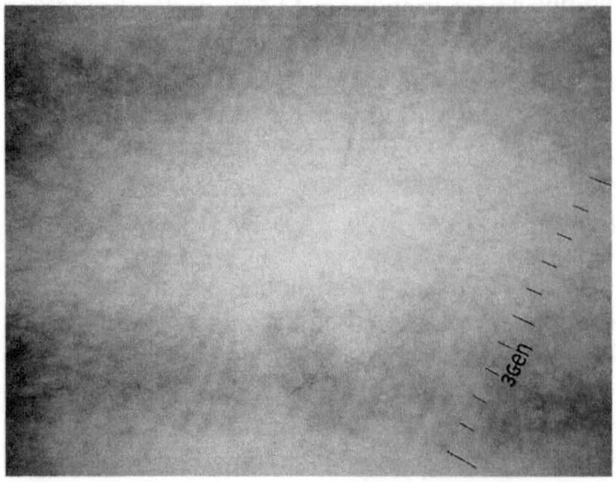

Fig. 4. Dermatoscopy of granuloma annulare (interstitial histologic subtype). Faint linear-irregular vessels over a pinkish background; several white areas are also present, whereas no orangish areas are visible.

CUTANEOUS LEISHMANIASIS

The most common dermatoscopic findings of cutaneous leishmaniasis include diffuse erythema (prevalence rate 81.9%–100.0%) and vessels (prevalence rate 86.9%–100.0%), usually having a polymorphic pattern (combination of 2 or more different types of vessels) (**Fig. 5**).[3,20–24] In particular, possible shapes or appearance of vascular structures include irregular-linear, arborizing, hairpin, glomerular, dotted, crown-like, strawberry-like, comma, and corkscrew, with the first 3 morphologies usually the most frequent.[3,20–24] Not uncommonly, vessels in cutaneous leishmaniasis are surrounded by a whitish halo due to the presence of epidermal acanthosis.[3,20–24]

Even though observed less commonly (39.1%–59.0% of cases), whitish or yellowish follicular plugs with a roundish, oval, or tear-drop shape (sometimes referred as yellowish tears) are considered a peculiar (but not absolutely specific) finding of cutaneous leishmaniasis (especially in facial or neck lesions) (see **Fig. 5**).[3,20–24] White starburst-like pattern (peripheral white halo or radiating striae) is another characteristic feature of such a condition, albeit it is found only in 8.6% to 60.4% of cases; histologically, it corresponds to parakeratotic hyperkeratosis located around the erosion.[3,20–24]

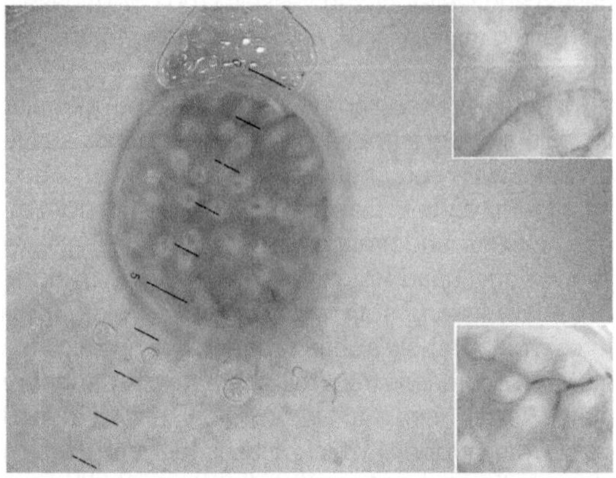

Fig. 5. Dermatoscopy of cutaneous leishmaniasis. Whitish or yellowish, follicular, keratotic plugs having a roundish, oval, and tear-drop (*yellowish tears*) appearance over a yellowish-orange or reddish background; both linear-irregular (*upper right box*) and branching (*lower right box*) vessels are also evident.

Notably, unlike other CGDs, cutaneous leishmaniasis is often characterized by epidermal or surface changes (especially advanced lesions), including hyperkeratosis, yellow or white scaling, central erosion, or ulceration and crusts.[3,20–24] The common presence of these findings may explain the low prevalence (13.1%–15.7%) of orange or salmon-colored ovoid areas (see **Fig. 5**) corresponding to the dermal granulomatous infiltrate because they are covered or masked by epidermal changes.[3,20–24]

Other possible dermatoscopic features of cutaneous leishmaniasis include thrombotic vessels, yellowish hue, white scarring areas, milia-like cysts, and pustules.[3,20–24]

LUPUS VULGARIS

Dermatoscopic appearance of lupus vulgaris is highly similar to that of cutaneous sarcoidosis, with the most common findings (prevalence rate 93.8%–100.0%) being yellowish-orange structureless areas and linear branching vessels (usually well-focused).[3,11,25] Even though differentiation between such conditions is usually impossible on dermatoscopic examination, granulomatous areas of lupus vulgaris often have a more yellowish hue compared with sarcoidosis (dull orange), likely because of the possible presence of caseation necrosis (which make granulomas less compact) or lipid deposition within the multinucleate Langerhans giant cells in the former.[3,11,25]

Additional dermatoscopic findings include whitish reticular streaks, milia-like cysts, white scales, pigmentation structures, and follicular plugs.[3,11,25]

OTHER GRANULOMATOUS DERMATOSES

Granulomatous Rosacea

Similar to other granulomatous dermatoses, granulomatous rosacea is characterized by the presence of focal (more common) or diffuse orangish structureless areas histologically corresponding to granulomas in the dermis (**Fig. 6**).[3,11] However, different from all the other CGDs, granulomatous rosacea also displays characteristic linear reddish or purple vessels arranged in a polygonal network (vascular polygons) (see **Fig. 6**).[3,11] Additional, less common, dermatoscopic findings include radially disposed linear and hairpin vessels and rosettes (using polarized-light devices).[3,11,26]

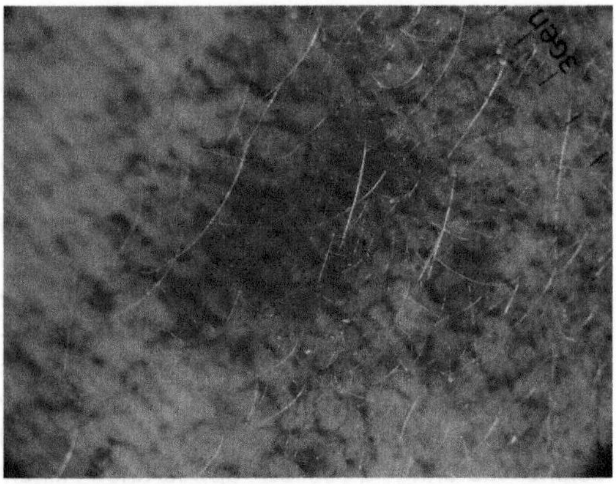

Fig. 6. Dermatoscopy of granulomatous rosacea. Multifocal orangish areas along with characteristic linear reddish or purple vessels arranged in a polygonal network (vascular polygons).

Acne Agminata (Lupus Miliaris Disseminatus Faciei)

The most characteristic dermatoscopic feature of acne agminata is discrete (nonconfluent) focal orangish structureless areas located around follicular openings, which are often filled with roundish or elongated, whitish or yellowish keratotic plugs (**Fig. 7**).[27] Such a pattern is due to the peculiar histologic background of this dermatosis, with perifollicular granulomatous infiltrate along with follicular hyperkeratosis.[27] Linear and hairpin-like vessels and central ulceration are other less common or less specific dermatoscopic findings.[27]

Leprosy

Borderline tuberculoid leprosy is the most studied form of leprosy.[28] In a recent study of 12 subjects, white areas (corresponding to a decreased number of melanocytes) and decreased density of hairs turned out to be the 2 most common dermatoscopic findings, with the former being present in

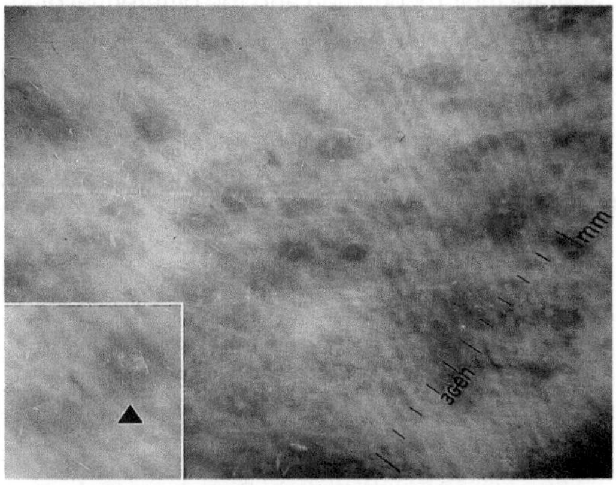

Fig. 7. Dermatoscopy of acne agminata (lupus miliaris disseminatus faciei). Discrete (nonconfluent) focal orangish structureless areas located around follicular openings, which are filled with roundish or elongated, whitish keratotic plugs (more visible in the *box; arrowhead*).

100% of cases.[28] Additionally, yellowish or orangish globules histologically representing dermal granulomas were found in 66.7% of subjects, whereas decreased white dots (sweat duct openings) and branching vessels were noted in 50% and 33.3% of cases, respectively.[28]

Interestingly, some dermatoscopic findings of borderline tuberculoid leprosy may vary according to the lesions localization (facial vs extrafacial areas), with vessels being evident only in facial lesions (because of the richer vascularity of this area and more marked destruction of vessels by granuloma in extrafacial sites) and hairs of facial lesions featuring a coiled appearance (likely because of involvement of hair shaft of vellus hairs).[28] Furthermore, yellow or orangish globules are not observed in all lesions but they are more common or prominent in more infiltrated areas (due to the higher density of granulomas in the dermis) and in facial areas (likely because epidermis is thinner in these sites, with subsequent increase in their visibility).[28] No dermatoscopic differences according to disease duration have been reported.[28]

A single report on histoid leprosy showed a central whitish-yellow structureless area along with peripheral brownish pigmentation as possible dermatoscopic features of this rare variant of leprosy.[29] It is likely that the whitish hue of this form of leprosy is due to whorled arrangement of spindle-shaped histiocytes in the context of granulomas.[29]

SUMMARY

Granulomatous dermatoses commonly show characteristic dermatoscopic features that may facilitate their recognition and the differential diagnosis with similar nongranulomatous skin conditions.[4,30] Although many of these features are shared by most cutaneous granulomatous diseases, due to their similar histologic background, an accurate analysis of these findings (eg, shape, color, and arrangement), along with the detection of peculiar additional dermatoscopic features, may sometimes be helpful even for distinguishing between the various forms.

REFERENCES

1. Tronnier M, Mitteldorf C. Histologic features of granulomatous skin diseases. Part 1: non-infectious granulomatous disorders. J Dtsch Dermatol Ges 2015;13:211–6.
2. Mitteldorf C, Tronnier M. Histologic features of granulomatous skin diseases. J Dtsch Dermatol Ges 2016;14:378–88.
3. Errichetti E, Stinco G. Dermoscopy in general dermatology: a practical overview. Dermatol Ther (Heidelb) 2016;6:471–507.
4. Errichetti E, Stinco G. The practical usefulness of dermoscopy in general dermatology. G Ital Dermatol Venereol 2015;150:533–46.
5. Avilés-Izquierdo JA, Parra Blanco V, Alfageme Roldán F. Dermoscopic features of cutaneous Rosai-Dorfman disease. Actas Dermosifiliogr 2012; 103:446–8.
6. Song M, Kim SH, Jung DS, et al. Structural correlations between dermoscopic and histopathological features of juvenile xanthogranuloma. J Eur Acad Dermatol Venereol 2011;25:259–63.
7. Errichetti E, Lacarrubba F, Micali G, et al. Differentiation of pityriasis lichenoides chronica from guttate psoriasis by dermoscopy. Clin Exp Dermatol 2015; 40:804–6.
8. Errichetti E, Lacarrubba F, Micali G, et al. Dermoscopy of Zoon's plasma cell balanitis. J Eur Acad Dermatol Venereol 2016;30:e209–10.
9. Errichetti E, Stinco G. Dermoscopy in differentiating palmar syphiloderm from palmar papular psoriasis. Int J STD AIDS 2017;28:1461–3.
10. Errichetti E, Piccirillo A, Viola L, et al. Dermoscopy of subacute cutaneous lupus erythematosus. Int J Dermatol 2016;55:e605–7.
11. Lallas A, Argenziano G, Apalla Z, et al. Dermoscopic patterns of common facial inflammatory skin diseases. J Eur Acad Dermatol Venereol 2014;28:609–14.
12. Ramadan S, Hossam D, Saleh MA. Dermoscopy could be useful in differentiating sarcoidosis from necrobiotic granulomas even after treatment with systemic steroids. Dermatol Pract Concept 2016;6:17–22.
13. Pellicano R, Tiodorovic-Zivkovic D, Gourhant JY, et al. Dermoscopy of cutaneous sarcoidosis. Dermatology 2010;221:51–4.
14. Vazquez-Lopez F, Palacios-Garcia L, Gomez-Diez S, et al. Dermoscopy for discriminating between lichenoid sarcoidosis and lichen planus. Arch Dermatol 2011;147:1130.
15. Pellicano R, Caldarola G, Filabozzi P, et al. Dermoscopy of necrobiosis lipoidica and granuloma annulare. Dermatology 2013;226:319–23.
16. Lallas A, Zaballos P, Zalaudek I, et al. Dermoscopic patterns of granuloma annulare and necrobiosis lipoidica. Clin Exp Dermatol 2013;38:425–7.
17. Vázquez-López F, Kreusch J, Marghoob AA. Dermoscopic semiology: further insights into vascular features by screening a large spectrum of nontumoral skin lesions. Br J Dermatol 2004;150:226–31.
18. Conde-Montero E, Avilés-Izquierdo JA, Mendoza-Cembranos MD, et al. Dermoscopy of necrobiosis lipoidica. Actas Dermosifiliogr 2013;104:534–7.
19. Errichetti E, Lallas A, Apalla Z, et al. Dermoscopy of granuloma annulare: a clinical and histological correlation study. Dermatology 2017;233:74–9.

20. Yücel A, Günaşti S, Denli Y, et al. Cutaneous leishmaniasis: new dermoscopic findings. Int J Dermatol 2013;52:831–7.
21. Taheri AR, Pishgooei N, Maleki M, et al. Dermoscopic features of cutaneous leishmaniasis. Int J Dermatol 2013;52:1361–6.
22. Ayhan E, Ucmak D, Baykara SN, et al. Clinical and dermoscopic evaluation of cutaneous leishmaniasis. Int J Dermatol 2015;54:193–201.
23. Llambrich A, Zaballos P, Terrasa F, et al. Dermoscopy of cutaneous leishmaniasis. Br J Dermatol 2009;160:756–61.
24. Caltagirone F, Pistone G, Arico M, et al. Vascular patterns in cutaneous leishmaniasis: a videodermatoscopic study. Indian J Dermatol Venereol Leprol 2015;81:394–8.
25. Brasiello M, Zalaudek I, Ferrara G, et al. Lupus vulgaris: a new look at an old symptom–the lupoma observed with dermoscopy. Dermatology 2009; 218:172–4.
26. Rubegni P, Tataranno DR, Nami N, et al. Rosettes: optical effects and not dermoscopic patterns related to skin neoplasms. Australas J Dermatol 2013;54: 271–2.
27. Ayhan E, Alabalik U, Avci Y. Dermoscopic evaluation of two patients with lupus miliaris disseminatus faciei. Clin Exp Dermatol 2014;39:500–2.
28. Ankad BS, Sakhare PS. Dermoscopy of borderline tuberculoid leprosy. Int J Dermatol 2018;57:74–6.
29. Ankad BS, Sakhare PS. Dermoscopy of histoid leprosy: a case report. Dermatol Pract Concept 2017;7. 63–5.78.
30. Micali G, Verzì AE, Lacarrubba F. Alternative uses of dermatoscopy in daily clinical practice: an update. J Am Acad Dermatol 2018 Jun 16. pii: S0190-9622(18)32143-1. [Epub ahead of print].

Dermoscopy of Lymphomas and Pseudolymphomas

Caterina Bombonato, MD[a], Riccardo Pampena, MD[a], Aimillios Lallas, MD, MSc, PhD[b], Pellacani Giovanni, MD[c,*], Caterina Longo, MD, PhD[a,c]

KEYWORDS

• Cutaneous lymphomas • Pseudolymphomas • Dermoscopy

KEY POINTS

- Cutaneous lymphomas are rare entities whose diagnosis is based on a cellular level (cytologic assessment, immunophenotyping, and molecular studies for clonality).
- Cutaneous lymphomas and pseudolymphomas are a heterogeneous group with distinct variability in clinical presentation. For this reason, diagnosis is not always easy.
- Although the dermoscopic framework is not always specific, in some cases it can help us in the differential diagnosis.

INTRODUCTION

With the term cutaneous lymphomas and pseudolymphomas, the authors refer to a heterogeneous group of diseases whose classification is an ongoing process as new technologies are changing the diagnostic and therapeutic approach (**Box 1**). The diagnosis can be difficult because of the rarity of these entities and because of the similarity with many other more common skin diseases, from infections, to autoimmune or hypersensitive reactions. The most frequent clinical forms of cutaneous lymphomas and their dermoscopic features are described in this article.

PRIMARY CUTANEOUS T-CELL LYMPHOMAS

Most lymphomas in the skin have a T-cell origin. This is logical, because T cells normally traffic through the skin and are important in "skin-associated lymphoid tissue." They represent approximately 80% of all cutaneous lymphomas. The most common forms are mycosis fungoides (MF) and Sézary syndrome (SS),[1] which represent about 65% of all cutaneous T-cell lymphomas (CTCLs), with an annual incidence of 5 new cases per million people. The second most common group is constituted by primary cutaneous CD30 + lymphoproliferative disorders that represent approximately 27% of CTCLs. This group includes the following: primary cutaneous anaplastic large cell lymphomas (pcALCL), lymphomatoid papulosis (LyP), and borderline cases. A summary of clinical and dermoscopic features of CTCL subtypes is reported in **Table 1**.

Mycosis Fungoides

Clinical features

MF is the most common type of CTCL, usually arising in mid-to-late adulthood (median age at diagnosis: 55–60 years; male-to-female

Disclosure: This work was partially funded by Research Project NET (2011-02347213), Italian Ministry of Health.
[a] Dermatology and Skin Cancer Unit, Arcispedale Santa Maria Nuova, IRCCS, Viale Risorgimento 80, Reggio Emilia 42123, Italy; [b] First Department of Dermatology, Aristotle University, Hospital of Skin and Venereal Diseases, 124 Delfon Street, Thessaloniki 54643, Greece; [c] Dermatology Department, University of Modena and Reggio Emilia, via del Pozzo 71, Modena 41124, Italy
* Corresponding author.
E-mail address: pellacani.giovanni@gmail.com

Dermatol Clin 36 (2018) 377–388
https://doi.org/10.1016/j.det.2018.05.005

Box 1
WHO-EORTC classification of cutaneous lymphomas with primary cutaneous manifestations

Cutaneous T-cell and NK-cell lymphomas

Mycosis fungoides

MF variants and subtypes

- Folliculotropic MF
- Pagetoid reticulosis
- Granulomatous slack skin

Sézary syndrome

Adult T-cell leukemia/lymphoma

Primary cutaneous CD30 + lymphoproliferative disorders

- Primary cutaneous anaplastic large cell lymphoma
- Lymphomatoid papulosis

Subcutaneous panniculitis-like T-cell lymphoma

Extranodal NK/T-cell lymphoma, nasal type

Primary cutaneous peripheral T-cell lymphoma, unspecified

- Primary cutaneous aggressive epidermotropic CD8+ T-cell lymphoma (provisional)
- Cutaneous γ/δ T-cell lymphoma (provisional)
- Primary cutaneous CD4+ small/medium-sized pleomorphic T-cell lymphoma (provisional)

Cutaneous B-cell lymphomas

Primary cutaneous marginal zone B-cell lymphoma

Primary cutaneous follicle center lymphoma

Primary cutaneous diffuse large B-cell lymphoma, leg type

Primary cutaneous diffuse large B-cell lymphoma, other

Intravascular large B-cell lymphoma

Precursor hematologic neoplasm

CD4+/CD56+ hematodermic neoplasm (blastic NK-cell lymphoma)

Abbreviations: MF, mycosis fungoides; NK, natural killer.

Data from Willemze R, Jaffe E, Burg G, et al. WHO-EORTC classification for cutaneous lymphomas. Blood 2005;105:3769.

Table 1
Summary of clinical and dermoscopic characteristics for various CTCL subtypes

	MF	pcALCL	LyP
Epidemiology	Mean age of onset 55–60 y; M > F	Adults 45–60 y; M:F = 2–3:1	Mean age of onset 45 y; M:F = 1.5:1
Clinical features	Patches, plaques, tumors	Solitary firm nodule that rapidly grows and often ulcerates	Recurrent papular, papulonecrotic, and/or nodular lesions
Dermoscopy	Fine short linear vessels, dotted vessels, spermatozoa-like structures, orange-yellowish patchy areas	Pink-to-yellow structureless areas, polymorphous vessels	Different in the different stages of the disease

Abbreviations: MF, Mycosis Fungoides; pcALCL, Primary Cutaneous CD30+ Anaplastic Large-Cell Lymphoma; LyP, Lymphomatoid Papulosis.

ratio: 1.6–2.0:1), but may also occur in children and adolescents.[2,3] The term should only be used for the classic "Alibert-Bazin" type characterized by the evolution of patches, plaques, and tumors, or for variants showing a similar course. MF is most often an indolent disease with slow progression over years or sometimes decades, from patches to more infiltrated plaques and eventually to tumors, but patients may simultaneously have more than one type of lesion. In the early patch-stage of MF there are single or multiple erythematous, scaly (cigarette paperlike wrinkly scale) macules and patches that vary from orange to a dusky violet-red and may be round to oval or serpiginous in appearance (**Fig. 1**A, B, D). They are located on the buttocks and other sun-protected areas. In advanced stages, patients present with patches, plaques, and tumors that often show ulceration when they are very large (**Fig. 2**A, B). In these cases, extracutaneous involvement may occur, with spreading to regional or distant lymph nodes, bone marrow, and other organs. Peripheral blood involvement may also occur at different disease stages and has a bearing on prognosis and treatment. Late progression of MF is often characterized by a progressive decrease in the functional immunity of the patient.

Differential diagnosis

In early patch stage, the diagnosis of MF may be very challenging. In fact, skin lesions may mimic chronic dermatitis (with some scales, but despite the itching, scratch marks and lichenification are usually absent), psoriasis, parapsoriasis, contact dermatitis, or tinea corporis. However, when dealing with plaques and tumors, other forms of lymphoreticular malignancies, sarcoidosis, deep fungal infections, atypical mycobacterial infections, leprosy, leishmaniasis, and metastases should be taken under consideration.

Dermoscopy

Dermoscopic patterns of MF have been described in a series of 32 cases of early stage MF consisting of fine short linear and dotted vessels, along with orange-yellowish patchy areas (**Fig. 1**C).[4] In this

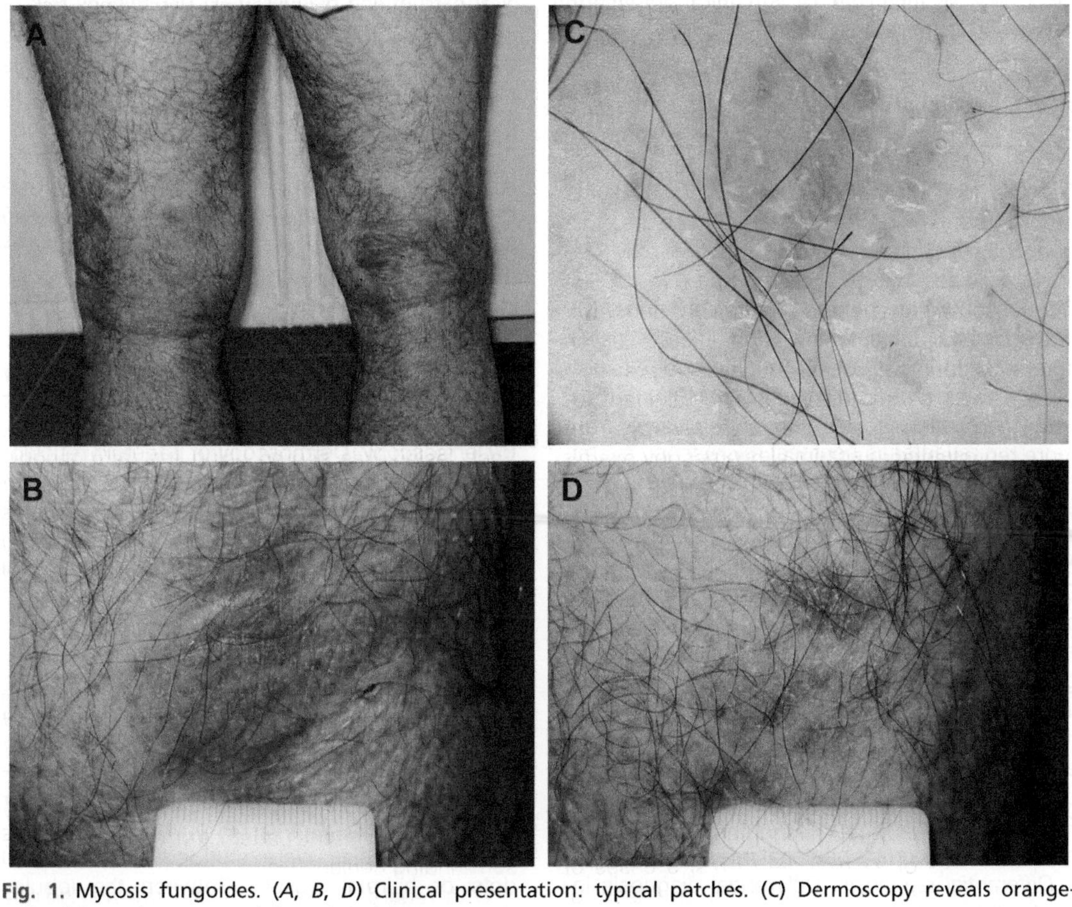

Fig. 1. Mycosis fungoides. (*A, B, D*) Clinical presentation: typical patches. (*C*) Dermoscopy reveals orange-yellowish patchy areas and dotted vessels.

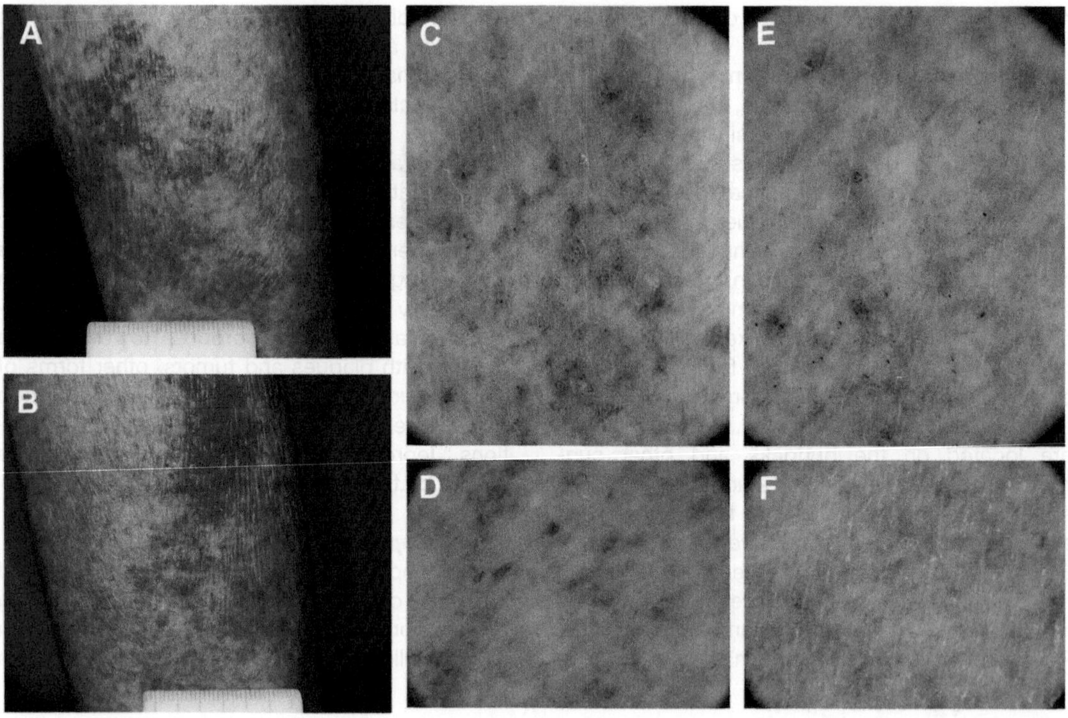

Fig. 2. Mycosis fungoides. (*A, B*) Clinical presentation: typical patches and plaques. (*C–F*) Dermoscopy reveals dotted and spermatozoa-like vessels.

article, the authors also emphasize the presence of a characteristic vascular structure resembling spermatozoa as a highly specific marker of MF. Bosseila and colleagues,[5] in a series of 25 patients with MF, confirmed the dotted pattern as the most frequently encountered vascular pattern of MF lesions, followed by the linear pattern (**Fig. 2**C–F). Dermoscopy can help us to differentiate MF from eczema. In fact, fine short linear vessels, spermatozoa-like structures, and orange yellowish patchy areas are more frequent in MF, whereas, white and yellow scales and dotted vessels are more represented in eczema lesions.[6]

Mycosis Fungoides Variants and Subtypes

Folliculotropic mycosis fungoides

Clinical features. Folliculotropic MF occurs in male adults but may occasionally affect children and adolescents. Clinically it is characterized by grouped follicular papules, acneiform lesions, indurated plaques, and sometimes tumors in the head and neck areas.[7] Skin lesions can be associated with alopecia on the scalp and also eyebrows, the last sign being highly characteristic. Pruritus is frequent and severe and scratching can cause secondary bacterial infections.

Differential diagnosis. Differential diagnosis includes lichen nitidus.

Dermoscopy. Dermoscopy of folliculotropic MF has not been reported in literature.

Pagetoid reticulosis

Clinical features. Pagetoid reticulosis clinically resemble solitary, slowly progressive, psoriasiform or hyperkeratotic patch or plaque, usually localized on the extremities. In contrast with classic MF, extracutaneous dissemination or disease-related deaths have never been reported.[8]

Differential diagnosis. Differential diagnosis includes psoriasis and chronic dermatitis.

Dermoscopy. Dermoscopy of pagetoid reticulosis has not been reported in literature.

Poikilodermatous mycosis fungoides

Clinical features. Poikilodermatous MF, a rare variant of patch-stage MF, is characterized by red or brownish plaques with scaling, mottled pigmentation, atrophy, and telangiectasia affecting the trunk and the extremities.[9]

Dermoscopy. Xu and colleagues[10] described a case report in which they observed multiple polygonal structures consisting of lobule of white storiform streaks, with the highest tone in the center and the lowest in the periphery. The streak-intersected holes were studded with fine red dots or hairpin vessels. Between the lobules were septa of pigmented dots that were unevenly and intermittently distributed throughout. In addition, red and yellowish smudges were easily noticed. Bosselia and colleagues[5] in their paper observed a light brown focal hyperpigmentation as characteristic of poikilodermatous MF.

Granulomatous slack skin

Clinical features. Granulomatous slack skin (GSS) is an extremely rare variant of MF, which appears as circumscribed areas of pendulous lax skin generally located in the axillae and groins. An association with Hodgkin lymphoma and with classic MF has been reported.[11–13] Most patients have an indolent clinical course.

Dermoscopy. Dermoscopy of GSS has not been reported in literature.

Sézary Syndrome

Clinical features. SS is historically defined by the presence of erythroderma, generalized lymphadenopathy, and the presence of neoplastic T cells, also known as Sézary cells, in skin, lymph nodes, and peripheral blood.[14] New criteria approved by International Society of Cutaneous Lymphomas are required for the diagnosis and include one or more of the following: an absolute Sézary cell count of least 1000 cells/mm^3; demonstration of immunophenotypical abnormalities, or demonstration of a T-cell clone in the peripheral blood by molecular or cytogenetic methods.[15] Patients are typically 55 to 60 years old and present with erythroderma (>80% body surface area), which may be associated with marked exfoliation, edema, and lichenification. Pruritus is severe. We can also observe lymphadenopathy, alopecia, onichodystrophy and palmoplantar hyperkeratosis. Fever is also common. Median overall survival is 63 months, and 5-year survival may be as low as 28%.

Differential diagnosis. The erythroderma of SS must be distinguished from chronic lymphocytic leukemia, psoriasis, severe atopic dermatitis, photodermatitis, seborrheic dermatitis, contact dermatitis, drug eruption, and pityriasis rubra pilaris.

Dermoscopy. Dermoscopy of SS has not been reported in literature.

Primary Cutaneous CD30 + Anaplastic Large-Cell Lymphoma

Clinical features. pcALCL is a rare and indolent type of CTCL affecting mainly adults aged between 45 and 60 years with male/female ratio of 2 to 3:1. It usually presents as an asymptomatic solitary or localized firm nodule or tumor, and sometimes papule, that rapidly grows and often ulcerates.[16,17] In about 20% of cases multifocal lesions may be seen. The skin lesions may show partial or complete spontaneous regression. These lymphomas frequently relapse in the skin. An extracutaneous involvement, in particular in the regional lymph node, is uncommon (only 10% of cases).

Differential diagnosis. Skin lesion clinically resembles Sweet syndrome, pyoderma gangrenosum, halogenoderma, leishmaniasis, or deep fungal infection.

Dermoscopy. Uzuncakmak and colleagues presented a case report in which they described the dermoscopic aspect of nodular lesions with pink-to-yellow structureless areas and polymorphous vessels especially visible at the periphery.[18]

Lymphomatoid Papulosis

Clinical features. LyP generally occurs in adults (median age, 45 years) but may occur in children as well. It is a chronic, recurrent, self-healing disease, characterized by the presence of different lesions in different stages of development, localized on the trunk and limbs. We can observe papular, papulonecrotic, and/or nodular lesions. Lesions resolve within 3 to 12 weeks, and may leave behind superficial scars. The duration of the disease varies from several months to more than 40 years (**Fig. 3**A, B).

Dermoscopy. Moura and colleagues described the dermoscopic criteria of LyP[19] and the dermoscopic criteria associated with the different stages of the disease from erythematous papule to scarring lesion. The first lesions (papules) showed a vascular pattern of tortuous irregular vessels radiating from the center to the periphery of the lesions with a white structureless area around the vessels. In hyperkeratotic papules, a whitish structureless area was described at the center of the papule. The vascular pattern spared the middle of the lesion. In the third stage, the necrotic ulceration replaced the whitish structureless area. The vascular pattern was strictly limited to the extreme periphery of the lesion. On the center, a brown-greyish structureless area, corresponding to the fibronecrotic material, was described. In the scarring phase, there was no more residual of vessels and only a brown-greyish structureless mark persisted, suggesting postinflammatory pigmentation (**Fig. 3**C–F).

Subcutaneous Panniculitis-Like T-Cell Lymphoma

Clinical features. Subcutaneous panniculitis-like T-cell lymphoma (SPTL) occurs in adults as well as in young children, and both sexes are equally

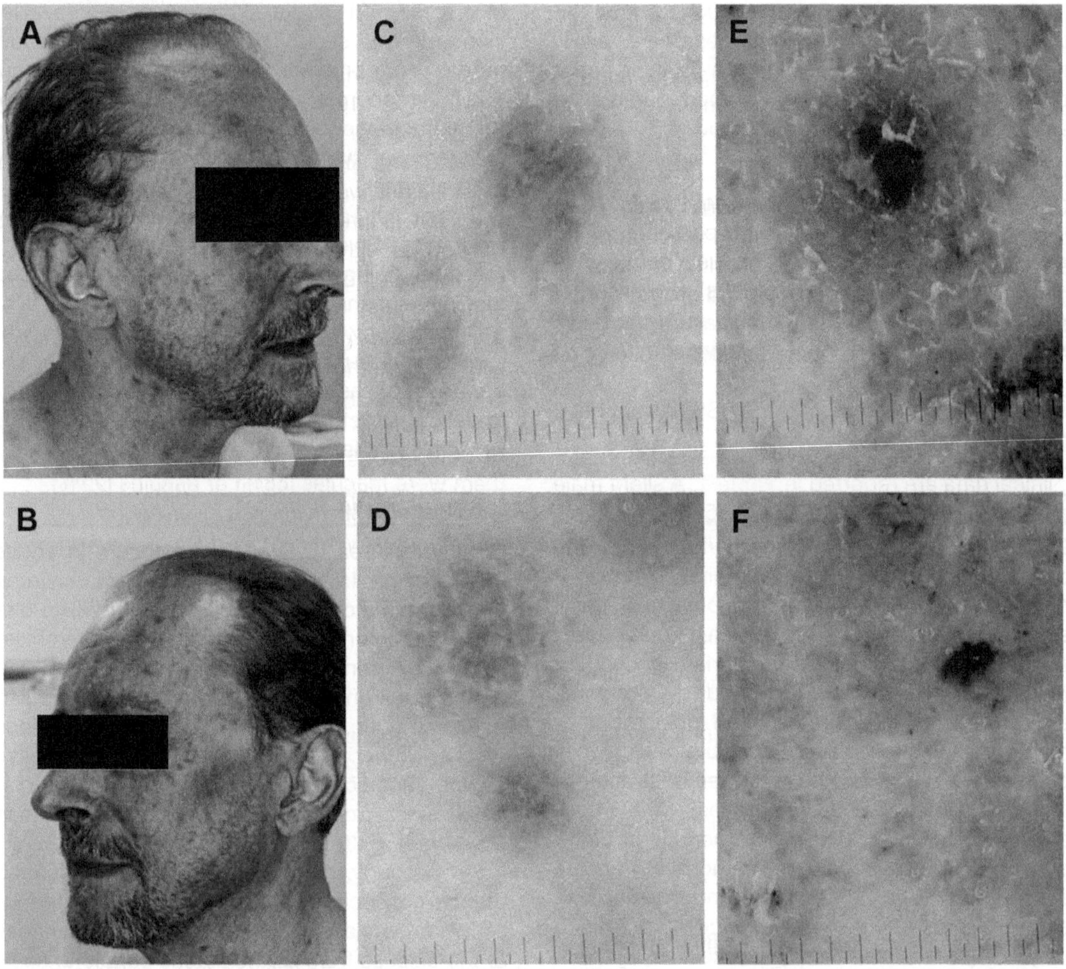

Fig. 3. Lymphomatoid papulosis. (*A, B*) Clinical presentation: papules and nodules. (*C–F*) Dermoscopy reveals tortuous irregular vessels.

affected. Patients generally present with solitary or multiple nodules and plaques, which mainly involve the legs. Systemic symptoms can be present and a dissemination to extracutaneous sites is rare. The disease may be complicated by a hemophagocytic syndrome, which is generally associated with a rapidly progressive course.[20]

Dermoscopy. Dermoscopy of SPTL has not been reported in literature.

Extranodal Natural Killer/T-Cell Lymphoma, Nasal Type

Clinical features. Patients are adults with a predominance of men. This type is more common in Asia and Central and South America and is related to Epstein–Barr (EBV) infection. It presents with multiple plaques or tumors preferentially on the trunk and extremities, or in the case of nasal type with a midfacial destructive tumor. Ulceration is common. Systemic symptoms may be present. The disease is closely related to aggressive natural killer (NK) cell leukemia, which may also have cutaneous manifestations and is also EBV associated.[21]

Dermoscopy. Dermoscopy of extranodal NK/T-cell lymphoma has not been reported in literature.

PRIMARY CUTANEOUS B-CELL LYMPHOMAS

Primary cutaneous B-cell lymphomas (PCBCLs) are a group of rare, malignant lymphoproliferative B-cell disorders that primarily affect the skin. They are approximately 20% to 25% of all cutaneous lymphomas and are classified into 3 major entities in the 2008 WHO-EORTC join classification: primary cutaneous follicle center cell lymphoma (PCFCL); primary cutaneous diffuse large B-cell lymphoma, leg type (PCDLBCL, LT); and primary cutaneous marginal zone lymphoma (PCMZL).[22] The incidence of cutaneous B-cell lymphomas (CBCLs) has been increasing in last decades and is currently 3.1 per million persons, with the highest incidence rates being reported among men, non-Hispanic whites, and adults older than 50 years.[23]

A summary of clinical and dermoscopic features of CBCL subtypes is reported in **Table 2**. A recent paper by Geller and colleagues observe that 2 dermoscopic features, salmon-colored area/background, and serpentine vessels are frequently seen in PCBCL lesions.[24]

Primary Cutaneous Follicle-Center Lymphoma

Clinical features. PCFCL is the most common CBCL. With a mean age of onset of 59 years, patients are a little older than those with PCMZL.[25] It often occurs as solitary or grouped plaques and tumors involving the scalp or forehead or the trunk.[26,27] Although grouped lesions may be observed, multifocal disease is less common. Particularly in the trunk, these tumors may be surrounded by erythematous papules and slightly indurated plaques, which may precede the development of tumorous lesions for months or even many years. In contrast to systemic follicular lymphomas, most PCFCLs do not harbor the t[14;18] translocation involving the bcl-2 locus and do not strongly express bcl-2 by immunohistochemistry, although weak expression may be observed in a minority of cases.[28]

Differential diagnosis. Differential diagnosis includes inflammatory lesions, arthropod bites, and other cutaneous neoplasm such as basal cell carcinoma, Merkel cell carcinoma, cutaneous lymphoid hyperplasia, and other non–B-cell cutaneous lymphomas (**Fig. 4**A, B).

Dermoscopy. Mascolo and colleagues reported a series of 10 PCBCLs among which 2 were PCFCL. They described the following dermoscopic criteria: white circle/areas, arborizing vessels, scales, salmon-colored background/area.[29] Recently, Geller and colleagues[24] reported that in 172 biopsy-proven B-cell lymphomas, 2 dermoscopic features, namely salmon-colored area and background and serpentine vessels, were frequently seen (**Fig. 4**C, D).

Primary Cutaneous Diffuse Large B-Cell Lymphoma, Leg Ttype

Clinical features. PCDLBCL, LT is an aggressive subtype of PCBCL that arises on the lower legs and commonly affects elderly women.[30–34] Patients present with generally rapidly growing red or bluish-red nodules, plaques, or tumor on one or both legs.[35] Approximately 10% of cases may involve other cutaneous sites apart from the lower legs. PCDLBCL, LT frequently disseminates to extracutaneous sites and has an unfavorable prognosis, with a 5-year survival rate of approximately 50%.

Dermoscopy. Mascolo and colleagues reported a series of 10 PCBCLs among which 2 were PCLBCL. They observed the following criteria: polymorphous vascular pattern, arborizing vessels, scales, white areas, and salmon-colored background/area.[30]

Primary Cutaneous Marginal-Zone B-Cell Lymphoma

Clinical features. PCMZL commonly affects middle-aged adults (mean age of onset is approximately 35–60 years) with men slightly more frequently affected than women. It presents as slowly growing infiltrated red to violaceous multifocal papules, plaques, or nodules involving the trunk and extremities, especially the arms, usually measuring less than 2 to 3 cm in size. In contrast to PCFCL, presentation with multifocal skin lesions is frequent. Ulceration is uncommon. Lesions have a tendency to locally recur, but extracutaneous

Table 2
Summary of clinical and dermoscopic characteristics for various CBCL subtypes

	PCFCL	PCLBCL, LT	PCMZL
Epidemiology	Mean age of onset 59 y, M = F	Mean age of onset 76 y, M < F	Mean age of onset 55 y, M = F/M > F
Clinical features	Solitary or multiple papules and plaques on the head, neck, thorax	Solitary or multiple papules and plaques on the legs	Solitary or multiple papules and plaques on trunk and extremities
Dermoscopy	White circles/areas, arborizing vessels, scales, salmon-colored background/area	Polymorphous vascular pattern and arborizing vessels, scales, salmon-colored background/area, white circles/areas	White circles/areas, polymorphous vascular pattern and arborizing vessels, scales, salmon-colored background/area

Abbreviations: PCFCL, Primary Cutaneous Follicle-center Lymphoma; PCLBCL LT, Primary Cutaneous diffuse Large B-Cell Lymphoma, Leg Type; PCMZL, Primary Cutaneous Marginal-Zone B-Cell Lymphoma.

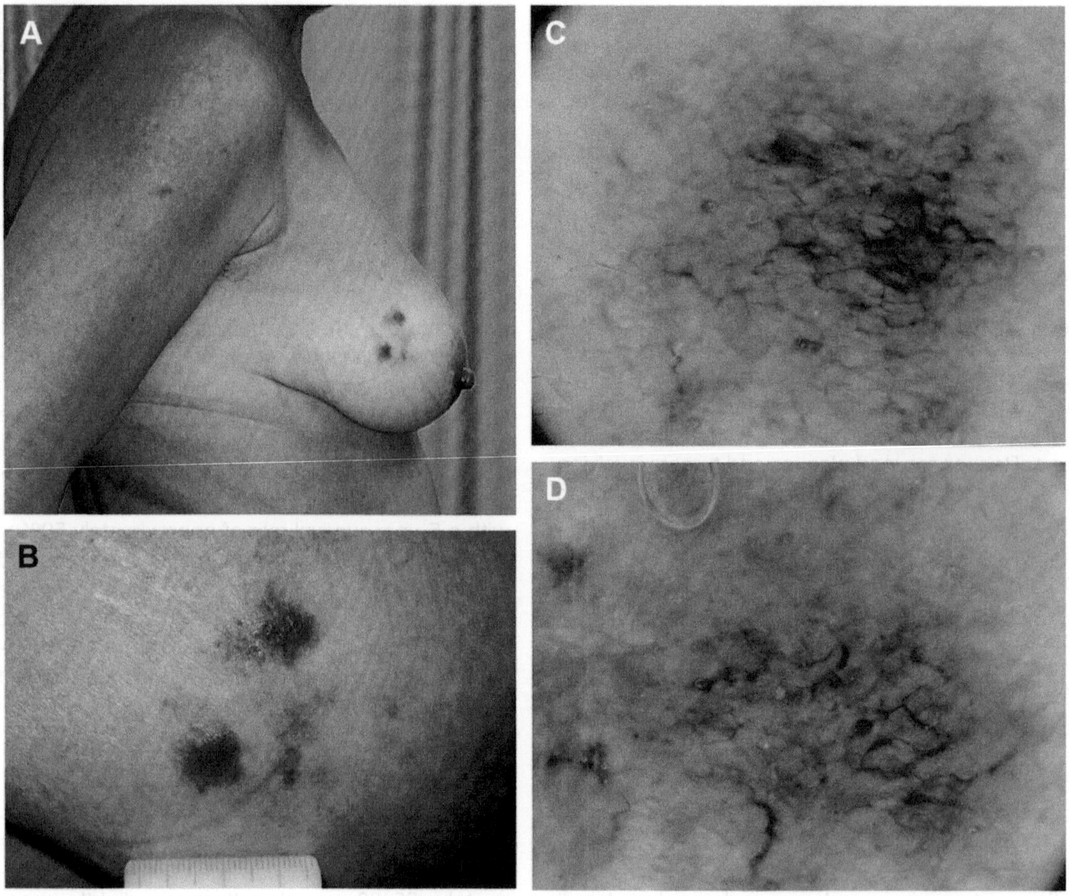

Fig. 4. Follicle center B-cell lymphoma. (*A, B*) Clinical presentation: red nodules. (*C, D*) Dermoscopy reveals arborizing vessels and white areas.

dissemination is rare.[35–37] In some cases, spontaneous resolution of the skin lesions may be observed. The development of anetoderma in spontaneously resolving lesions has been described (**Figs. 5**A and **6**A, B).[38] Although an association with *Borrelia burgdorferi* has been observed in Europe, it has not been reported in cases from the United States and Asia.

Diagnosis and disease classification is based on histologic examination and immunohistochemical staining of an appropriate skin biopsy and an appropriate staging evaluation to exclude systemic disease.[39]

Differential diagnosis. Differential diagnosis includes arthropod bites, urticaria, leukemia cutis, and medication-induced pseudolymphoma.

Dermoscopy. Piccolo and colleagues[40] reported 2 cases of PCMZL, showing a similar pattern with subtle arborizing vessels, salmon-colored background, and white areas/circle. Mascolo and colleagues,[29] in their paper describe 6 cases of PCMZL; dermoscopic appearance was characterized by the presence of white circles with salmon-colored background/areas, scales, arborizing vessels, or a polymorphous vascular pattern (**Figs. 5**B–E and **6**C).

CUTANEOUS PSEUDOLYMPHOMAS

Cutaneous pseudolymphomas are benign reactive lymphoid proliferation in the skin that simulate cutaneous lymphomas clinically, histologically, or both. The term includes various reactive conditions with a varied cause, pathogenesis, clinical presentation, histology, and behavior. To reach a correct diagnosis, it is necessary to contrast clinical, histologic, immunophenotypic, and molecular findings, and even with these data in some cases only the clinical course will confirm the diagnosis, making follow-up essential.[41]

Because the group includes a great variety of entities here the authors report only the variants with dermoscopic features described in literature.

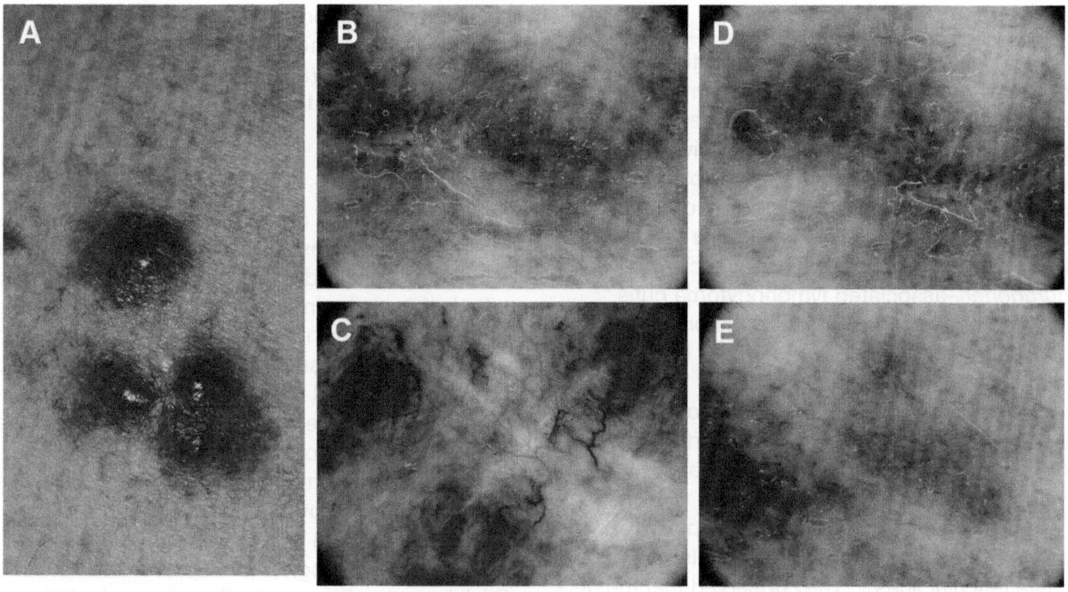

Fig. 5. Marginal zone B-cell lymphoma. (*A*) Clinical presentation: multiple red-pinkish nodules on the back. (*B–E*) Dermoscopy reveals scales, white areas, and polymorphous vascular pattern.

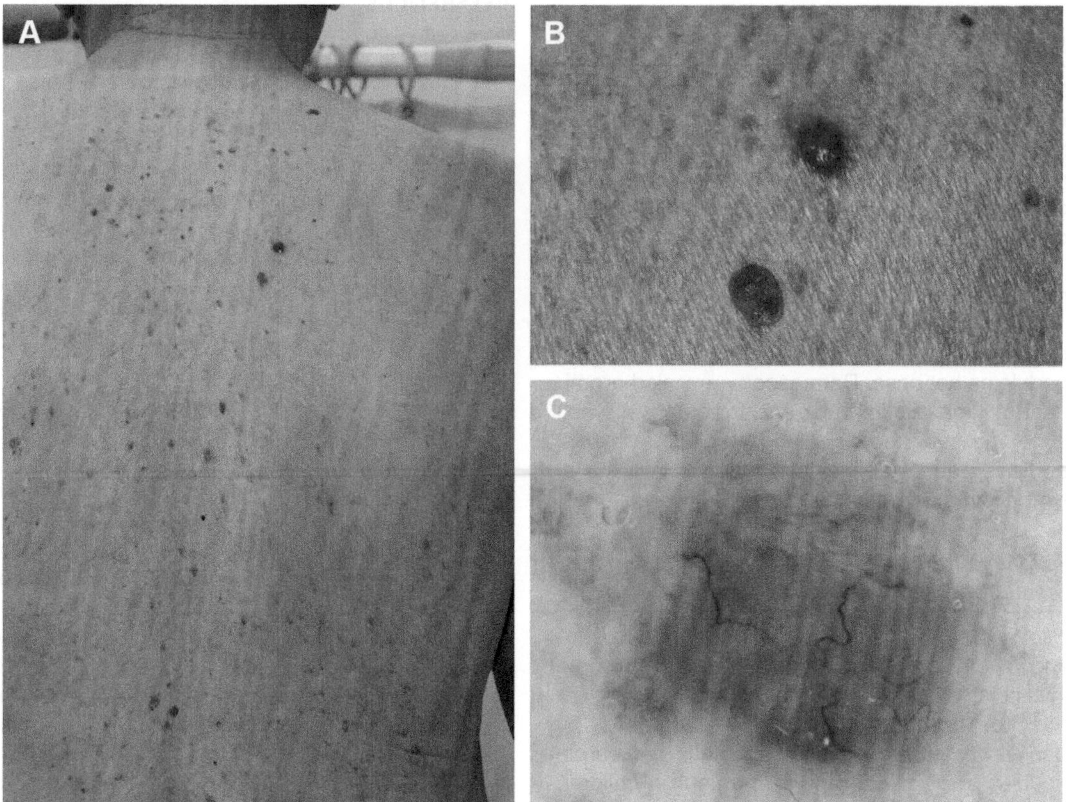

Fig. 6. Marginal zone B-cell lymphoma. (*A*, *B*) Clinical presentation: typical well delimited, red-pinkish nodule, on the back. (*C*) Dermoscopy reveals salmon-colored background/area and polymorphous vascular pattern.

Lymphocytoma Cutis

Clinical features. Lymphocytoma cutis is the prototype of cutaneous B-cell pseudolymphoma and the most common variant. It represents an exaggerated local immune response to diverse stimuli, in particular by arthropod bites. It presents as a solitary reddish nodule or plaques or crops of papules on face and neck. Lesions on the earlobe, nipples, and scrotum are highly associated with *B burgdorferi*–associated lymphocytoma cutis.[42]

Differential diagnosis. It includes primary malignant cutaneous B-cell lymphomas, inflammatory skin disease, and arthropod bites.

Dermoscopy. Only one dermoscopic description has been published to date. In that report, the investigators report a case of a 69-year-old man with a red nodule on his cheek. Dermoscopy revealed white reticular lines on a pinkish background and some fine linear vessels across the white reticular lines.[42] They observed that the dermoscopic pattern with linear vessels across white reticular line reflects the histopathologic architecture of dilated blood vessels and thin fibrous septa. For this reason, this combination of dermoscopic features may be a clue for the accurate diagnosis of lymphocytoma cutis.

Pseudolymphomatous Folliculitis

Clinical features. Pseudolymphomatous folliculitis is a rare variant, characterized by hyperplastic hair follicles with a lymphoid infiltrate that can mimic cutaneous lymphoma. It appears as a single dome-shaped or nodular lesion on the face, scalp, or trunk.[43]

Differential diagnosis. It includes primary malignant cutaneous lymphomas.

Dermoscopy. Fujimura and colleagues[44] described a case of a 45-year-old woman with a nodule on her nose. Dermoscopy revealed prominent multiple perifollicular and follicular yellowish spots, follicular red dots, and arborizing vessels, and this pattern suggests the dense infiltrate of lymphocytic cells around the hair follicles.

Acral Pseudolymphomatous Angiokeratoma/ Small Popular Pseudolymphoma

Clinical features. It is a rare benign condition of unknown cause and pathogenesis although some investigators believe it is a hypersensitivity reaction to insect bites. It is characterized by papules or clusters of asymptomatic red-purple nodules at acral site and is frequent in children and adolescent.[45]

Dermoscopy. Tokuda and colleagues[46] described a case with punctate vessels, irregular linear vessels, and whitish-pink areas without structures. In another report, the most representative finding was a rainbow pattern located mainly in the periphery of the lesions.[47]

SUMMARY

Dermoscopy may add useful information in the evaluation of these entities although further studies are needed to define specific diagnostic criteria for each single variant.[4,40,48] A good rule of thumb is to maintain alertness for features that do not follow the usual clinical and histopathologic patterns described for these entities. When diagnostic features are not clear, a comprehensive approach is to perform a skin biopsy and to always ensure clear communication between Clinicians and Pathologists by offering clinical and dermoscopic information for an optimal reappraisal.[49] When histopathologic features are also unclear, Clinicians should consider the option of additional biopsies over time, in particular when clinical and dermoscopic aspects change, because this might suggest an evolution toward a clearer diagnostic phenotype.

REFERENCES

1. Litvinov IV, Tetzlaff MT, Rahme E, et al. Demographic patterns of cutaneous T-cell lymphoma incidence in Texas based on two different cancer registries. Cancer Med 2015;4(9):1440–7.
2. Scarisbrick JJ, Prince M, Vermeer MH, et al. Cutaneous Lymphoma International Consortium study of outcome in advanced stages of mycosis fungoides and Sézary Syndrome: effect of specific prognostic markers on survival and development of a prognostic model. J Clin Oncol 2015;33(32): 3766–73.
3. Quaglino P, Pimpinelli N, Berti E, et al. Time course, clinical pathways, and long-term hazards risk trends of disease progression in patients with classic mycosis fungoides: a multicenter, retrospective follow-up study from the Italian Group of Cutaneous Lymphomas. Cancer 2012;118(23):5830–9.
4. Lallas A, Apalla Z, Lefaki I, et al. Dermoscopy of early stage mycosis fungoides. J Eur Acad Dermatol Venereol 2013;27:617–21.
5. Bosseila M, Sayed KS, El-Din Sayed SS, et al. Evaluation of angiogenesis in early mycosis fungoides patients: dermoscopic and immunohistochemical study. Dermatology 2015;231:82–6.
6. Vazquez-Loèez F, Kreusch J, Marghoob AA. Dermoscopic semiology: further insights into vascular features by screening a large spectrum of nontumoral skin lesions. Br J Dermatol 2004; 150:226–31.

7. van Doorn R, Scheffer E, Willemze R. Follicular mycosis fungoides: a distinct disease entity with or whitout associated follicular mucinosis. Arch Dermatol 2001;138:191–8.
8. Mielke V, Wolff HH, Winzer M, et al. Localized and disseminated pagetoid reticulosis: diagnostic immunophenotypical findings. Arch Dermatol 1989;125: 402–6.
9. Abbott RA, Sahni D, Robson A, et al. Poikilodermatous mycosis fungoides: a study of its clinicopathological, immunophenotypic, and prognostic features. J Am Acad Dermatol 2011;65:313–9.
10. Xu P, Tan C. Dermoscopy of poikilodermatous mycosis fungoides (MF). J Am Acad Dermatol 2016;74:45–7.
11. LeBoit PE. Granulomatous slack skin. Dermatol Clin 1994;12:375–89.
12. van Haselen CW, Toonstra J, van der Putte SJ, et al. Granulomatous slack skin: report of three patients with an updated review of the literature. Dermatology 1998;196:382–91.
13. Clarijs M, Poot F, Laka A, et al. Granulomatous slack skin: treatment with extensive surgery and review of the literature. Dermatology 2003;206:393–7.
14. Wieselthier JS, Koh HK. Sézary syndrome: diagnosis, prognosis and critical review of treatment options. J Am Acad Dermatol 1990;22:381–401.
15. Vonderheid EC, Bernengo MG, Burg G, et al. Update on erythrodermic cutaneous T-cell lymphoma: report of the International Society for Cutaneous Lymphomas. J Am Acad Dermatol 2002;46:95–106.
16. Bekkenk M, Geelen FAMJ, van Voorst Vader PC, et al. Primary and secondary cutaneous CD30-positive lymphoproliferative disorders: long term follow-up data of 219 patients and guidelines for diagnosis and treatment: a report from the Dutch Cutaneus Lymphoma Group. Blood 2000;95: 3653–61.
17. Liu HL, Hoppe RT, Kohler S, et al. CD30+ cutaneous lymphoproliferative disorders: the Stanford experience in lymphomatoid papulosis and primary cutaneous anaplastic large cell lymphoma. J Am Acad Dermatol 2003;49:1049–58.
18. Uzuncakmak TK, Akdeniz N, Karadag AS, et al. Primary cutaneous CD30 (+) ALK (-) anaplastic large cell lymphoma with dermoscopic findings: a case report. Dermatol Pract Concept 2017;7(1):12.
19. Moura FN, Thomas L, Balme B, et al. Dermoscopy of Lymphomatoid papulosis. Arch Dermatol 2009; 145(8):966–7.
20. Marzano AV, Berti E, Paulli M, et al. Cytophagocytic histiocytic panniculitis and subcutaneous panniculitis-like T-cell lymphoma. Arch Dermatol 2000;136:889–96.
21. Cheung MMC, Chan JKC, Lau WH, et al. Primary non-Hodgkin lymphoma of the nose and nasopharynx: clinical features, tumor immunophenotype, and treatment outcome in 113 patients. J Clin Oncol 1998;16:70–7.
22. Willemze R, Jaffe ES, Burge G, et al. WHO-EORTC classification for cutaneous lymphomas. Blood 2005;105:3768–85.
23. Bradford PT, Devesa SS, Anderson WF, et al. Cutaneous lymphoma incidence in the United States: a population-based study of 3884 cases. Blood 2009;113:5064–73.
24. Geller S, Marghoob AA, Scope A, et al. Dermoscopy and the diagnosis of primary cutaneous B-cell lymphoma. J Eur Acad Dermatol Venereol 2018;32(1): 53–6.
25. Lima M. cutaneous primary B-cell lymphomas: from diagnosis to treatment. An Bras Dermatol 2015;90: 687–706.
26. Selva R, Violetti SA, Delfino C, et al. A literature revision in primary cutaneous B-cell lymphoma. Indian J Dermatol 2017;62(2):146–57.
27. Santucci M, Grandi V, Maio V, et al. Indolent cutaneous B-cell lymphoma: diagnosis and treatment 2012. G Ital Dermatol Venereol 2012;147(6): 581–8.
28. Kodama K, Massone C, Chott A, et al. Primary cutaneous large B-cell lymphomas: clinicopathologic features, classification, and prognostic factors in a large series of patients. Blood 2005;106(7):2491–7.
29. Mascolo M, Piccolo V, Argenziano G, et al. Dermoscopy pattern, Histopathology and immunophenotype of primary cutaneous B-cell lymphomas presenting as a solitary skin nodule. Dermatology 2016;232:203–7.
30. Vermeer MH, Geelen FAMJ, van Haselen CW, et al. Primary cutaneous large B-cell lymphomas ofthe legs: a distinct type of cutaneous B-cell lymphomas with an intermediate prognosis. Arch Dermatol 1996; 132:1304–8.
31. Grange F, Bekkenk MW, Wechsker J, et al. Prognostic factors in primary cutaneus large B-cell lymphomas: a European multicenter study. J Clin Oncol 1998;16:2080–5.
32. Goodlad JR, Krajewski AS, Batstone PJ, et al. Primary cutaneous diffuse large B-cell lymphoma: prognostic significance and clinicopathologic subtypes. Am J Surg Pathol 2003;27:1538–45.
33. Grange F, Beylot-Barry M, Courville P, et al. Primary cutaneous diffuse large B-cell lymphomas, leg type: clinicopathologic features and prognostic analysis in 60 cases. Arch Dermatol 2007;143:1144–50.
34. Senff NJ, Hoefnagel JJ, Jansen PM, et al. Reclassification of 300 primary cutaneous B-cell lymphomas according to the new WHO-EORTC classification for cutaneous lymphomas: comparison with previous classification and identification of prognostic markers. J Clin Oncol 2007;25:1581–7.
35. Li C, Inagaki H, Kuo TT, et al. Primary cutaneous marginal zone B-cell lymphoma: a molecular and

clinicopathologic study of 24 Asian cases. Am J Surg Pathol 2003;27:1061–9.
36. Cerroni L, Signoretti S, Hofler G, et al. Primary cutaneous marginal zone B-cell lymphoma: a recently described entity of low-grade malignant cutaneous B-cell lymphoma. Am J Surg Pathol 1997;21:1307–15.
37. Bailey EM, Ferry JA, Harris NL, et al. Marginal zone lymphoma (low-grade B-cell lymphoma of mucosa-associated lymphoid tissue type) of skin and subcutaneous tissue: a study of 15 patients. Am J Surg Pathol 1996;20:1011–23.
38. Child FJ, Woollons A, Prince ML, et al. Multiple cutaneous immunocytoma with secondary anetoderma: report of two cases. Br J Dermatol 2000; 143:165–70.
39. Kim YH, Willemze R, Pimpinelli N, et al. TNM classification system for primary cutaneous lymphomas other than mycosis fungoides and Sezary syndrome: a proposal of the International Society for Cutaneous Lymphomas (ISCL) and the Cutaneous Lymphomas Task Force of the European Organization of Research and Treatment of Cancer (EORTC). Blood 2007;110:479–84.
40. Piccolo V, Mascolo M, Russo T, et al. Dermoscopy of primary cutaneous B-cell lymphomas (PCBCL). J Am Acad Dermatol 2016;75(4):e137–9.
41. Romero-Pérez D, Blanes Martìnez M, Encabo-Dùran B. Cutaneous pseudolymphomas. Actas Dermosifiliogr 2016;107(8):640–51.
42. Namiki T, Miura K, Tokoro S, et al. Dermoscopic features of lymphocytoma cutis: a case report of a representative dermoscopic feature. J Dermatol 2016;43(11):1367–8.
43. Kakizaki A, Fujimura T, Numata I, et al. Pseudolymphotous folliculitis on the nose. Case Rep Dermatol 2012;4:27–30.
44. Fujimura T, Hidaka T, Hashimoto A, et al. Dermoscopy findings of pseudolymphomatous folliculitis. Case Rep Dermatol 2012;4:154–7.
45. Hussein MR. Cutaneous pseudolymphomas: inflammatory reactive proliferations. Expert Rev Hematol 2013;6:713–33.
46. Tokuda Y, Arakura F, Murata H, et al. Acral pseudolymphomatous angiokeratoma of children; a case report with immunohistochemical study of antipodoplanin antigen. Am J Dermatopathol 2012;34: e128–32.
47. Pinos Leòn VH, Granizo Rubio JD. Acral pseudolymphomatous angiokeratoma of children with rainbow pattern: a mimicker of Kaposi sarcoma. J Am Acad Dermatol 2017;76(2S1):S25–7.
48. Micali G, Verzì AE, Lacarrubba F. Alternative uses of dermatoscopy in daily clinical practice: an update. J Am Acad Dermatol 2018 Jun 16. pii: S0190-9622(18)32143-1. [Epub ahead of print].
49. Longo C, Piana S, Lallas A, et al. Routine clinicalpathologic correlation of pigmented skin tumors can influence patient management. PLoS One 2015;10(9): e0136031.

Dermatoscopy of Vascular Lesions

Vincenzo Piccolo, MD[a,*], Teresa Russo, MD[a], Elvira Moscarella, MD[a], Gabriella Brancaccio, MD[a], Roberto Alfano, MD[b], Giuseppe Argenziano, MD, PhD[a]

KEYWORDS

• Dermatoscopy • Dermoscopy • Vascular lesions • Angioma • Hemangioma • Kaposi sarcoma

KEY POINTS

- The correct identification of vascular lesions through dermoscopy is important in avoiding useless excisions and ruling out aggressive malignant tumors.
- With dermoscopy, most vascular lesions exhibit lacunae; that is, well-demarcated, variably colored areas, corresponding to the vascular proliferation of the lesions.
- When no specific dermoscopic features are detectable, biopsy is mandatory for the diagnosis to exclude malignancies.

INTRODUCTION

The evaluation of vessels through dermoscopy plays a key role in the correct recognition of skin tumors, infections, and inflammatory diseases.[1] The adequate interpretation of the shapes and distribution of vascular structures is definitely among the most important steps in the diagnostic pathway. With dermoscopy, it seems obvious that skin diseases that originate from cutaneous vessels are expected to show predominant vascular structures that, if promptly recognized, lead the observer to the right diagnosis. In practice, the correct identification through dermoscopy of vascular tumors (VTs) is highly important to avoid inopportune excisions and to rule out aggressive malignant tumors mimicking VTs and lacking specific dermoscopic features, such as amelanotic melanoma, poorly differentiated squamous cell carcinoma, Merkel cell carcinoma, dermatofibrosarcoma protuberans, and primary cutaneous B-cell lymphoma.[2–8]

Vascular lesions (VLs) refer to all the cutaneous diseases that either originate from or affect vessels, both blood and lymphatic, including benign and malignant tumors, malformations, and inflammatory diseases.

This article reviews the literature concerning the dermoscopic features of VLs and provides an easy, practical guide. **Table 1** lists the dermoscopic features of the VLs described in this article.

INFANTILE HEMANGIOMA AND CHERRY ANGIOMA

Infantile hemangiomas (IHs) and cherry angiomas (CAs) are benign tumors that develop from blood vessels; they can be considered the most common VTs observed in children and adults, respectively. Although different in clinical presentation and biological behavior, IHs and CAs are described together because they share common dermoscopic features. Lacunae (or lagoons) are well-demarcated round or oval areas in which the color can range from red to reddish-brown or reddish-blue, and the size can vary within the lesion. Their presence is a quite constant dermoscopic finding in IH and CA[9,10] (**Figs. 1–3**). Additional features, such as a variably colored background (red, red-blue, and red-white

Disclosure: None.

[a] Dermatology Unit, University of Campania Luigi Vanvitelli, Via Pansini 5, Naples 80131, Italy; [b] Department of Anesthesiology, Surgery and Emergency, University of Campania Luigi Vanvitelli, Via Pansini 5, Naples 80131, Italy

* Corresponding author. c/o Il Policlinico, Edificio 9, Primo piano, Via Pansini 5, Napoli 80131, Italy.
E-mail address: piccolo.vincenzo@gmail.com

Dermatol Clin 36 (2018) 389–395
https://doi.org/10.1016/j.det.2018.05.006

Table 1
Dermoscopy features commonly seen in vascular lesions

VLs	Dermoscopic Features
Infantile hemangioma and cherry angioma	• Variably colored lacunae and background • Isolated vessels • Jet-black area (thrombosed hemangioma)
Angiokeratoma	• Dark lacunae • Blue-whitish veil • Ulceration • Rainbow pattern
Pyogenic granuloma	• Reddish homogeneous areas • White rail lines • White collarette • Ulceration • Vessels
Targetoid hemosiderotic hemangioma	• Lacunae • Ecchymotic ring • Peripheral network • Shiny lines
Angioma serpiginosum	• Small multiple round to oval lacunae
Microvenular hemangioma	• Small regular red globules • Fine pigment network
Port-wine stain	• Superficial port-wine stain: dotted or globular vessels • Deep port-wine stain: linear or tortuous vessels, gray-whitish veil, pale circular areas surrounding brownish dots
Lymphangioma circumscriptum	• Variably colored lacunae • Vascular structures • Hypopyon sign • Scales
Kaposi sarcoma	• Variably colored lacunae • Rainbow pattern • Scales • White collarette • Structureless areas • Vascular structures
Angiosarcoma	• Reddish or purple structureless areas • White lines (nodular part)
Pigmented purpuric dermatoses	• Coppery-red background • Round to oval dots • Gray dots • Network

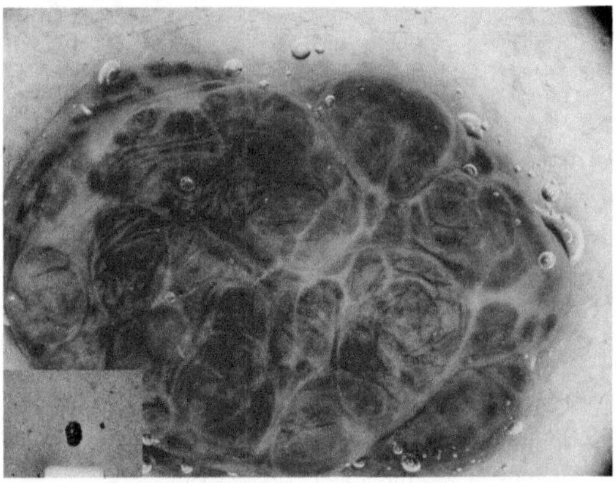

Fig. 1. Dermoscopy of cherry angioma showing red whitish lacunae and scattered vessels (original magnification ×10). In the inset the clinical presentation as red nodule of the back.

homogeneous) and isolated dilated vessels or vascular network can be found. In most cases, angiomas are easily diagnosed but differential diagnosis between thrombosed hemangioma (TH) and melanoma may be challenging. With dermoscopy, TH usually shows a sharply demarcated jet-black area corresponding to the thrombus and associated with the classic lacunae[11] (**Fig. 4**).

ANGIOKERATOMA

Angiokeratomas are acquired benign vascular proliferations histologically characterized by a combination of dilated subepidermal vessels with epidermal acanthosis and hyperkeratosis. Angiokeratoma can present as isolated or multiple, blue-violaceous to black or red, 2 to 10 mm papules or plaques with a scaly surface. At least 5 different types have been described, including angiokeratoma of Mibelli, solitary angiokeratoma, angiokeratoma corporis diffusum (usually

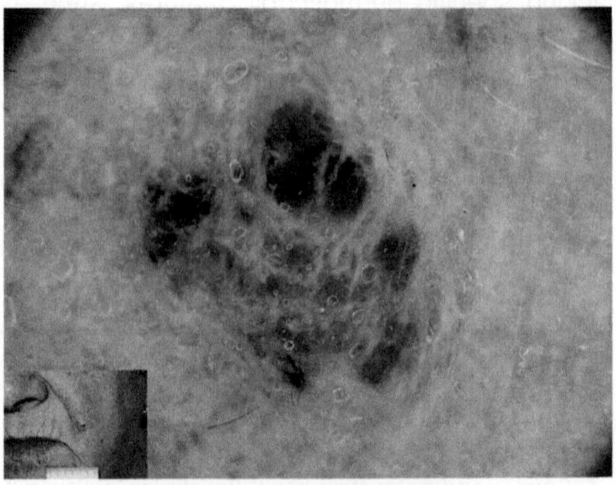

Fig. 2. Dermoscopy of angioma showing blue lagoons (original magnification ×10). The lesion presented clinically as a bluish nodule of the face (see inset).

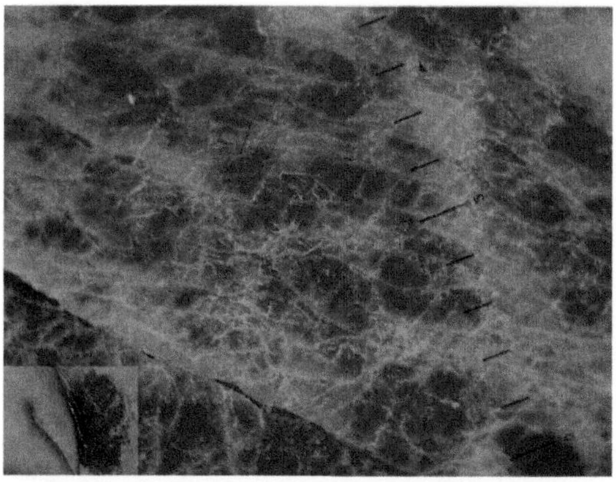

Fig. 3. Dermoscopy of infantile hemangiomas does not significantly differ from cherry angioma, showing multiple well demarcated red lacunae (original magnification x10). In the inset the clinical presentation as a reddish plaque of the left groin.

associated with Fabry disease), angiokeratoma of Fordyce, and angiokeratoma circumscriptum naeviforme. Different from angioma, solitary angiokeratoma often clinically present as a dark papule or nodule, making the differential diagnosis with other benign or malignant cutaneous tumors challenging. In particular, it may be difficult to distinguish it from melanocytic nevi, Spitz-Reed nevi, malignant melanomas, pigmented basal cell carcinomas, seborrheic keratoses, or dermatofibromas, as well as other VLs, such as hemangiomas or pyogenic granulomas (PGs).[12]

Dermoscopy of angiokeratoma shows quite constant features, such as dark lacunae, described as well-demarcated dark blue, dark violaceous, or black; round or ovoid structures; with a blue whitish veil, ulceration, and (occasionally) a rainbow pattern[12] (**Fig. 5**).

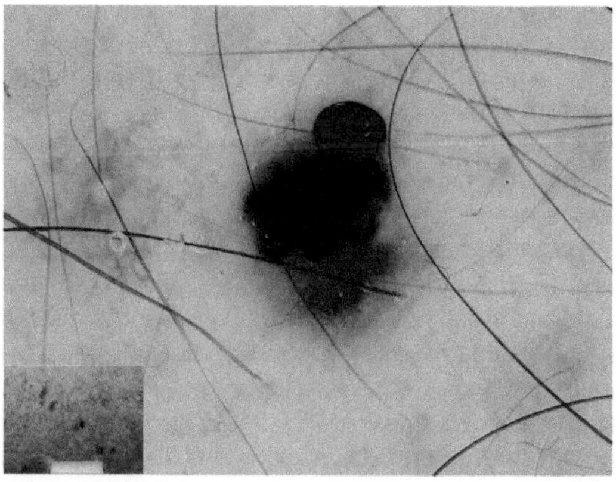

Fig. 4. Dermoscopy of thrombosed hemangioma showing Jet-black areas (original magnification ×10). Clinically, the lesion presented as a small bluish papule located on the back (see the inset).

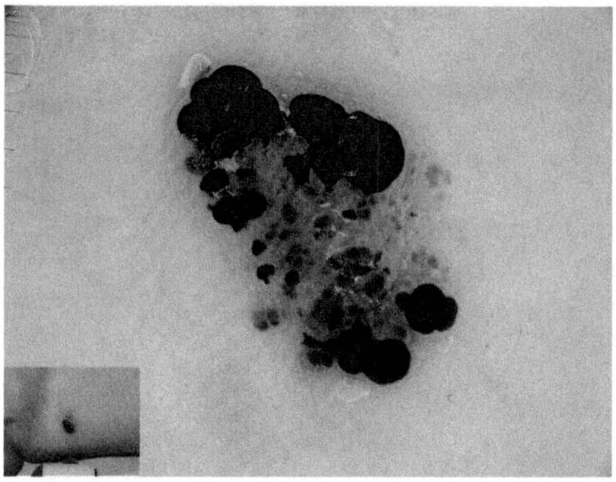

Fig. 5. Typical dermoscopic appearance of solitary angiokeratoma showing dark lacunae and blue-whitish veil. Angiokeratoma often presents as a dark lesion of the skin, clinically misdiagnosed as melanocytic lesion (see inset).

PYOGENIC GRANULOMA

PG or telangiectatic granuloma is a benign acquired VL of the skin or mucosa. It usually occurs in children or in adults as a rapidly growing, red, often easily bleeding, papule or nodule; this is a matter of concern for patients. PG can be associated with a trauma, infection, pregnancy, or medications, such as retinoids or docetaxel. Because malignant tumors, such as amelanotic melanoma, can be misdiagnosed as PG, histopathology is mandatory for the correct diagnosis, even though dermoscopy can play a primary role in the prompt recognition of PG, showing highly repetitive patterns that can support the diagnosis.[13]

In particular, the presence of reddish homogeneous area, white collarette, or white rail lines (even more so when associated together) are strongly suggestive of PG[13] (**Figs. 6** and **7**). On

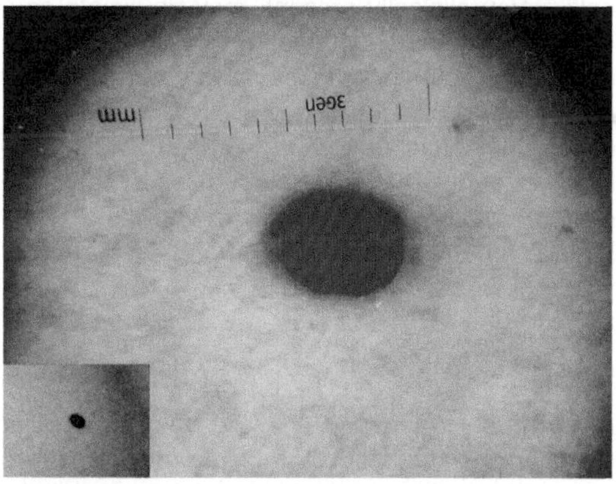

Fig. 6. Dermoscopy of pyogenic granuloma showing reddish homogeneous areas associated with white rail lines (original magnification ×10). The inset shows the typical clinical presentation in a child.

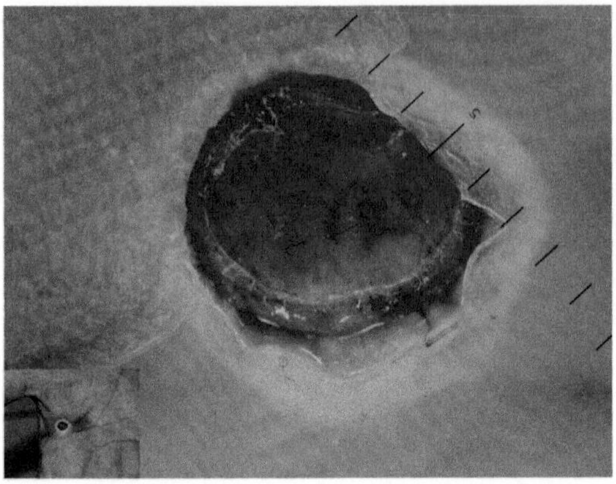

Fig. 7. Dermoscopy of pyogenic granuloma of the palmar area: the white collarette is the most striking feature (original magnification ×10). in the inset, the clinical presentation as an erosive nodule.

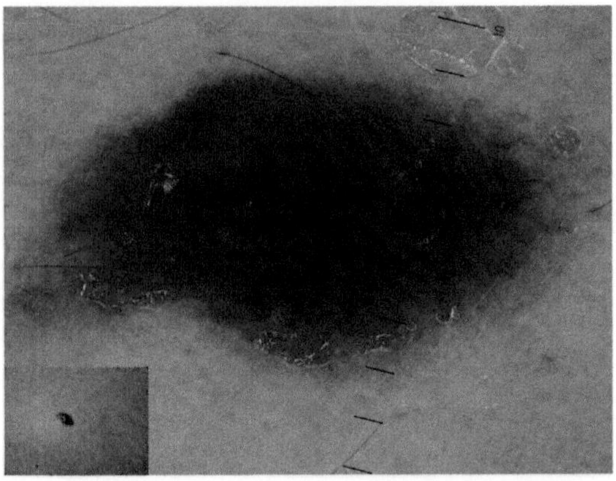

Fig. 8. Dermoscopy of targetoid hemosiderotic hemangioma: it may mimic melanoma, showing shiny lines and peripheral network (original magnification ×10). A small red-brownish nodule of the thigh in a young woman is shown in the inset.

the other hand, with dermoscopy, it is not uncommon to detect ulceration and vascular structures that do not rule out malignancies.

TARGETOID HEMOSIDEROTIC HEMANGIOMA

Targetoid hemosiderotic hemangioma (THH), also known as hobnail hemangioma, is a benign VT, probably originating from lymphatic vessels, usually presenting as a single papular or nodular lesion, typically surrounded a pale halo, in turn circumscribed by a peripheral ecchymotic ring. A cyclic changing in size and color of the lesion is typically reported by the patients, mainly women during menstrual cycles. In its classic presentation, recognition can be easy but THH may be sometimes confused with amelanotic melanoma and other cutaneous malignancies. Dermoscopy usually shows red or dark lacunae in the center surrounded by an ecchymotic area. The pale halo, when clinically present, may be visible as a circular homogeneous area. THH can sometimes show a homogeneous ecchymotic area covering all of the lesions, rendering the diagnosis more difficult. Different patterns of presentations have been described that are characterized by the presence of peripheral pigment network and shiny lines, sometimes making the differential diagnosis with melanoma challenging[14,15] (**Fig. 8**).

ANGIOMA SERPIGINOSUM

Angioma serpiginosum (AS) is a benign vascular disorder characterized by multiple minute, red to purple, grouped macules in serpiginous and gyrate fashion and histopathologically by ectatic dilatation of capillaries. AS is often confused with hematological disorders or chronic purpuric dermatoses. With dermoscopic examination AS typically shows numerous small, round to oval, red lacunae.[16]

MICROVENULAR HEMANGIOMA

Microvenular hemangioma is a rare, asymptomatic, slowly growing, benign VT usually presenting in young or middle-aged adults as purple red papule or plaque, measuring from 0.5 to 2 cm, and occurring on the trunk or the extremities. Its name derives from histologic findings typically showing a dermal proliferation of small, irregular, branching capillaries and venules with inconspicuous lumina. There is an anecdotal report of diffuse erythema with multiple, well-defined, small, regular, red globules associated with a peripheral fine pigment network.[17]

PORT-WINE STAIN

Port-wine stain (PWS) is a capillary malformation present since birth and persisting for life. It usually appears as a reddish patch that progressively assumes a port-wine color and may develop nodular areas within the context of the main lesion. It is important to promptly recognize PWS in infants and to distinguish them from IHs because of the different treatments required. With dermoscopy, it is possible to distinguish superficial PWS, typically showing red, dotted or globular vessels, from deep PWS, typically showing dilated linear and tortuous vessels, a gray-whitish veil, and a pale circular area surrounding a central brownish dot[18] (**Figs. 9** and **10**). Obviously, mixed findings are possible when a combination of superficial and deep PWS is seen.

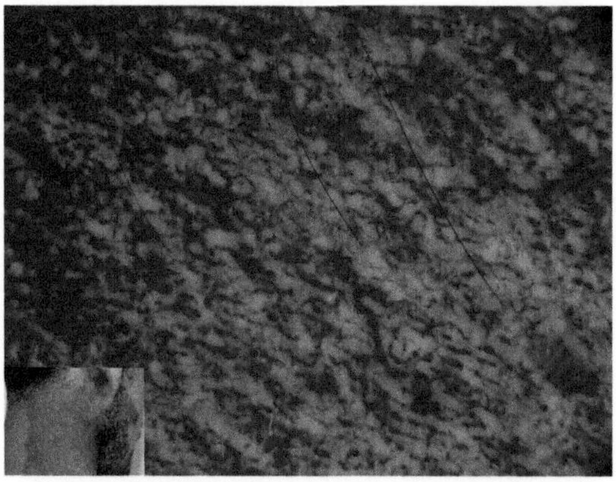

Fig. 9. Dermoscopy of port-wine stain of the neck (see the inset) showing multiple tortuous vessels (original magnification ×10).

LYMPHANGIOMA CIRCUMSCRIPTUM

Lymphangioma circumscriptum (LC) is a benign vascular malformation originating from lymphatic vessels, clinically presenting as a plaque constituted by multiple, grouped, vesicle-like lesions with the so-called frogspawn appearance, differentiating it from cystic lymphangioma, which is a deep dermal and subcutaneous lymphatic malformation. Different studies have investigated dermoscopy of LC, finding that variably colored (dark, yellowish, whitish, multicolored) lacunae seem to be the most common detectable feature, followed by vascular structures, white lines, the so-called hypopyon sign or 2-tone lacunae (as a result a half blood-filled lacunae resembling the hypopyon in the eye), and scales[19] (**Fig. 11**).

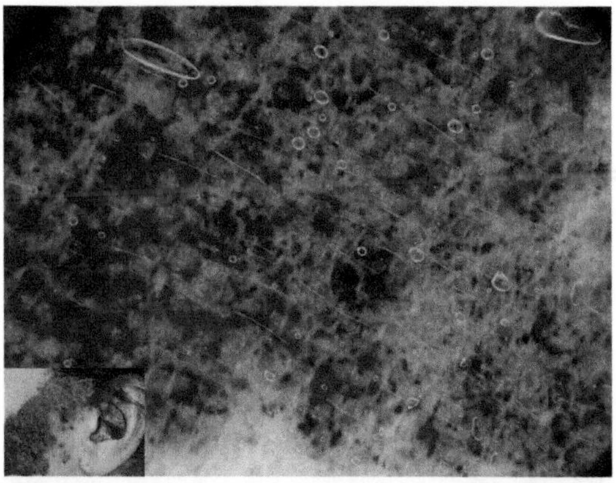

Fig. 10. Dermoscopy of port-wine stain: in deeper lesions, tortuous vessels, a gray-whitish veil, and pale circular areas surrounding brownish dots are seen (original magnification ×10). In the inset, the clinical presentation on the face.

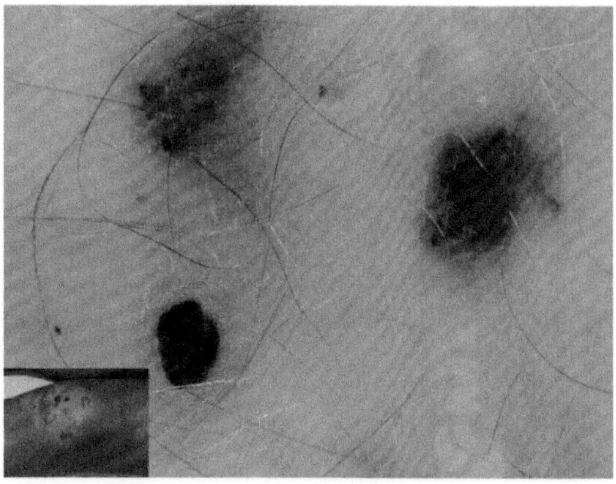

Fig. 11. Dermoscopy of lymphangioma circumscriptum showing variably colored lacunae (original magnification ×10). The inset shows a complex lesion characterized by multiple red to bluish papules of the knee.

KAPOSI SARCOMA

KS is a low-grade, malignant, spindle-cell tumor deriving from endothelial cell lineage and thought to be related to human herpesvirus-8 infection. KS is classified into 4 subtypes: epidemic or AIDS-related, immunocompromised, classic or sporadic, and endemic (African). Clinical presentation is extremely variable, ranging from isolated red to purple papules of the extremities to large plaques or disseminated forms. The role of dermoscopy is important in the early diagnosis of KS, in particular when it presents with isolated lesions, whose differential diagnosis from other benign and malignant skin tumors can be challenging. Currently, there are no specific dermoscopic patterns described for KS but several findings can be considered highly suggestive. The most common feature is the homogeneous pattern, which is characteristically variably colored in different lesions of the same patient, with the color ranging from reddish to bluish, pinkish, whitish, or violaceous. Formerly considered pathognomonic, the rainbow-like pattern is the most striking dermoscopic sign of KS. It is characterized by the presence of multicolored areas, romantically compared with the rainbow spectrum, in the same lesion. Additional features, including scales, white collarette, structureless areas, and vascular structures may be detectable[20,21] (**Figs. 12** and **13**).

ANGIOSARCOMA

Angiosarcoma is a malignant VT with a very aggressive behavior and tendency to metastasize rapidly to regional lymph nodes and lungs. Three types have been identified: angiosarcoma of the head and scalp, radiation-induced angiosarcoma,

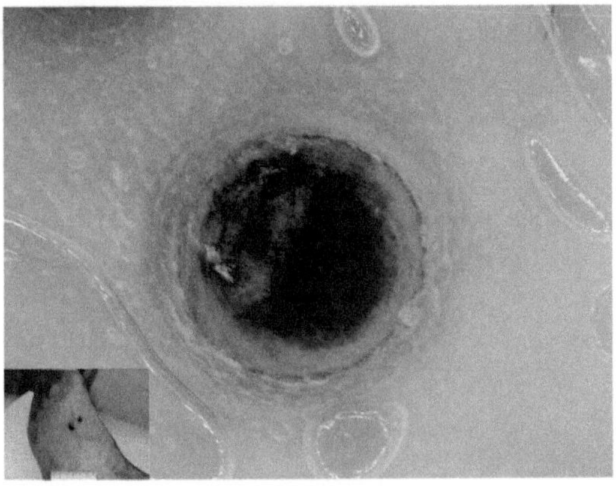

Fig. 12. Dermoscopy of Kaposi sarcoma showing central reddish lacunae surrounded by collarette (original magnification ×10). In the inset, multiple nodules of the sole in a 72-year-old man.

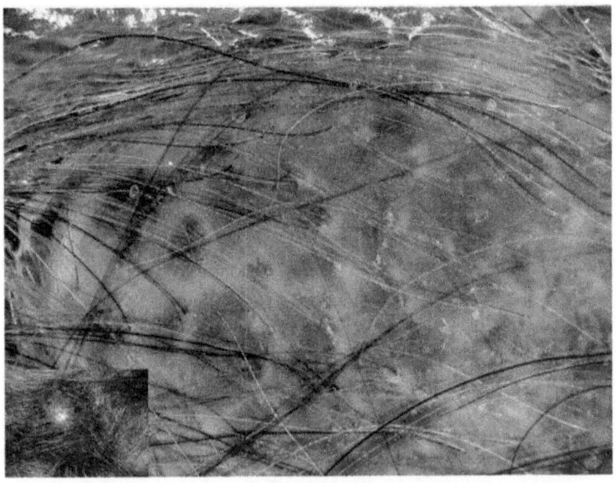

Fig. 14. Dermoscopy of the nodular part of angiosarcoma showing structureless areas and white lines (original magnification ×10). The inset shows an infiltrated plaque of the scalp.

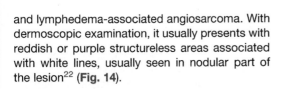

and lymphedema-associated angiosarcoma. With dermoscopic examination, it usually presents with reddish or purple structureless areas associated with white lines, usually seen in nodular part of the lesion[22] (**Fig. 14**).

PIGMENTED PURPURIC DERMATOSES

Pigmented purpuric dermatoses (PPDs) are a complex group of cutaneous diseases, in which the clinical hallmark is the cayenne pepper–like discoloration of the skin deriving from extravasation of erythrocytes in the skin with marked hemosiderin deposition. PPDs include progressive pigmentary dermatosis (Schamberg disease), purpura annularis telangiectodes of Majocchi, lichen aureus, itching purpura, eczematoid-like purpura of Doucas and Kapetanakis, and the pigmented purpuric lichenoid dermatosis of Gougerot and Blum, with each subtype showing distinctive clinical features. PPDs are often misdiagnosed as vasculitides and are a matter of concern among patients affected by these cutaneous diseases. A few studies have shown how dermoscopy can be useful in the prompt recognition of PPDs by detecting several findings, such as a coppery-red background, round to oval dots, gray dots, and a network of brownish to gray interconnected lines[23] (**Fig. 15**). An attempt at classification of purpuric lesions based on dermoscopic findings has been made with the recognition of 4 specific patterns, each of them corresponding to a group of diseases. In particular, a homogeneous pattern is associated with bleeding diathesis and steroid-induced or senile purpura, a mottled pattern has been described in PPD and leukocytoclastic vasculitis, a perifollicular pattern is found only in scurvy, and an

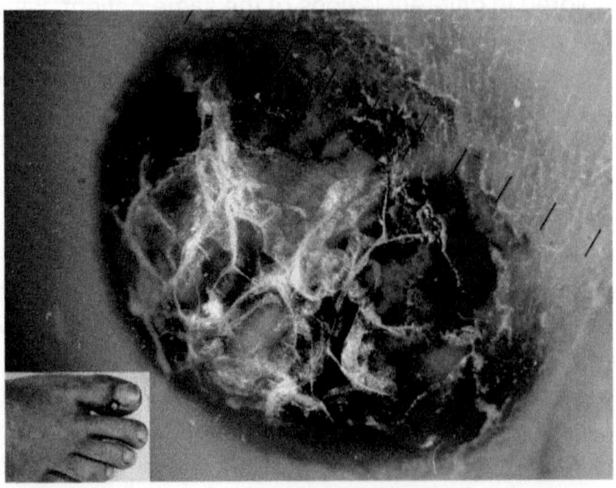

Fig. 13. Dermoscopy of Kaposi sarcoma showing a typical rainbow pattern with scales (original magnification ×10). In the inset the clinical presentation as a single nodule of the big toe.

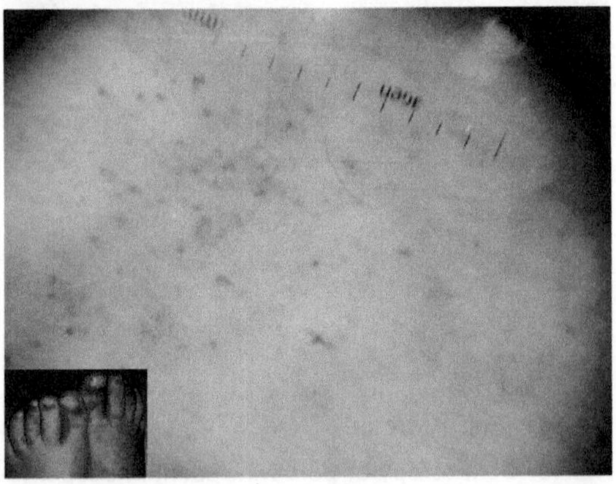

Fig. 15. Dermoscopy of lichen aureus in a child showing red, round dots associated with red coppery background (clinical appearance is shown in the inset).

epidermal purpuric pattern is seen in subungual or subcorneal hemorrhages.[24]

REFERENCES

1. Argenziano G, Zalaudek I, Corona R, et al. Vascular structures in skin tumors: a dermoscopy study. Arch Dermatol 2004;140:1485–9.
2. Russo T, Piccolo V, Lallas A, et al. Dermoscopy of malignant skin tumours: what's new? Dermatology 2017;233:64–73.
3. Costa C, Cappello M, Argenziano G, et al. Dermoscopy of uncommon variants of dermatofibrosarcoma protuberans. J Eur Acad Dermatol Venereol 2017;31:e366–8.
4. Russo T, Piccolo V, Lallas A, et al. Recent advances in dermoscopy. F1000Res 2016;5 [pii:F1000 Faculty Rev-184].
5. Piccolo V, Mascolo M, Russo T, et al. Dermoscopy of primary cutaneous B-cell lymphoma (PCBCL). J Am Acad Dermatol 2016;75:e137–9.
6. Mascolo M, Piccolo V, Argenziano G, et al. Dermoscopy pattern, histopathology and immunophenotype of primary cutaneous B-cell lymphoma presenting as a solitary skin nodule. Dermatology 2016;232:203–7.
7. Piccolo V, Mascolo M, Russo T, et al. A solitary fast growing red nodule of the abdomen. J Dtsch Dermatol Ges 2014;12:1147–8.
8. Baroni A, Piccolo V. Images in clinical medicine. Red melanoma. N Engl J Med 2013;368(16):1536.
9. Oiso N, Kawada A. The dermoscopic features in infantile hemangioma. Pediatr Dermatol 2011;28:591–3.
10. Grazzini M, Stanganelli I, Rossari S, et al. Dermoscopy, confocal laser microscopy, and hi-tech evaluation of vascular skin lesions: diagnostic and therapeutic perspectives. Dermatol Ther 2012;25: 297–303.
11. Moscarella E, Zalaudek I, Buccini P, et al. Dermoscopy and confocal microscopy of thrombosed hemangiomas. Arch Dermatol 2012;148:410.
12. Zaballos P, Daufí C, Puig S, et al. Dermoscopy of solitary angiokeratomas: a morphological study. Arch Dermatol 2007;143:318–25.
13. Zaballos P, Carulla M, Ozdemir F, et al. Dermoscopy of pyogenic granuloma: a morphological study. Br J Dermatol 2010;163:1229–37.
14. Zaballos P, Llambrich A, Del Pozo LJ, et al. Dermoscopy of targetoid hemosiderotic hemangioma: a morphological study of 35 cases. Dermatology 2015;231:339–44.
15. Piccolo V, Russo T, Mascolo M, et al. Dermoscopic misdiagnosis of melanoma in a patient with targetoid hemosiderotic hemangioma. J Am Acad Dermatol 2014;71:e179–81.
16. Ohnishi T, Nagayama T, Morita T, et al. Angioma serpiginosum: a report of 2 cases identified using epiluminescence microscopy. Arch Dermatol 1999; 135:1366–8.
17. Scalvenzi M, De Natale F, Francia MG, et al. Dermoscopy of microvenular hemangioma: report of a case. Dermatology 2007;215:69–71.
18. Vázquez-López F, Coto-Segura P, Fueyo-Casado A, et al. Dermoscopy of port-wine stains. Arch Dermatol 2007;143:962.
19. Gencoglan G, Inanir I, Ermertcan AT. Hypopyon-like features: new dermoscopic criteria in the differential diagnosis of cutaneous lymphangioma circumscriptum and haemangiomas? J Eur Acad Dermatol Venereol 2012;26:1023–5.
20. Cheng ST, Ke CL, Lee CH, et al. Rainbow pattern in Kaposi's sarcoma under polarized dermoscopy: a dermoscopic pathological study. Br J Dermatol 2009;160:801–9.
21. Vázquez-López F, García-García B, Rajadhyaksha M, et al. Dermoscopic rainbow pattern in non-Kaposi sarcoma lesions. Br J Dermatol 2009;161:474–5.
22. Zalaudek I, Gomez-Moyano E, Landi C, et al. Clinical, dermoscopic and histopathological features of spontaneous scalp or face and radiotherapy-induced angiosarcoma. Australas J Dermatol 2013; 54:201–7.
23. Zaballos P, Puig S, Malvehy J. Dermoscopy of pigmented purpuric dermatoses (lichen aureus): a useful tool for clinical diagnosis. Arch Dermatol 2004; 140:1290–1.
24. Vazquez-Lopez F, García-García B, Sanchez-Martin J, et al. Dermoscopic patterns of purpuric lesions. Arch Dermatol 2010;146:938.

Dermoscopy of Adnexal Tumors

Pedro Zaballos, MD, PhD[a,*], Ignacio Gómez-Martín, MD[a], José María Martin, MD, PhD[b], José Bañuls, MD, PhD[c]

KEYWORDS

• Dermoscopy • Adnexal tumors • Sebaceous tumors • Follicular tumors • Eccrine and apocrine tumors

KEY POINTS

- Many uncommon adnexal tumors have been described only sporadically.
- Arborizing telangiectasias are common in adnexal tumors.
- Adnexal tumors are usually mimickers of basal cell carcinomas.
- Yellow structures are very suggestive of sebaceous tumors.
- Sweat gland tumors usually display great dermoscopic variability.

INTRODUCTION

Cutaneous adnexal tumors are classified according to their adnexal differentiation as sebaceous, follicular, eccrine, and apocrine. These tumors often cause immense diagnostic difficulty. Dermoscopy is a noninvasive technique that has greatly improved the diagnostic accuracy of pigmented and nonpigmented skin tumors. In this article, we provide a review of the literature on the dermoscopic structures and patterns associated with adnexal tumors along with representative examples from our database.

DERMOSCOPY OF SEBACEOUS TUMORS

Sebaceous tumors are traditionally classified as sebaceous nevus, sebaceous hyperplasia, sebaceous adenoma, sebaceoma, and sebaceous carcinoma.

Sebaceous Nevus

Sebaceous nevus is considered a complex hamartoma that presents at birth and commonly affects the head and neck, particularly the scalp. The natural history of sebaceous nevus is traditionally divided into 3 evolutionary and overlapping stages.

The first is the infancy and childhood stage, characterized by underdeveloped adnexal structures and, clinically, by the presence of a round, oval, or linear smooth, yellowish patch or plaque of alopecia.[1–3] Bright yellow dots not associated with hair follicles (**Fig. 1**), corresponding to incipient sebaceous glands, may be seen on dermoscopy at this stage.[1–3] This finding can be very useful in differentiating sebaceous nevus from aplasia cutis congenital in newborns.[1]

The second stage or the puberty stage is characterized by proliferative lesions involving adnexal and epidermal structures, in which the lesion transforms from a smooth into an incipient verrucous plaque. At this stage, dermoscopy reveals yellowish globules that can be arranged in cobblestone pattern (see **Fig. 1**) that correspond to dermal conglomerations of numerous, hyperplastic sebaceous glands in the histopathology.[1–3]

Disclosure: None.

[a] Dermatology Department, Hospital Sant Pau i Santa Tecla, C/ Joan Fuster s/n, 43007 Tarragona, Spain; [b] Dermatology Department, Hospital Clínico Universitario, Avenida Blasco Ibáñez 17, 46010 Valencia, Spain; [c] Dermatology Department, Hospital General Universitario de Alicante, ISABIAL, C/Maestro Alonso 109, 03010 Alicante, Spain
* Corresponding author. Dermatology Department, Hospital Sant Pau i Santa Tecla, Rambla Vella, 14, Tarragona 43003, Spain.
E-mail address: pzaballos@aedv.es

Dermatol Clin 36 (2018) 397–412
https://doi.org/10.1016/j.det.2018.05.007

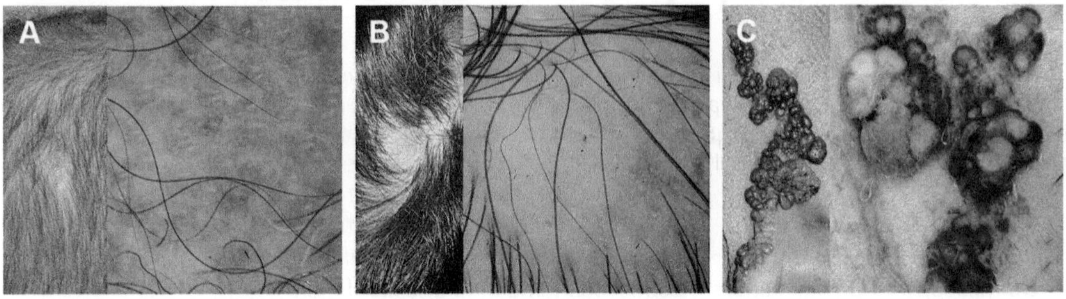

Fig. 1. Evolutionary stages of sebaceous nevus. (*A*) In the dermoscopic view, we can find a pattern composed of bright yellow dots (infancy and childhood stage). (*B*) Yellowish globules (puberty stage). (*C*) Yellowish-brown globules and exophytic papillary structures (post pubertal stage).

And finally, the third stage or post pubertal stage is characterized by more verrucous sebaceous nevi and the appearance of benign or malignant neoplasms.[4–6] Dermoscopically, sebaceous nevus is characterized by the presence of yellowish-brown globules, fissures, and ridges that can be arranged in "cerebriform pattern" (see **Fig. 1**), comedolike openings, and milialike cysts.[2–6] At this stage, it is estimated that approximately 10% to 20% of nevus sebaceous are complicated by benign or malignant epidermal, adnexal, or mesenchymal tumors.[6] Trichoblastoma and syringocystadenoma papilliferum are the 2 most frequent benign tumors to develop in nevus sebaceous, and basal cell carcinoma (BCC) is the most common malignant neoplasm.[4–6] The adnexal tumors arising in sebaceous nevus are discussed in depth later in this article.

Sebaceous Hyperplasia

Sebaceous hyperplasia is the most common proliferative abnormality of the sebaceous glands. It most often presents on the face of older adults, particularly men. The classic appearance of sebaceous hyperplasia on physical examination reveals whitish-yellow or skin-colored, normally umbilicated, papules that are soft and vary in size from 2 to 9 mm.

Dermoscopically, sebaceous hyperplasia shows a pattern composed of the presence of aggregated white-yellowish globules in the center of the lesions with a surrounding crown of vessels (**Fig. 2**).[7–10] The central aggregated white-yellowish structures or globules, showing a sharp difference from surrounding skin, were defined by Bryden and colleagues,[7] in a descriptive way as "cumulus sign," because these structures resemble the cumulus clouds and correspond histopathologically to hyperplastic sebaceous glands. Bryden and colleagues[7] and Oztas and colleagues[9] observed these structures in 100% of the sebaceous hyperplasias of their studies. Sometimes the ostium of the gland is visible as a small crater or umbilication in the center of these yellowish structures. Oztas and colleagues[9] named the association of the

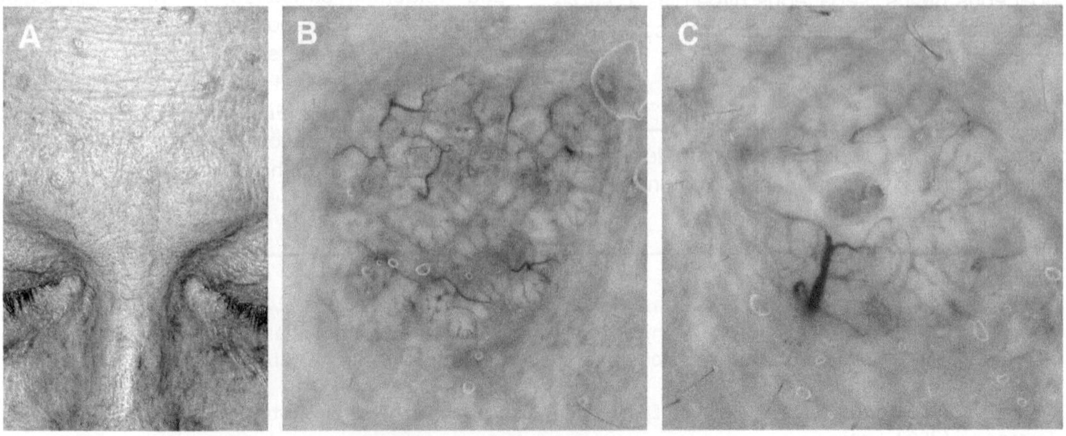

Fig. 2. Dermoscopy of 2 sebaceous hyperplasias. (*A*) Clinical view. (*B*) Dermoscopic pattern composed of the presence of aggregated white-yellowish globules in the center of the lesions with a surrounding crown of vessels. (*C*) Dermoscopic pattern called "Bonbon Toffee sign."

central umbilication surrounded by cumulus sign as "Bonbon Toffee sign" (see **Fig. 2**) and found this pattern in 80% of sebaceous hyperplasias. Regarding vascular structures that we can find at the periphery of sebaceous hyperplasias, the most common ones are the "crown vessels."[7–10] These vascular structures have been defined as groups of orderly, bending, scarcely branching vessels located along the border of the lesion.[11] These vessels may extend toward the center but never cross it. Argenziano and colleagues[11] found crown vessels in 83.3% of sebaceous hyperplasias and Oztas and colleagues[9] found them in 86.7% of cases. Other vascular structures that we can observe are arborizing vessels in 16.7% of cases according to Argenziano and colleagues.[11] Brown dots and globules, some of them with ringlike appearance, and milialike cysts are less common features that we can see in a few sebaceous hyperplasias.

Sebaceous Adenoma/Sebaceoma

Sebaceous adenoma and sebaceoma are benign neoplasms with sebaceous differentiation that may occur isolated or as part of Muir-Torre syndrome.[12–17] Both tumors present clinically as solitary or multiple (especially sebaceous adenoma), skin-colored, yellowish or reddish nodules, sometimes with multilobulated surface, ranging in size from 0.5 to 5.0 cm, preferentially involving the head and neck area.[12–17] Both lesions present histopathologically as well-circumscribed tumors composed of multiple lobules of sebaceous cells. The proportion of mature sebaceous cells over basaloid germinative cells distinguishes sebaceous adenoma (where mature cells predominate) from sebaceoma (where basaloid germinative cells predominate). Although there are usually other differences in the silhouette of both tumors (sebaceous adenoma usually connects to the epidermis, whereas sebaceoma do not), there are many cases of benign sebaceous neoplasms with overlapping cytologic and architectural features, suggesting a possible morphologic spectrum.[12–17]

Dermoscopically, differentiating between sebaceous adenoma and sebaceoma is not achievable and 2 main patterns have been described in both lesions.[12–17] First, tumors with a central crater are dermoscopically characterized by elongated radial telangiectasias (crown vessels) that embrace an opaque structureless ovoid white-yellow center, which are at times covered by blood crusts.[13] Second, tumors without a central crater reveal dermoscopically branching but unfocussed arborizing vessels over a white to yellow background and few, loosely arranged, yellow comedolike globules (**Fig. 3**).[13] The yellow ovoid structures correspond histopathologically to dermal conglomerations of enlarged sebaceous glands.

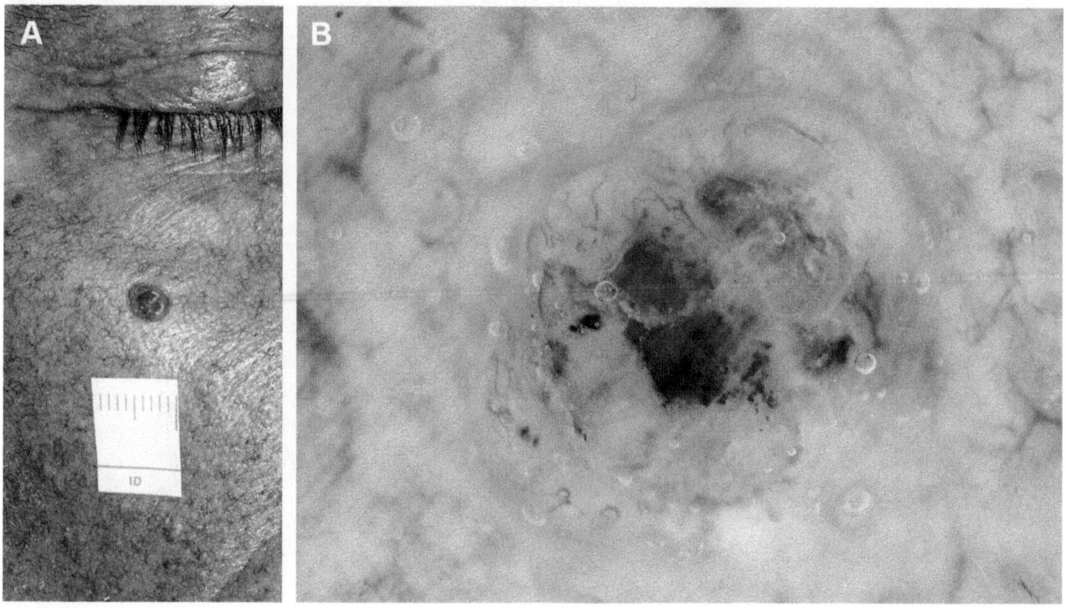

Fig. 3. Dermoscopy of a sebaceous adenoma. (*A*) Clinical view. (*B*) In the dermoscopic view, we can find a pattern composed of elongated radial telangiectasias (crown vessels) that embrace ovoid yellowish structures covered by blood crusts.

Sebaceous Carcinoma

Sebaceous carcinoma is a rare adenocarcinoma with variable degrees of sebaceous differentiation. They have traditionally been classified into periocular and extraocular subtypes. It can occur in isolation or as part of the Muir-Torre syndrome. Sebaceous carcinoma has a 30% to 40% risk for local tumor recurrence, 20% to 25% for distant metastases, and 10% to 20% for tumor-related mortality.[18] Its clinical presentation is notoriously varied and it is often mistaken for other lesions. On histologic examination, they are typically poorly circumscribed, asymmetric, infiltrative, and the individual cells are pleomorphic with atypical nuclei, mitoses, and coarsely vacuolated cytoplasm.

Sebaceous carcinoma is an uncommon tumor and its dermoscopic pattern has been described only sporadically.[15,19] However, dermoscopy of sebaceous carcinoma usually reveals the pattern composed of polymorphous atypical vessels, homogeneous yellowish background and, in many cases, ulceration (**Fig. 4**).[15,19] The term "polymorphous atypical vessels" is used when 2 or more types of vessel morphologies are detected in the same lesion. The polymorphic vascular pattern and ulceration should suggest malignancy, and juxtaposed with a variably yellow background may alert the dermoscopist to the possibility of the diagnosis of sebaceous carcinoma.[15,19]

DERMOSCOPY OF FOLLICULAR TUMORS

Follicular tumors encompass a large and heterogeneous group of neoplasms. In this article, we emphasize those that have dermoscopic description.

Nevus Comedonicus

Nevus comedonicus manifests as multiple, grouped dilated follicular openings with dark keratin plugs resembling comedones. Most cases are isolated, but may be part of nevus comedonicus syndrome. The typical dermoscopic findings described include multiple, well-defined, light and dark brown, circular or barrel-shaped homogeneous areas with prominent keratin plugs.[20–23]

Basaloid Follicular Hamartoma

Basaloid follicular hamartoma is a rare, acquired or hereditary (basaloid follicular hamartoma syndrome, Gorlin syndrome, Bazex-Dupré-Christol syndrome) benign adnexal tumor that presents as an asymptomatic, stable, small lesion (macule/papule/nodule/plaque/skin tag) typically located on the head. Dermoscopically it has

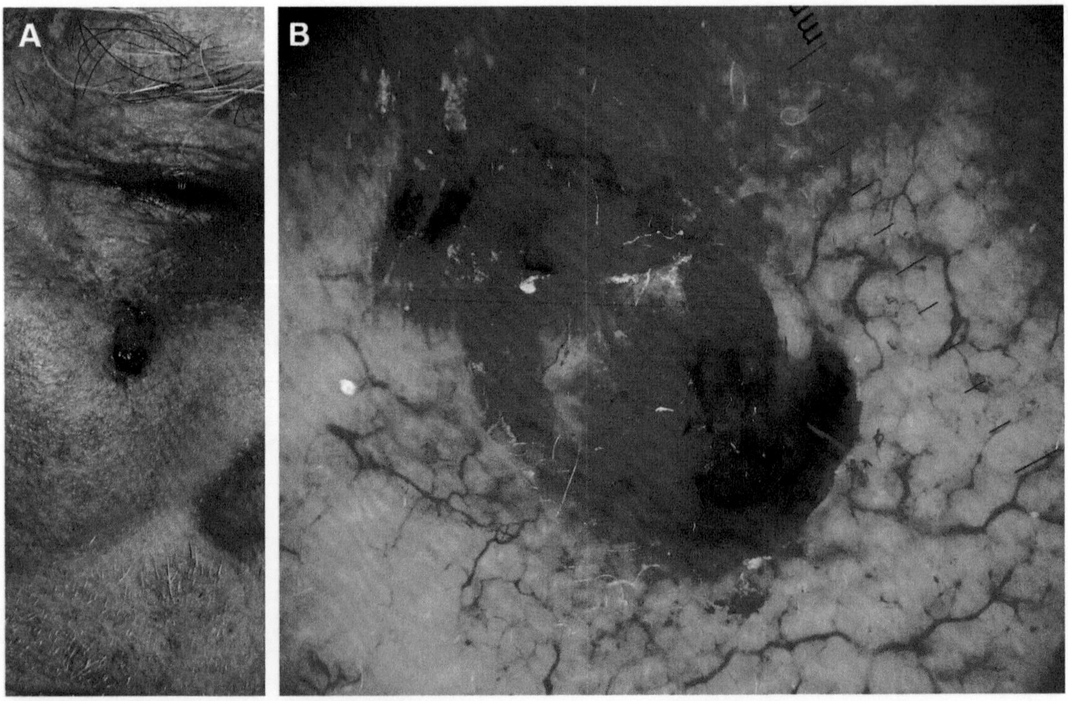

Fig. 4. Dermoscopy of a sebaceous carcinoma. (*A*) Clinical view. (*B*) In the dermoscopic view, we can find a pattern composed of polymorphous atypical vessels, homogeneous yellowish background, and ulceration. (*Courtesy of* Luis Javier del Pozo, MD, Illes Balears, Spain.)

been described as a structureless bluish macule[24] or as a lesion with globular pattern; white, pink, and gray areas; and the presence of comedolike openings and milialike cysts.[25]

Trichilemmoma

Trichilemmomas present as well-defined, asymptomatic, flesh-colored papules or verrucous growths, typically located on the head. If multiple trichilemmomas are present, Cowden disease should be suspected. Dermoscopy of trichilemmoma typically shows radial linear vessels (and occasionally hairpin vessels) with distal thickening adopting a triangular form in the periphery of the lesion (red irislike structure), white shiny areas surrounding those vessels, a whitish keratin mass, and also may exhibit a central hyperkeratotic crust.[14,26,27] The keratin mass and the whitish areas are correlated with the squamous lobes of the neoplasm on histopathologic examination.[27] Dermoscopic examination of desmoplastic trichilemmoma revealed crown vessels and unspecific ill-defined white areas, probably reflecting the presence of desmoplasia, and a hyperkeratotic central depression.[28]

Inverted Follicular Keratosis

Inverted follicular keratosis is a rare, benign tumor that possibly originates from the follicular infundibulum. It usually presents as an asymptomatic, solitary, white-pink nodular or verrucous lesion smaller than 1 cm, typically located on the head of older men. Dermoscopically, there are 2 main patterns: the keratoacanthomalike pattern (the most common) composed of central keratin surrounded by hairpin vessels with a white halo in a radial arrangement (**Fig. 5**), and the other pattern characterized by a yellowish-white, homogeneous, amorphous, central area surrounded by hairpin vessels with a white halo, in a radial arrangement.[29,30] The central keratin correlates histopathologically with hyperkeratosis and parakeratosis, whereas the amorphous whitish central area correlates with the tumor lobules of the inverted follicular keratosis.[30] Vascular structures are commonly present (monomorphic more often than polymorphic), especially hairpin vessels surrounded by a whitish halo, which is indicative of epithelial differentiation. Arborizing vessels, glomerular vessels, linear irregular vessels, corkscrew vessels, and milky-red globules can be present in some cases.[30] There is only 1 case reported as a rare pigmented inverted follicular keratosis mimicking a melanoma, with variegated pigmentation, featureless areas, and black dots on dermoscopy.[31]

Pilomatricoma

Benign tumor, with tendency toward calcification, that usually presents as a single, firm, dermal

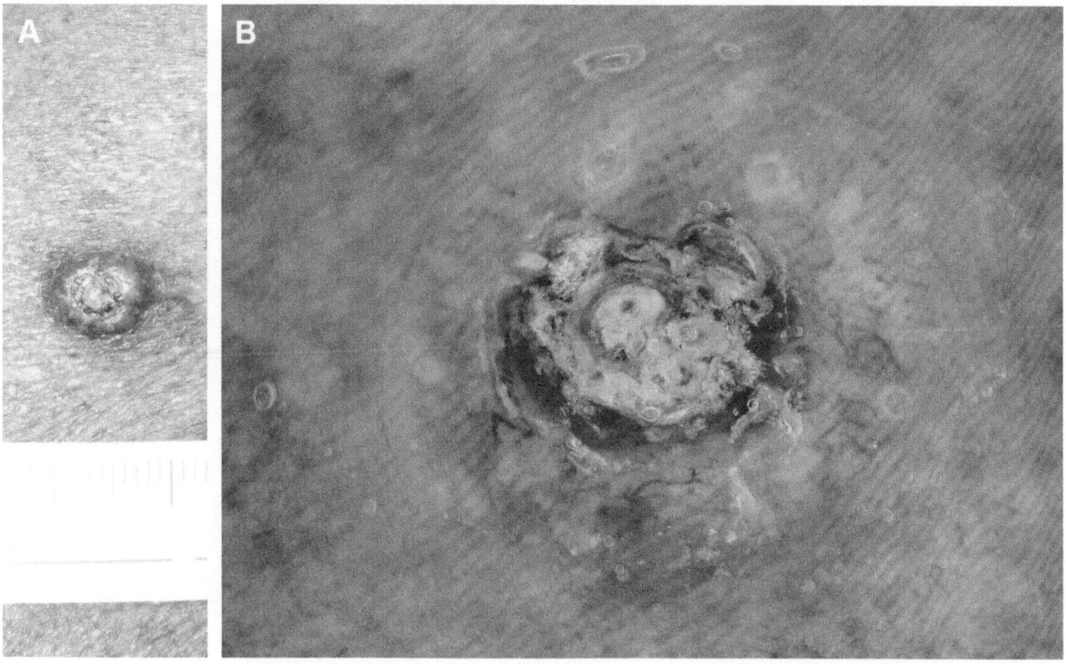

Fig. 5. Dermoscopy of an inverted follicular keratosis. (*A*) Clinical view. (*B*) In the dermoscopic view, we can find a keratoacanthomalike pattern (central keratin surrounded by polymorphous atypical vessels with a white halo in a radial arrangement; we can also see comedolike openings).

nodule, often on the head or neck of children or adolescents. Multiple pilomatricomas may be associated with myotonic dystrophy, Gardner syndrome, or Turner syndrome. White and/or yellow homogeneous areas shaped and distributed irregularly (corresponding histopathologically to calcification or keratin masses), white streaks, reddish homogeneous areas, hairpin vessels, and linear irregular vessels represent the most frequent dermoscopic features of pilomatricoma, whereas ulceration, dotted vessels, and structureless blue-gray areas are common additional findings (**Fig. 6**).[14,32–35] Specific dermoscopic criteria for melanocytic or nonmelanocytic tumors are absent.

Trichofolliculoma

Trichofolliculoma is an uncommon, benign hair follicle hamartoma that typically presents in adulthood as a solitary, facial or scalp papule that occasionally presents a central dilated pore with a small tuft of hairs, which corresponds on histology to the central primary follicle with secondary vellus hair follicles emerging from it.[36–38] Dermoscopically, Panasiti and colleagues[39] described one case with a "firework" pattern consisting of a central, brown zone with radial, dark brown projections. Jégou-Penouil and colleagues[40] reported a trichofolliculoma that presented as a pinkish papule with a central disruptor and fine peripheral serpiginous vascularization with centripetal disposition. Recently, Garcia-Garcia and colleagues[41] defined a trichofolliculoma as a well-defined, firm, bluish nodule with a white-pink central area, shiny white structures, dotted vessels, and a central scale.

Trichoblastoma

Trichoblastoma is a rare, benign skin tumor of rudimentary hair follicles that typically appears as a solitary, skin-colored papule on the scalp or face. It may develop in isolation or arise within a sebaceous nevus. When multiple, it may be associated with Brooke-Spiegler syndrome. Dermoscopically, trichoblastomas are usually difficult to differentiate from BCC, because they share dermoscopic features, such as blue-gray ovoid nests and arborizing vessels (although less branching than in BCC).[6,14,42–46] Ghigliotti and colleagues[42] compared 19 primitive trichoblastomas with 19 trichoblastic BCC (tBCC) and observed that arborizing vessels were present in both groups but with a lower frequency in the tBCC group. Additionally, the main dermoscopic difference was

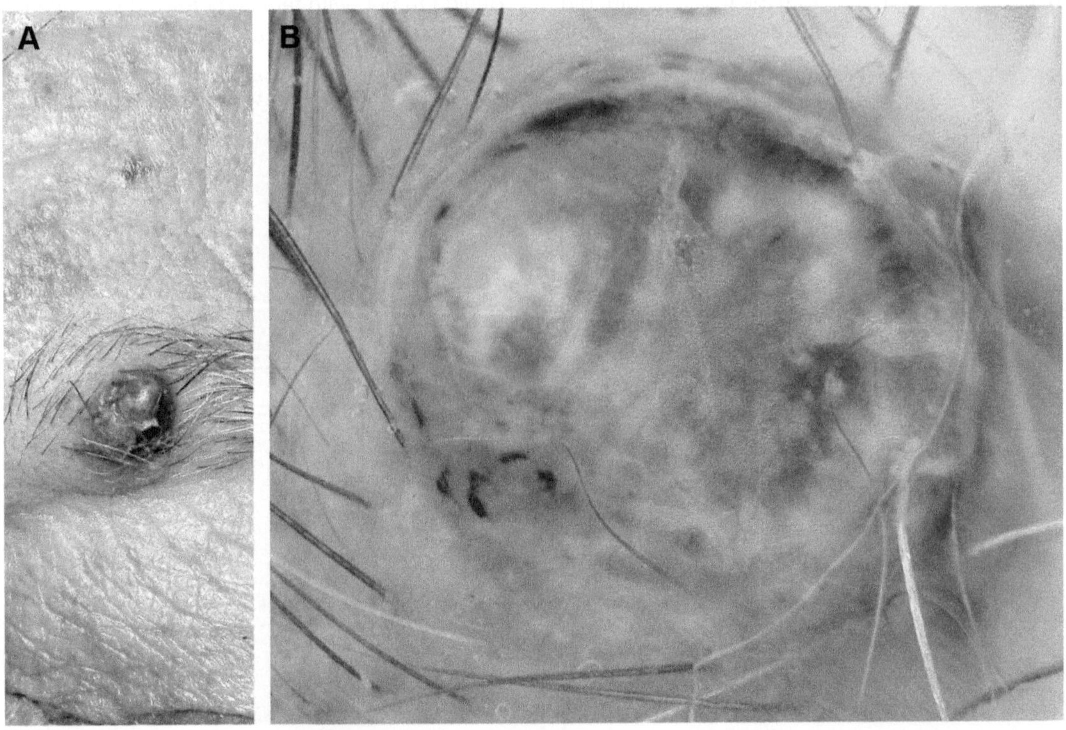

Fig. 6. Dermoscopy of a pilomatricoma. (*A*) Clinical view. (*B*) In the dermoscopic view, we can find a pattern composed of whitish-yellow homogeneous areas shaped and distributed irregularly, violaceous homogeneous areas, and peripheral linear irregular vessels.

that blue-gray ovoid nests and blue-gray globules were more frequently found (but not exclusively) in tBCC. Zaballos and colleagues[6] collected 58 tumors (23 trichoblastomas) arising in sebaceous nevus and observed that (1) 87% of trichoblastomas were symmetric (whereas BCCs were mainly asymmetric) and presented a "total large blue-gray ovoid nest" that occupied the whole lesion (the most common structure in trichoblastomas); (2) arborizing vessels were found in 61% of lesions; and (3) white structures (including shiny white streaks) were observed in almost 70% of cases (**Fig. 7**). Other dermoscopic structures found in trichoblastomas were large blue-gray ovoid nests, multiple blue-gray globules, and leaflike structures. This study concluded that the pattern composed of a symmetric total large blue-gray ovoid nest, arborizing telangiectasias, and white structures was characteristic of well-established trichoblastoma, and the presence of an isolated symmetric total large blue-gray ovoid nest was characteristic of incipient trichoblastoma. The histopathologic correlation of blue-gray structures was the pigmented basaloid nodules and the white structures corresponded to their densely fibrous stroma.[6,43] The adamantinoid variant of trichoblastoma (previously called cutaneous lymphadenoma) was described as a pink papule with arborizing vessels on an orange background and peripheral dotted and glomerular vessels.[47]

Trichoepithelioma

Trichoepithelioma is currently considered a superficial trichoblastoma with prominent infundibulocystic differentiation (cribiform trichoblastoma). It usually appears as single or multiple (Brooke-Spiegler syndrome, multiple familial trichoepithelioma, Rombo syndrome) skin-colored papules smaller than 1 cm on the central face. Dermoscopically, it is characterized by small, thin, in-focus arborizing vessels, shiny white areas/background (**Fig. 8**) and milialike cysts (keratin cysts on histology).[14,43,48–50] Rosettes, blue-gray dots, and yellowish-brown background color have been reported sporadically.[49–51] Desmoplastic trichoepithelioma (columnar trichoblastoma) commonly presents as a solitary, firm, skin-colored to erythematous facial plaque with raised margins and depressed center varying in size from 3 to 20 mm. Dermoscopic examination typically reveals an ivory-white background color throughout the entire lesion (desmoplastic stroma seen under histology) with arborizing vessels and sometimes keratin cysts or shiny white streaks.[14,43,48,52,53]

Fibrofolliculoma/Trichodiscoma

Fibrofolliculoma and trichodiscoma are benign, clinically indistinguishable connective tissue tumors that may be solitary or multiple (hallmark of Birt-Hogg-Dubé syndrome). They are small

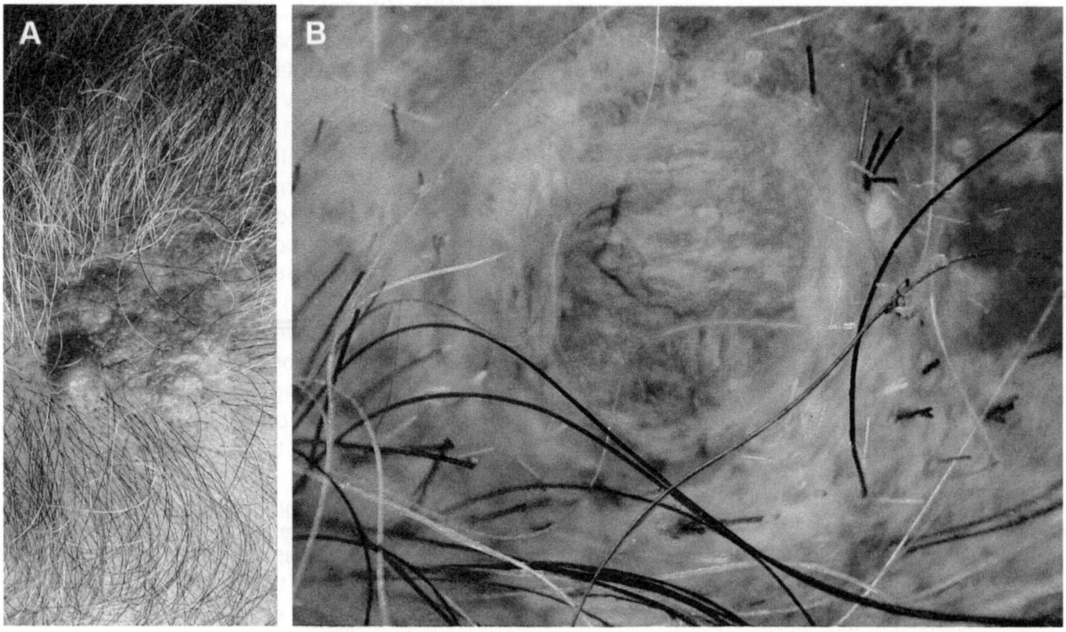

Fig. 7. Dermoscopy of a trichoblastoma arising in a sebaceous nevus. (*A*) Clinical view. (*B*) In the dermoscopic view, we can find a pattern composed of a total large blue-gray ovoid nest that occupies the whole lesion, arborizing telangiectasias and white structures.

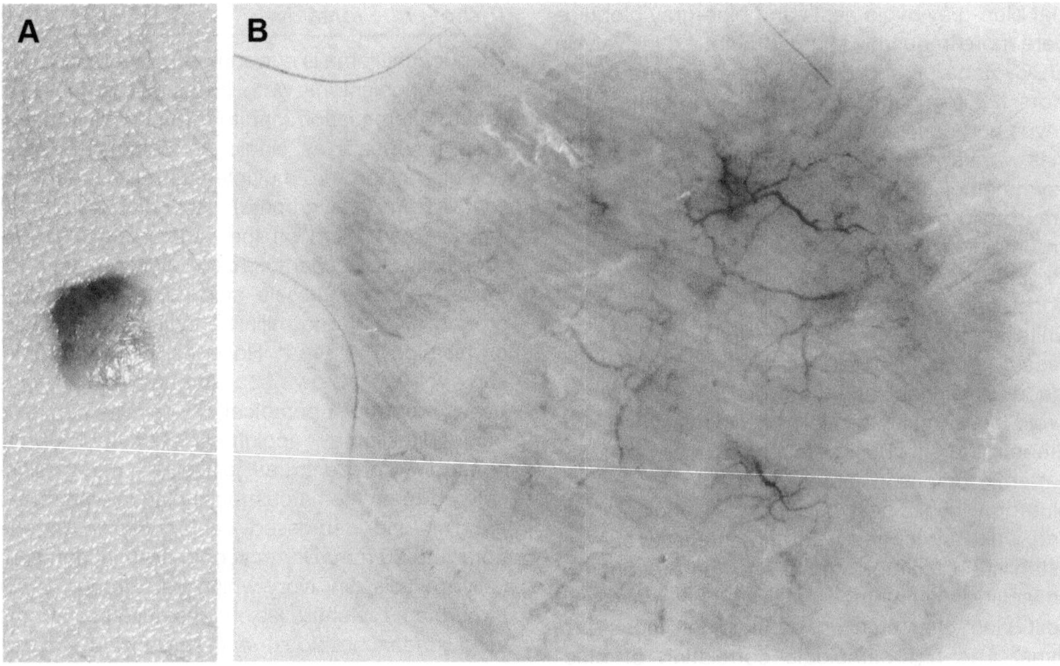

Fig. 8. Dermoscopy of a trichoepithelioma. (*A*) Clinical view. (*B*) In the dermoscopic view, we can find a pattern composed of small, thin, in-focus arborizing vessels and shiny white areas in a pinkish background.

(2–4 mm), white-to-flesh-colored papules distributed predominately over the head, neck, and upper trunk. Dermoscopically, fibrofolliculomas show well-demarcated areas/globules of whitish coloration (epithelial strands with a fibrous sheath and normal connective tissue on histologic examination) with a central yellowish-brown spot (follicular opening that may correlate histologically with an enlarged infundibular portion of the hair follicle).[54,55] Recently, fibrofolliculomas with central open comedo were described as a diagnostic clue to Birt-Hogg-Dubé syndrome.[56] Additionally, fibrofolliculomas may present a prominent vascular component, such as curvilinear vessels connecting red dots and globules.[57] Trichodiscomas reveal dermoscopically whitish globular structures, blue-gray nests, and blurred linear vessels.[14]

Others

Pilar sheath acanthoma is a rare, benign tumor that typically presents as an asymptomatic, facial (upper lip) papule or plaque with a central opening/pore. Dermoscopy may show papillomatous projections toward the center of the lesion, linear vessels on the periphery, and a depressed central area with rests of yellowish keratin.[58,59]

Trichilemmal carcinoma is a rare malignant tumor that frequently appears on the face and ears of elderly patients. Dermoscopically, it is characterized by polymorphous vascular pattern, white-yellowish areas, and ulceration.[14]

DERMOSCOPY OF ECCRINE AND APOCRINE TUMORS

Apocrine Hidrocystomas

Apocrine hidrocystomas are benign, cystic lesions of apocrine sweat glands, usually found on the head and neck. They present as an intradermal translucent nodule.[60] Dermoscopy of apocrine hidrocystomas was studied by Zaballos and colleagues[61] in 22 lesions, and they observed in all cases a central homogeneous area, translucent to opaque, which occupied the whole lesion. That area was skin-colored (31.8%), yellowish (31.8%), blue (22.7%), or less frequently pinkish-blue or gray. There were also vascular structures (81.8%), usually arborizing vessels, and whitish structures (22.7%) (**Fig. 9**). The histopathological correlation was the presence of a large cystic space situated within the dermis.

Eccrine Hidrocystomas

Eccrine hidrocystomas are benign tumors of the eccrine sweat glands that arise from cystic dilatation of the excretory duct. They are translucent, skin-colored vesicular-papular lesions, mainly localized on the face.[62] Its dermoscopic characteristics have been described only in 6

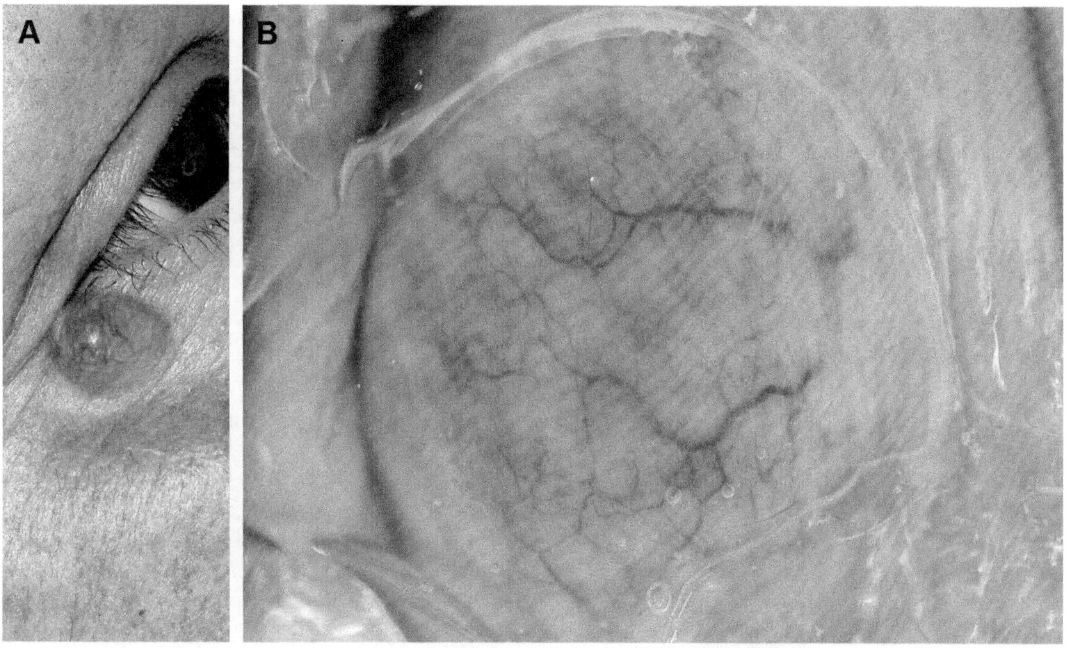

Fig. 9. Dermoscopy of an apocrine hidrocystoma. (*A*) Clinical view. (*B*) In the dermoscopic view, we can find a pattern composed of arborizing vessels in a pinkish background.

patients.[62–64] A central homogeneous area with a skin-colored[62] or bluish hue[63,64] sometimes surrounded by a pale halo has been observed.[64]

Syringocystadenoma Papilliferum

Syringocystadenoma papilliferum is an uncommon benign sweat glandular tumor, frequently seen in association with other adnexal tumors. It is the second most common benign neoplasm occurring in sebaceous nevus after trichoblastoma.[61] Its dermoscopic features have been described in several studies mainly associated with sebaceous nevus[6,45,65–67] and only one solitary case has been reported.[68] The largest series was published by Zaballos and colleagues[6] and they found that the most common pattern consisted of a quite symmetric, erythematous lesion with exophytic papillary structures, ulceration, and vessels. The histologic correlation was cystic spaces open to skin corresponding to the dermoscopic central ulceration or depression.[60] Other investigators have observed that the flatter lesions (or "plaquelike lesions") did not show papillary structures, but a pinkish-white or yellowish structureless central area with irregular vessels.[65–67]

Nodular Hidradenoma

Nodular hidradenoma is an uncommon, benign, slowly growing benign tumor of mostly apocrine origin.[60] It usually presents as a solitary, nodular, cystic, or pedunculated lesion. The dermoscopic features of nodular hidradenoma have been described by Serrano and colleagues.[69] They found that the most frequent pattern in these lesions consisted of a homogeneous area, which occupied the whole lesion with vascular and white structures. The color of this homogeneous area was pinkish in nonpigmented hidradenomas (42.8% of cases) (**Fig. 10**), bluish, or less commonly brownish in pigmented hidradenomas (39.3% of cases) and pink-bluish in the rest of the cases. A large proportion of hidradenomas appeared highly vascular, with arborizing telangiectasias, polymorphous atypical vessels, and linear irregular vessels being the 3 most common vascular structures.[69,70] They concluded that these vascular patterns are not specific of hidradenomas and these have been published in association with other benign or malignant tumors, including BCCs and melanomas.[69] They also described a lesion that showed a total delicate pigment network on dermoscopy without any additional features and, for that, it had been diagnosed dermoscopically as a dermatofibroma.[69] The histopathological correlation of this homogeneous area was the presence of large lobulated masses of cells and abundant cystic spaces located in the upper and middermis.[60]

Cylindroma and Spiradenoma

Cylindroma is a benign tumor that mainly occurs on the head as slowly growing, solitary pink or

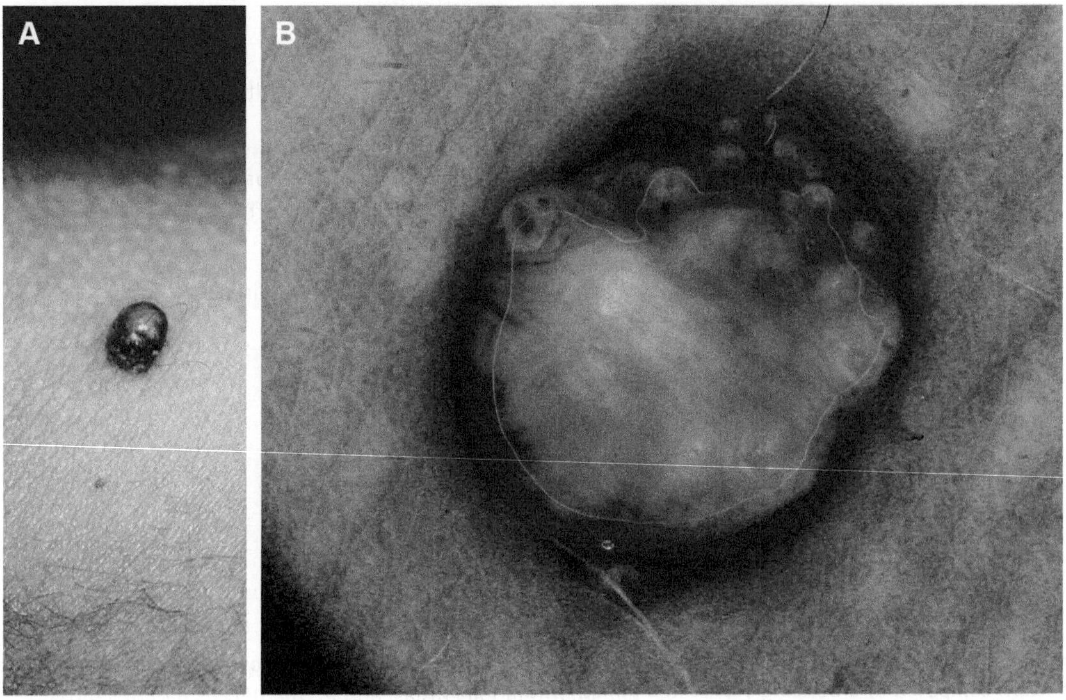

Fig. 10. Dermoscopy of a nodular hidradenoma. (*A*) Clinical view. (*B*) In the dermoscopic view, we can find a pattern composed of a pinkish homogeneous area that occupies the whole lesion with peripheral arborizing telangiectasias and central white structures.

red dermal nodules.[60] Spiradenoma is a benign tumor that usually presents as solitary, intradermal, round oval, and blue or pink.[60] Familiar cases of cylindroma have been described and in Brooke-Spiegler syndrome may be associated with trichoepitheliomas and spiradenomas.[60,71–73] Dermoscopy descriptions of both tumors are similar, and reports of 1 or 2 cases have been described.[72–77] A homogeneous pink[72–76] or pink orange[77] area with arborizing telangiectasias (**Fig. 11**) is observed.[72–77] In some of them, blue ovoid nests or blue globules can be seen.[73–75] The histopathological correlation of this homogeneous area is the presence of multiple lobules arranged in a compact jigsaw pattern in cylindroma or 1 or 2 lobules in the case of spiradenoma.[60]

Syringoma

Syringomas are common tumors that usually present as multiple small papules on the lower eyelids, and less frequently on other locations.[60] An eruptive variant on the anterior surfaces of young people has been described.[60] There are few dermoscopic reports of syringomas. Corazza and colleagues[78] described an isolated lesion on the vulva with a homogeneous pinkish central area with multiple round yellow-whitish structures. Hayashi and colleagues[79] observed, in a linear unilateral syringoma, a central homogeneous light brownish area with a delicate pigment network at the periphery. In 2 reported cases of eruptive syringoma, a pigment network with hypopigmented areas was seen.[80,81]

Poroma

Poromas are uncommon benign tumors that clinically simulate other neoplasms. Its classical description consists of a solitary reddish nodule on the soles or palms; however, multiple lesions, pigmented variants, and different localizations also have been reported.[60] Approximately 20 case reports about dermoscopy of poromas have been published.[82–100] Because of its large number of forms, poroma has been called the great dermoscopic imitator.[82] Recently, a cross-sectional study of 113 poromas and 106 matched controls has been conducted.[101] In this study, dermoscopic features associated with poromas included white interlacing areas around vessels (odds ratio [OR] 7.9), yellow structureless areas (OR 2.5), milky-red globules (OR 3.9), and vessels poorly visualized (OR 33.3). These investigators found 4 patterns in almost 77% of the cases, and the rest (23%) remained nonclassified. Pattern 1 (23.9% of the cases) consisted of pinkish oval or round tumors commonly located on hands and

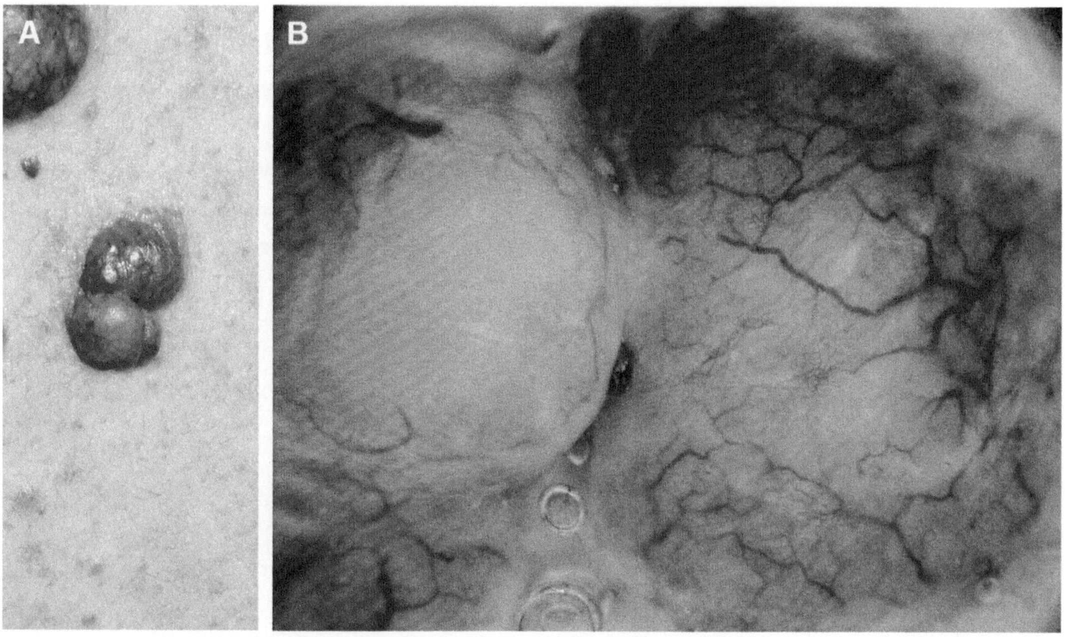

Fig. 11. Dermoscopy of cylindromas. (*A*) Clinical view. (*B*) In the dermoscopic view, we can see a pinkish homogeneous area with arborizing telangiectasias and white structures.

feet and often had a collarette. These lesions had some of the following dermoscopic characteristics, from higher to lower frequency: blood spots, yellow structureless areas, milky-red globules, milky-red areas, and branched vessels with rounded endings (**Fig. 12**). This pattern appeared to be the most similar to the classical descriptions of poromas. Pattern 2 (17.7% of the cases) consisted of pinkish tumors of irregular shape with polymorphous vessels simulating a vascular tumor. Pattern 3 (25.7% of the cases) comprised small-size pink tumors, occurring anywhere on the body, often without vessels and sometimes having branched vessels with rounded endings. Although lesions with this pattern clinically simulated nodular BCCs, arborizing vessels were rare. Pattern 4 (9.7% of the cases) consisted of lesions larger in size, usually pigmented, occurring anywhere on the body, with frequent blood spots, keratin, and sometimes atypical hairpin vessels suggesting a keratinizing or pseudoepitheliomatous tumor.[101]

Hidroacanthoma Simplex

Hidroacanthoma simplex is a benign intraepidermal neoplasm derived from the acrosyringium and usually clinically misdiagnosed as a seborrheic keratosis, BCC, or Bowen disease.[60] There are few dermoscopic descriptions of this entity.[102–105] Although it is considered as an intraepidermal poroma, this location gives the hidroacanthoma simplex special dermatoscopic characteristics other than dermal poromas. These lesions had a pinkish, whitish, or brownish background with black dots/globules,[102–105] black lines,[102–105] whitish globular structures,[105] scales,[102–105] and dotted vessels.[102,103]

Porocarcinoma

Porocarcinoma is the most frequent malignant sweat gland neoplasm.[60] It commonly occurs on the lower extremities of elderly individuals and usually has the appearance of a pink nodule with occasional ulceration.[60,106] There are some dermoscopic reports of it.[93,103,106–112] The lesions had a pink, whitish, or brown background and presented vascular structures.[93,103,106–112] There were also white-to-pink halos around the vascular structures,[93,103,107,108,112] round or oval structureless areas,[93,107,110] hemorrhage,[93,103,108,110,112] and ulceration.[93,103,108,109]

Others

There are some skin glandular tumors with very few dermoscopic descriptions (3 or less), and they are the following.

Accessory nipples, on dermoscopy, resemble dermatofibromas, with a peripheral delicate pigment network corresponding histopathologically to the areolar epidermal hyperplasia and a central white scarlike area.[113–115]

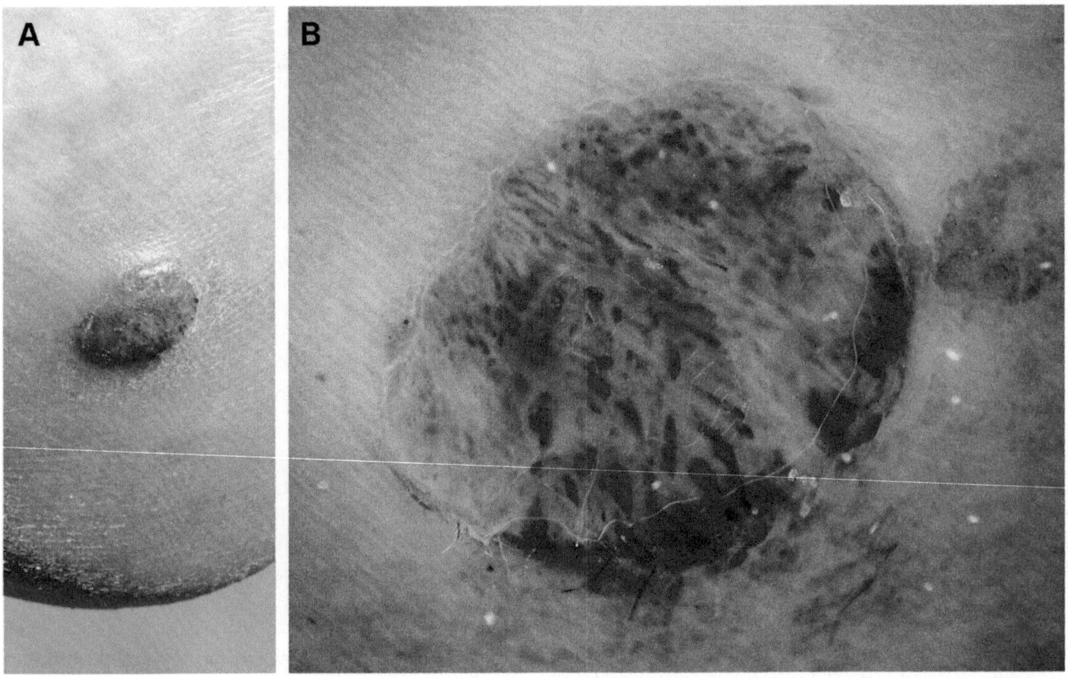

Fig. 12. Dermoscopy of a poroma. (*A*) Clinical view. (*B*) In the dermoscopic view, we can find a pattern composed of a pinkish oval tumor with a collarette, large amount of vessels with rounded endings, yellow structureless areas, and some milky-red globules.

Hidradenoma papilliferum is a rare, slow-growing benign tumor with apocrine differentiation, usually localized in the anogenital area.[60] The only one dermoscopic description of hidradenoma papilliferum has been in an ectopic form, which showed a diffuse, homogeneous, blue pigmentation.[116]

Nipple adenoma is a very uncommon, benign tumor of lactiferous ducts of the nipple, which can clinically mimic the presentation of mammary Paget disease of the nipple. The 2 dermoscopic descriptions so far showed a light red background with irregular vascular structures.[117,118]

Tubular apocrine adenoma is a rare benign tumor, typically presenting as a red to brownish nodule on the scalp.[60] The only dermoscopic description revealed oval bluish areas with short fine telangiectasias and large blue-gray ovoid nests very similar to BCC.[119]

Microcystic adnexal carcinoma is a locally aggressive malignant adnexal tumor displaying sweat duct and follicular differentiation, and it presents on the head and neck.[60] There are only 3 dermoscopic reports, which showed a white[120] or orange[120,121] background with prominent arborizing vessels, and 2 of the cases exhibited white small dots that might represent keratinous cysts.[120–122]

Malignant nodular hidradenoma or hidroadenocarcinoma is a rare sweat gland neoplasm.[60] The only dermoscopic description was about a fast-growing facial nodule and it showed a round lesion with a whitish pink background and, scattered around, pinpoint, linear irregular, hairpin, and glomerular vessels. These features were quite unspecific; therefore, the authors made a dermoscopic diagnosis of amelanotic melanoma versus poroma or carcinoma.[123]

REFERENCES

1. Neri I, Savoia F, Giacomini F, et al. Usefulness of dermatoscopy for the early diagnosis of sebaceous naevus and differentiation from aplasia cutis congenita. Clin Exp Dermatol 2009;34:e50–2.
2. Ankad BS, Beergouder SL, Domble V. Trichoscopy: the best auxiliary tool in the evaluation of nevus sebaceous. Int J Trichology 2016;8:5–10.
3. Donati A, Cavelier-Balloy B, Reygagne P. Histologic correlation of dermoscopy findings in a sebaceous nevus. Cutis 2015;96:E8–9.
4. Cribier B, Scrivener Y, Grosshans E. Tumors arising in nevus sebaceus: a study of 596 cases. J Am Acad Dermatol 2000;42:263–8.
5. Idriss MH, Elston DM. Secondary neoplasms associated with nevus sebaceus of Jadassohn: a study of 707 cases. J Am Acad Dermatol 2014;70:332–7.

6. Zaballos P, Serrano P, Flores G, et al. Dermoscopy of tumours arising in naevus sebaceous: a morphological study of 58 cases. J Eur Acad Dermatol Venereol 2015;29:2231–7.
7. Bryden AM, Dawe RS, Fleming C. Dermatoscopic features of benign sebaceous proliferation. Clin Exp Dermatol 2004;29:676–7.
8. Zaballos P, Ara M, Puig S, et al. Dermoscopy of sebaceous hyperplasia. Arch Dermatol 2005;141:808.
9. Oztas P, Polat M, Oztas M, et al. Bonbon toffee sign: a new dermatoscopic feature for sebaceous hyperplasia. J Eur Acad Dermatol Venereol 2008;22:1200–2.
10. Kim NH, Zell DS, Kolm I, et al. The dermoscopic differential diagnosis of yellow lobularlike structures. Arch Dermatol 2008;144:962.
11. Argenziano G, Zalaudek I, Corona R, et al. Vascular structures in skin tumors: a dermoscopy study. Arch Dermatol 2004;140:1485–9.
12. Marques-da-Costa J, Campos-do-Carmo G, Ormiga P, et al. Sebaceous adenoma: clinics, dermatoscopy, and histopathology. Int J Dermatol 2015;54:e200–2.
13. Moscarella E, Argenziano G, Longo C, et al. Clinical, dermoscopic and reflectance confocal microscopy features of sebaceous neoplasms in Muir-Torre syndrome. J Eur Acad Dermatol Venereol 2013;27:699–705.
14. Lallas A, Moscarella E, Argenziano G, et al. Dermoscopy of uncommon skin tumours. Australas J Dermatol 2014;55:53–62.
15. Satomura H, Ogata D, Arai E, et al. Dermoscopic features of ocular and extraocular sebaceous carcinomas. J Dermatol 2017;44:1313–6.
16. Coppola R, Carbotti M, Zanframundo S, et al. Use of dermoscopy in the diagnosis of sebaceoma. J Am Acad Dermatol 2015;72:e143–5.
17. Nomura M, Tanaka M, Nunomura M, et al. Dermoscopy of rippled pattern sebaceoma. Dermatol Res Pract 2010;2010:140486.
18. Moreno C, Jacyk WK, Judd MJ, et al. Highly aggressive extraocular sebaceous carcinoma. Am J Dermatopathol 2001;23:450–5.
19. Coates D, Bowling J, Haskett M. Dermoscopic features of extraocular sebaceous carcinoma. Australas J Dermatol 2011;52:212–3.
20. Vano-Galvan S, Hernández-Martín A, Colmenero I, et al. Disseminated congenital comedones. Pediatr Dermatol 2011;28:58–9.
21. Kaliyadan F, Bhimji SS. Nevus comedonicus. StatPearls. Treasure Island (FL): StatPearls Publishing; 2017. Last Update: June 12, 2017. Available at: https://www.ncbi.nlm.nih.gov/books/NBK441903/.
22. Vora RV, Kota RS, Sheth NK. Dermoscopy of nevus comedonicus. Indian Dermatol Online J 2017;8:388–9.
23. Kamińska-Winciorek G, Spiewak R. Dermoscopy on nevus comedonicus: a case report and review of the literature. Postepy Dermatol Alergol 2013;30:252–4.
24. Choi E, Liau M, Huang J, et al. Basaloid follicular hamartoma: clinical, dermoscopic, and histopathological characteristics of case. Dermatol Online J 2017;23 [pii:13030/qt3xn054wf].
25. Mauleón C, Valdivielso M, Chavarría E, et al. Simultaneous presentation of localized basaloid follicular hamartoma and epithelioid blue nevus in a 44-year-old patient. Actas Dermosifiliogr 2011;102:233–5.
26. Horcajada-Reales C, Avilés-Izquierdo JA, Ciudad-Blanco C, et al. Dermoscopic pattern in facial trichilemmomas: red iris-like structure. J Am Acad Dermatol 2015;72:S30–2.
27. Lozano-Masdemont B, Lara Simón IM, López LG. Dermoscopic features of facial trichilemmoma. Actas Dermosifiliogr 2017;108:863–4.
28. Navarrete-Dechent C, Uribe P, Gonzalez S. Desmoplastic trichilemmoma dermoscopically mimicking molluscum contagiosum. J Am Acad Dermatol 2017;76:S22–4.
29. Armengot-Carbo M, Abrego A, Gonzalez T, et al. Inverted follicular keratosis: dermoscopic and reflectance confocal microscopic features. Dermatology 2013;227:62–6.
30. Llambrich A, Zaballos P, Taberner R, et al. Dermoscopy of inverted follicular keratosis: study of 12 cases. Clin Exp Dermatol 2016;41:468–73.
31. Thom GA, Quirk CJ, Heenan PJ. Inverted follicular keratosis simulating malignant melanoma. Australas J Dermatol 2004;45:55–7.
32. Zaballos P, Llambrich A, Puig S, et al. Dermoscopic findings of pilomatricomas. Dermatology 2008;217:225–30.
33. Alarcon I, Malvehy J, Puig S. Rapidly growing nodule on the cheek of a 12-year-old boy. J Am Acad Dermatol 2014;70:e11–3.
34. Ayhan E, Ertugay O, Gundogdu R. Three different dermoscopic view of three new cases with pilomatrixoma. Int J Trichology 2014;6:21–2.
35. Martínez-Morán C, Echeverría-García B, Nájera L, et al. A tumor in images: anetodermic pilomatrixoma. Actas Dermosifiliogr 2015;106:241–3.
36. Gokalp H, Gurer MA, Alan S. Trichofolliculoma: a rare variant of hair follicle hamartoma. Dermatol Online J 2013;19:19264.
37. Singh N, Kumar N, Chandrashekar L, et al. Umbilicated nodule over eyebrow. Dermatol Online J 2013;19:19622.
38. Romero-Pérez D, García-Bustinduy M, Cribier B. Clinicopathologic study of 90 cases of trichofolliculoma. J Eur Acad Dermatol Venereol 2017;31:e141–2.
39. Panasiti V, Roberti V, Lieto P, et al. The "firework" pattern in dermoscopy. Int J Dermatol 2013;52:1158–9.

40. Jégou-Penouil MH, Bourseau-Quetier C, Cajanus S, et al. Trichofolliculoma: a retrospective review of 8 cases. Ann Dermatol Venereol 2015;142:183–8.
41. Garcia-Garcia SC, Villarreal-Martinez A, Guerrero-Gonzalez GA, et al. Dermoscopy of trichofolliculoma: a rare hair follicle hamartoma. J Eur Acad Dermatol Venereol 2017;31:e123–4.
42. Ghigliotti G, De Col E, Parodi A, et al. Trichoblastoma: is a clinical or dermoscopic diagnosis possible? J Eur Acad Dermatol Venereol 2016;30: 1978–80.
43. Pitarch G, Botella-Estrada R. Dermoscopic findings in trichoblastoma. Actas Dermosifiliogr 2015; 106:e45–8.
44. Kitamura S, Hata H, Imafuku K, et al. Basal cell carcinoma or trichoblastoma? Dermoscopic examination of black macules developing in the same nevus sebaceus. Case Rep Oncol 2016;9:143–7.
45. De Giorgi V, Massi D, Trez E, et al. Multiple pigmented trichoblastomas and syringocystadenoma papilliferum in naevus sebaceous mimicking a malignant melanoma: a clinical dermoscopic-pathological case study. Br J Dermatol 2003;149: 1067–70.
46. Picard A, Tsilika K, Cardot-Leccia N, et al. Trichoblastoma with dermoscopic features of a malignant tumor: three cases. J Am Acad Dermatol 2014;71: e63–4.
47. Pitarch G, Botella-Estrada R. Dermoscopy of adamantinoid trichoblastoma. J Eur Acad Dermatol Venereol 2016;30:345–6.
48. Ardigo M, Zieff J, Scope A, et al. Dermoscopic and reflectance confocal microscope findings of trichoepithelioma. Dermatology 2007;215:354–8.
49. Navarrete-Dechent C, Bajaj S, Marghoob AA, et al. Multiple familial trichoepithelioma: confirmation via dermoscopy. Dermatol Pract Concept 2016;6:51–4.
50. Huet P, Barnéon G, Cribier B. Trichoblastoma: dermatopathology-dermatoscopy correlation. Ann Dermatol Venereol 2017;144:462–5.
51. Lazaridou E, Fotiadou C, Patsatsi A, et al. Solitary trichoepithelioma in an 8-year-old child: clinical, dermoscopic and histopathologic findings. Dermatol Pract Concept 2014;4:55–8.
52. Khelifa E, Masouyé I, Kaya G, et al. Dermoscopy of desmoplastic trichoepithelioma reveals other criteria to distinguish it from basal cell carcinoma. Dermatology 2013;226:101–4.
53. López-Navarro N, Alcaide A, Gallego, et al. Dermatoscopy in the diagnosis of combined desmoplastic trichoepithelioma and naevus. Clin Exp Dermatol 2009;34:e395–6.
54. Jarrett R, Walker L, Side L, et al. Dermoscopic features of Birt-Hogg-Dubé syndrome. Arch Dermatol 2009;145:1208.
55. Iwabuchi C, Ebana H, Ishiko A, et al. Skin lesions of Birt-Hogg-Dubé syndrome: clinical and histopathological findings in 31 Japanese patients who presented with pneumothorax and/or multiple lung cysts. J Dermatol Sci 2017;89:77–84.
56. Aivaz O, Berkman S, Middelton L, et al. Comedonal and cystic fibrofolliculomas in Birt-Hogg-Dube syndrome. JAMA Dermatol 2015;151:770–4.
57. Criscito MC, Mu EW, Meehan SA, et al. Dermoscopic features of a solitary fibrofolliculoma on the left cheek. J Am Acad Dermatol 2017;76:S8–9.
58. Rodriguez-Lojo R, Castiñeiras I, Robles O, et al. Lesión cribiforme en la cara de un varón de 44 años de edad. Dermatol Online J 2017;23 [pii: 13030/qt42k1c7z1].
59. Iino Y, Ito S. A case of pilar sheath acanthoma with a characteristic pattern on dermoscopy. J-STAGE Home 2014;76:199–201.
60. Kazacov DV, Michal M, Kacerovska D, et al. Lesions with predominant apocrine and eccrine differentiation. In: Kazakov DV, Michal M, Kacerovska D, et al, editors. Cutaneous adnexal tumors. 1st edition. Philadelphia: Wolters Klumer Health/Lippincott Williams & Wilkins; 2012. p. 1–172.
61. Zaballos P, Bañuls J, Medina C, et al. Dermoscopy of apocrine hidrocystomas: a morphological study. J Eur Acad Dermatol Venereol 2014;28:378–81.
62. Correia O, Duarte AF, Barros AM, et al. Multiple eccrine hidrocystomas—from diagnosis to treatment: the role of dermatoscopy and botulinum toxin. Dermatology 2009;219:77–9.
63. Kluger N, Monthieu JY, Gil-Bistes D, et al. A bluish pigmented cystic lesion of the nose. Acta Derm Venereol 2010;90:555–6.
64. Duman N, Duman D, Sahin S. Pale halo surrounding a homogeneous bluish-purplish central area: dermoscopic clue for eccrine hidrocystoma. Dermatol Pract Concept 2015;5:43–5.
65. Lombardi M, Piana S, Longo C, et al. Dermoscopy of syringocystadenoma papilliferum. Australas J Dermatol 2017. https://doi.org/10.1111/ajd.12654.
66. Bruno CB, Cordeiro FN, Soares FE, et al. Dermoscopic aspects of syringocystadenoma papilliferum associated with nevus sebaceus. An Bras Dermatol 2011;86:1213–6.
67. Duman N, Ersoy-Evans S, Erkin Özaygen G, et al. Syringocystadenoma papilliferum arising on naevus sebaceus: a 6-year-old child case described with dermoscopic features. Australas J Dermatol 2015;56:e53–4.
68. Shindo M, Yamada N, Yoshida Y, et al. Syringocystadenoma papilliferum on the male nipple. J Dermatol 2011;38:593–6.
69. Serrano P, Lallas A, Del Pozo LJ, et al. Dermoscopy of nodular hidradenoma, a great masquerader: a morphological study of 28 cases. Dermatology 2016;232:78–82.
70. Robles-Mendez JC, Martínez-Cabriales SA, Villarreal-Martínez A, et al. Nodular hidradenoma:

Dermoscopic presentation. J Am Acad Dermatol 2017;76:S46–8.
71. Mataix J, Bañuls J, Botella R, et al. Síndrome de Brooke-Spiegler: una entidad heterogénea. Actas Dermosifiliogr 2006;97:669–72.
72. Pinho AC, Gouveia MJ, Gameiro AR, et al. Brooke-Spiegler Syndrome—an underrecognized cause of multiple familial scalp tumors: report of a new germline mutation. J Dermatol Case Rep 2015;9:67–70.
73. Jarrett R, Walker L, Bowling J. Dermoscopy of Brooke-Spiegler syndrome. Arch Dermatol 2009;145:854.
74. Cohen YK, Elpern DJ. Dermatoscopic pattern of a cylindroma. Dermatol Pract Concept 2014;4:67–8.
75. Cabo H, Pedrini F, Cohen Sabban E. Dermoscopy of cylindroma. Dermatol Res Pract 2010;2010 [pii:285392].
76. Lallas A, Apalla Z, Tzellos T, et al. Dermoscopy of solitary cylindroma. Eur J Dermatol 2011;21:645–6.
77. Bañuls J, Arribas P, Berbegal L, et al. Yellow and orange in cutaneous lesions: clinical and dermoscopic data. J Eur Acad Dermatol Venereol 2015;29:2317–25.
78. Corazza M, Borghi A, Minghetti S, et al. Dermoscopy of isolated syringoma of the vulva. J Am Acad Dermatol 2017;76:S37–9.
79. Hayashi Y, Tanaka M, Nakajima S, et al. Unilateral linear syringoma in a Japanese female: dermoscopic differentiation from lichen planus linearis. Dermatol Reports 2011;3:e42.
80. Zhong P, Tan C. Dermoscopic features of eruptive milium-like syringoma. Eur J Dermatol 2015;25:203–4.
81. Sakiyama M, Maeda M, Fujimoto N, et al. Eruptive syringoma localized in intertriginous areas. J Dtsch Dermatol Ges 2014;12:72–3.
82. Lallas A, Chellini PR, Guimaraes MG, et al. Eccrine poroma: the great dermoscopic imitator. J Eur Acad Dermatol Venereol 2016;30:e61–3.
83. Kuo HW, Ohara K. Pigmented eccrine poroma: a report of two cases and study with dermatoscopy. Dermatol Surg 2003;29:1076–9.
84. Altamura D, Piccolo D, Lozzi GP, et al. Eccrine poroma in an unusual site: a clinical and dermoscopic simulator of amelanotic melanoma. J Am Acad Dermatol 2005;53:539–41.
85. Nicolino R, Zalaudek I, Ferrara G, et al. Dermoscopy of eccrine poroma. Dermatology 2007;215:160–3.
86. Ferrari A, Buccini P, Silipo V, et al. Eccrine poroma: a clinical-dermoscopic study of seven cases. Acta Derm Venereol 2009;89:160–4.
87. Aviles-Izquierdo JA, Velazquez-Tarjuelo D, Lecona-Echevarria M, et al. Dermoscopic features of eccrine poroma. Actas Dermosifiliogr 2009;100:133–6 [in Spanish].
88. Aydingoz IE. New dermoscopic vascular patterns in a case of eccrine poroma. J Eur Acad Dermatol Venereol 2009;23:725–6.
89. Nishikawa Y, Kaneko T, Takiyoshi N, et al. Dermoscopy of eccrine poroma with calcification. J Dermatol Case Rep 2009;3:38–40.
90. Minagawa A, Koga H, Takahashi M, et al. Dermoscopic features of nonpigmented eccrine poromas in association with their histopathological features. Br J Dermatol 2010;163:1264–8.
91. Minagawa A, Koga H. Dermoscopy of pigmented poromas. Dermatology 2010;221:78–83.
92. Shalom A, Schein O, Landi C, et al. Dermoscopic findings in biopsy-proven poromas. Dermatol Surg 2012;38:1091–6.
93. Sgouros D, Piana S, Argenziano G, et al. Clinical, dermoscopic and histopathological features of eccrine poroid neoplasms. Dermatology 2013;227:175–9.
94. Espinosa AE, Ortega BC, Venegas RQ, et al. Dermoscopy of non-pigmented eccrine poromas: study of Mexican cases. Dermatol Pract Concept 2013;3:25–8.
95. Almeida FC, Cavalcanti SM, Medeiros AC, et al. Pigmented eccrine poroma: report of an atypical case with the use of dermoscopy. An Bras Dermatol 2013;88:803–6.
96. Oiso N, Matsuda H, Kawada A. Biopsy-proven pigmented poroma with no vascular structure in dermoscopy. Int J Dermatol 2014;53:e334–5.
97. Dos Santos BS. Clinical and dermoscopic features of eccrine poroma. Indian J Dermatol Venereol Leprol 2015;81:308–9.
98. Bombonato C, Piana S, Moscarella E, et al. Pigmented eccrine poroma: dermoscopic and confocal features. Dermatol Pract Concept 2016;6:59–62.
99. Iwasaki J, Yoshida Y, Yamamoto O, et al. Poroma with sebaceous differentiation of the eyelid: a rare site of occurrence. Acta Derm Venereol 2008;88:166–7.
100. Brugués A, Gamboa M, Alós L, et al. The challenging diagnosis of eccrine poromas. J Am Acad Dermatol 2016;74:e113–5.
101. Marchetti MA, Marino ML, Virmani P, et al. Dermoscopic features and patterns of poromas: a multicenter observational case-control study conducted by the International Dermoscopy Society (IDS). J Eur Acad Dermatol Venereol 2017. https://doi.org/10.1111/jdv.14729.
102. Shiiya C, Hata H, Inamura Y, et al. Dermoscopic features of hidroacanthoma simplex: usefulness in distinguishing it from Bowen's disease and seborrheic keratosis. J Dermatol 2015;42:1002–5.
103. Dong H, Zhang H, Liu N, et al. Dermoscopy of a pigmented apocrine porocarcinoma arising from a pigmented hidroacanthoma simplex. Australas

J Dermatol 2017. https://doi.org/10.1111/ajd.12624.

104. Furlan KC, Kakizaki P, Chartuni JCN, et al. Hidroacanthoma simplex: dermoscopy and cryosurgery treatment. An Bras Dermatol 2017;92:253–5.
105. Sato Y, Fujimura T, Tamabuchi E, et al. Dermoscopy findings of hidroacanthoma simplex. Case Rep Dermatol 2014;6:154–8.
106. Edamitsu T, Minagawa A, Koga H, et al. Eccrine porocarcinoma shares dermoscopic characteristics with eccrine poroma: a report of three cases and review of the published work. J Dermatol 2016;43:332–5.
107. Godinez-Puig V, Martini MC, Yazdan P, et al. Dermoscopic findings in porocarcinoma. Dermatol Surg 2017;43:744–5.
108. Pinheiro R, Oliveira A, Mendes-Bastos P. Dermoscopic and reflectance confocal microscopic presentation of relapsing eccrine porocarcinoma. J Am Acad Dermatol 2017;76:S73–5.
109. Sawaya JL, Khachemoune A. Poroma: a review of eccrine, apocrine, and malignant forms. Int J Dermatol 2014;53:1053–61.
110. Blum A, Metzler G, Bauer J. Polymorphous vascular patterns in dermoscopy as a sign of malignant skin tumors. A case of an amelanotic melanoma and a porocarcinoma. Dermatology 2005; 210:58–9.
111. Johr R, Saghari S, Nouri K. Eccrine porocarcinoma arising in a seborrheic keratosis evaluated with dermoscopy and treated with Mohs' technique. Int J Dermatol 2003;42:653–7.
112. Suzaki R, Shioda T, Konohana I, et al. Dermoscopic features of eccrine porocarcinoma arising from hidroacanthoma simplex. Dermatol Res Pract 2010; 2010:192371.
113. Blum A, Roehm S. Accessory nipple looks like dermatofibroma in dermoscopy. Arch Dermatol 2003; 139:948–9.
114. Scope A, Benvenuto-Andrade C, Agero AL, et al. Nonmelanocytic lesions defying the two-step dermoscopy algorithm. Dermatol Surg 2006;32: 1398–406.
115. Oztas MO, Gurer MA. Dermoscopic features of accessory nipples. Int J Dermatol 2007;46:1067–8.
116. Panasiti V, Curzio M, Roberti V, et al. Ectopic hidradenoma papilliferum dermoscopically mimicking a blue nevus: a case report and review of the literature. Int J Dermatol 2014;53:e103–6.
117. Spohn GP, Trotter SC, Tozbikian G, et al. Nipple adenoma in a female patient presenting with persistent erythema of the right nipple skin: case report, review of the literature, clinical implications, and relevancy to health care providers who evaluate and treat patients with dermatologic conditions of the breast skin. BMC Dermatol 2016;16:4.
118. Takashima S, Fujita Y, Miyauchi T, et al. Dermoscopic observation in adenoma of the nipple. J Dermatol 2015;42:341–2.
119. Ito T, Nomura T, Fujita Y, et al. Tubular apocrine adenoma clinically and dermoscopically mimicking basal cell carcinoma. J Am Acad Dermatol 2014; 71:e45–6.
120. Inskip M, Magee J. Microcystic adnexal carcinoma of the cheek-a case report with dermatoscopy and dermatopathology. Dermatol Pract Concept 2015; 5:43–6.
121. Shinohara R, Ansai S, Ogita A, et al. Dermoscopic findings of microcystic adnexal carcinoma. Eur J Dermatol 2015;25:516–8.
122. Yoshida M, Kato H, Watanabe S, et al. A case of microcystic adnexal carcinoma complicated with sigmoid colon carcinoma. Rinsho Derma 2011;53: 389–92.
123. Bakar O, Ince U. A rare tumor of the face: malignant nodular hidradenoma with dermoscopic features mimicking amelanotic melanoma. J Cutan Med Surg 2011;15:167–71.

Trichoscopy Tips

Rodrigo Pirmez, MD[a,*], Antonella Tosti, MD[b]

KEYWORDS

• Trichoscopy • Dermoscopy • Alopecia • Hair • Lupus • Lichen planopilaris • Eyebrows • Scalp

KEY POINTS

- Trichoscopy is useful to diagnose early scarring alopecias and to select the optimal biopsy site in these patients.
- Trichoscopy can easily distinguish hair loss from hair breakage and provides good information on hair shaft damage.
- The pigmented scalp has unique trichoscopic features that make diagnosis of scarring alopecia more difficult.
- Be aware of possible pitfalls, including scalp staining and scalp and hair shaft deposits.

INTRODUCTION

Dermoscopy has only recently been introduced in the assessment of hair and scalp disorders. However, in the past few years, much attention has been given to the method, with many studies focusing on its applications in the field being published; to the point that many hair specialists now consider dermoscopy as an essential part of their dermatologic consultation. Dermoscopy allows visualization of morphologic structures that are not readily visible by the naked eye, including perifollicular and interfollicular features, as well as changes to hair shaft thickness and shape.[1] In 2006, the name *trichoscopy* was first proposed for the use of dermoscopy in the diagnosis of hair and scalp disorders[2] and is now widely adopted.[3] The aim of this article was not to make an extensive and overdetailed review of all trichoscopic signs, but rather to discuss topics that may be a source of doubt and to give tips that will help clinicians to better perform trichoscopy.

PERFORMING TRICHOSCOPY: THE BASICS

How to Evaluate My Patient

First, it is important to determine in which general group of hair loss your patient best fits: diffuse, patchy, or marginal alopecia. Examination of the scalp will depend on the type of hair loss presented by the patient.[4] In addition, examination of hair shafts and eyebrows may be decisive in some individuals.

Diffuse alopecia

In patients with diffuse hair loss, it is important to part the hair in the midline and to examine at least 3 sites: frontal and middle scalp and vertex. We recommend evaluating each one of the sites with at least 2 magnifications: first with a lower one (×10–20) and then with a higher magnification (×40–50). Hair diameter variability, a hallmark of androgenetic alopecia (AGA), may be better appreciated at higher magnifications (**Fig. 1**). Because the occipital scalp is commonly spared in patients with AGA, control pictures can be taken from this site for comparison.

Patchy alopecia

When patients present with patchy alopecia, both the center and the periphery of the alopecic patch should be checked. When examining the center of the lesion, it is important to establish whether hair follicle openings are present or not. Loss of follicular openings will guide the diagnosis toward a scarring

Disclosure Statement: None declared.

[a] Dermatology Department, Instituto de Dermatologia Professor Rubem David Azulay, Santa Casa de Misericórdia do Rio de Janeiro, Rua Visconde de Pirajá 330, sala 1001 22410-000, Rio de Janeiro, RJ, Brazil; [b] Department of Dermatology and Cutaneous Surgery, Miami Miller School of Medicine, University of Miami, 1295 NW 14th Street South Building Suites K-M, Miami, FL 33125, USA

* Corresponding author.

E-mail address: rodrigopirmez@gmail.com

Dermatol Clin 36 (2018) 413–420
https://doi.org/10.1016/j.det.2018.05.008

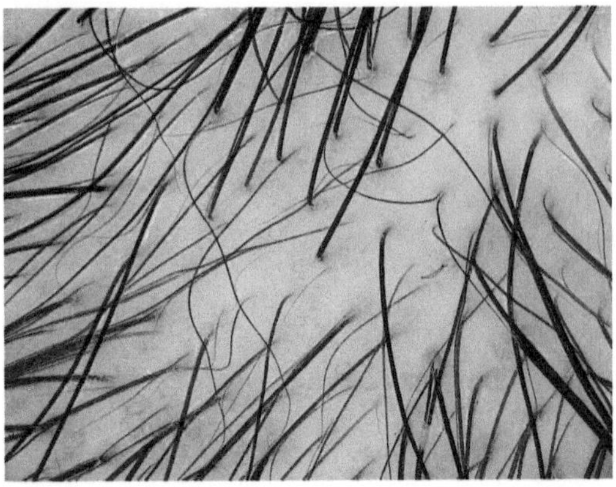

Fig. 1. Hair shaft variability: presence of more than 20% diversity in the hair shaft diameter is suggestive for a diagnosis of androgenetic alopecia.

condition. Signs of disease activity may be present either at the center or at the periphery of lesions, depending on the etiology. So, the latter should always be examined, as well. In addition, it is important to evaluate apparently normal scalp surrounding alopecic patches because early signs of disease activity may already be present in trichoscopy, even before hair loss becomes clinically evident.

Marginal alopecia

An important tip when evaluating a patient with marginal alopecia is to check if vellus hairs are present. Loss of vellus hairs in the hairline is a typical sign of frontal fibrosing alopecia (FFA) (**Fig. 2**).

"My hair does not grow"

This is a common complaint of patients with either congenital or acquired hair shaft disorders. In these cases, shafts should be directly examined and trichoscopy has satisfactorily replaced optical microscopy in most scenarios. For hair shafts, it's interesting to use polarized light, and higher magnifications are needed (at least ×70). Clinicians should look for causes of hair breakage, such as trichorrhexis nodosa (**Fig. 3**), commonly seen in hair weathering; or hair shaft defects that may signal a congenital condition, such as the typical constrictions of monilethrix (**Fig. 4**).[5,6]

Eyebrows

Hair disorders, such as alopecia areata (AA) and FFA, may also affect the eyebrows (**Fig. 5**). Trichoscopy may be quite useful, particularly in cases of atypical presentation or when the disease is limited to this area.[7] Of note, disorders or hair shaft formation, such as trichorrhexis invaginata, might be detectable only in the eyebrows.

Immersion Fluid: When to Use It

A few variables will determine whether immersion fluid should be used or not, when performing trichoscopy. A few simple points should be taken into account:

1. Contact dermoscopy always will be necessary if an immersion fluid is being used.
2. Devices with nonpolarized light will require the use of an immersion fluid to cancel out reflections from the stratum corneum.
3. Immersion fluids may hamper evaluation of scaling conditions and visualization of vellus and white hairs (as they "disappear" when a fluid is used).
4. "Elimination" of scaling with immersion fluid is sometimes desirable, as excessive scaling may interfere with visualization of underlying trichoscopic features.

As a general rule, we start the examination with dry dermoscopy and then use an immersion fluid if we judge necessary. The choice of the immersion fluid (eg, water, gel, alcohol) is a matter of personal choice.

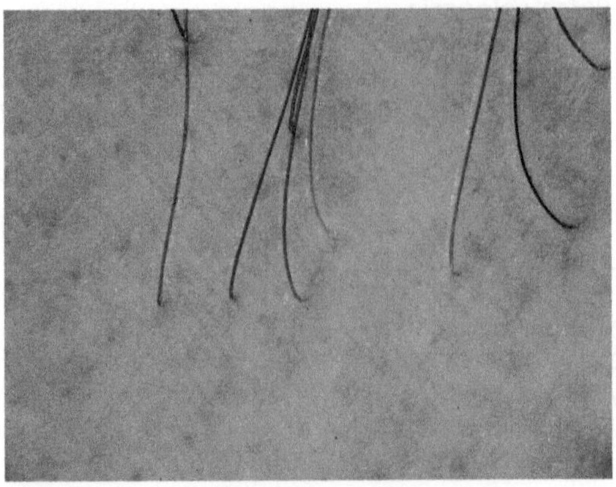

Fig. 2. Frontal fibrosing alopecia: the hairline has no vellus hair.

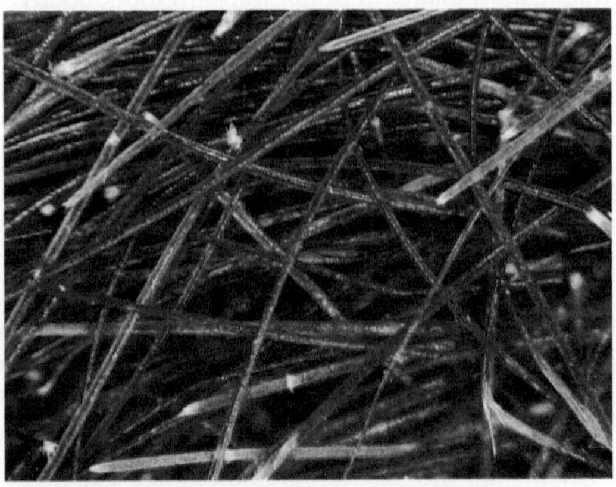

Fig. 3. Trichorrhexis nodosa.

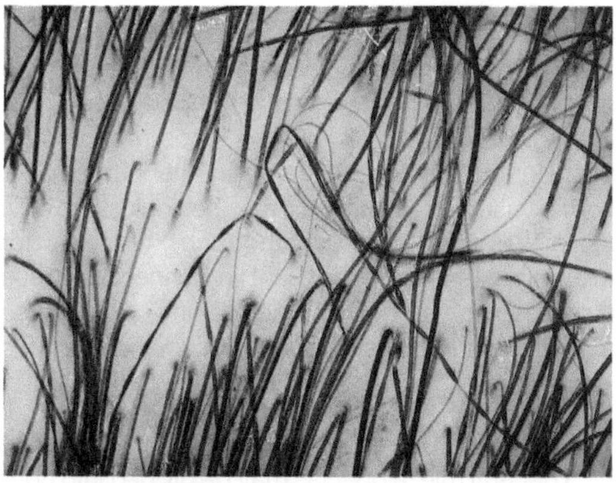

Fig. 4. Monilethrix.

Which Dermoscope Should I Use?

Each device has its advantages and drawbacks, and the clinician should opt for the one that will best fit his or her practice profile. Handheld portable dermoscopes usually allow a 10-fold magnification; which is quite satisfactory in daily practice. In addition, lower magnifications provide a better overview of a large scalp area.[8] Such dermoscopes are generally considered to be reasonably cost-effective. On the other hand, higher magnifications (20-fold to 100-fold and higher) provided by digital dermoscopes allow better visualization of fine details, specially hair shaft defects and changes in scalp vessels. Another advantage of this more expensive group of devices is that they are usually equipped with photo storage software, allowing comparison of "before and after" pictures, among other resources. Personally, we feel that showing patients their trichoscopic pictures helps them to understand their condition and to better appreciate the results of the treatment being used. A somewhat in-between and practical option are the mobile-connected dermoscopes, which allow photography usually at a magnification of ×10 to ×20. Recently, cheaper videodermatoscopes that can be connected to any computer via USB also became available. According to some investigators, these cheaper devices may have image quality drawbacks, when compared with the more expensive digital dermoscopes.[9]

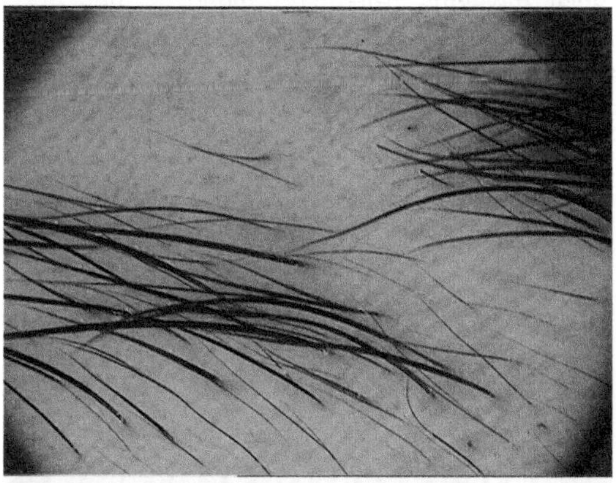

Fig. 5. Eyebrows from a patient with alopecia areata: note exclamation mark hairs.

IDENTIFYING BASIC STRUCTURES IN TRICHOSCOPY

A didactic way to learn the trichoscopic structures is to organize them in groups, according to their distribution on the scalp. In this regard, trichoscopic features could be divided into (1) follicular, (2) perifollicular and interfollicular; (3) vascular, and (4) hair shaft.[10] The following examples are not a comprehensive review of all trichoscopic structures, but illustrative of this classification. Hair shafts are discussed in the article by Lidia Rudnicka and colleagues, "Trichoscopy in Hair Shaft Disorders," elsewhere in this issue.

Follicular Structures

Because in trichoscopy we observe a 3-dimensional structure such as the skin as a 2-dimensional image, follicular structures will be seen as dots by the observer. A few examples include yellow, black, red, and white dots.

In case shafts break before scalp emergence, they will be perceived as black dots (Fig. 6). This may be due to weakening of shafts secondary to inflammation, such as seen in AA, or to mechanical trauma, as provoked by patients with trichotillomania.[11–13]

If a hair follicle loses its shaft, it becomes filled with sebum and keratin debris. This material gives a yellow hue to hair follicle openings and can be observed as a yellow dot (Fig. 7) under trichoscopy of patients with AGA or long-standing AA, for example.[14]

Follicular red dots (FRD) were described in active discoid lupus (DLE). They are a positive prognostic factor, representing a greater chance

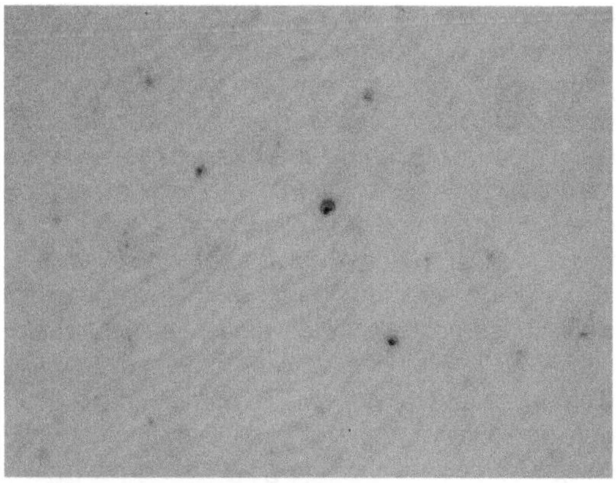

Fig. 6. Alopecia areata: black dots.

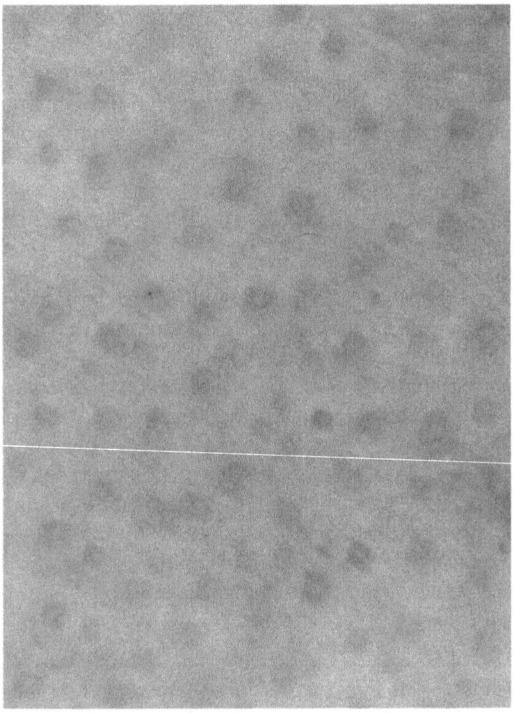

Fig. 7. Alopecia areata totalis: yellow dots.

of hair regrowth.[15] Because of vasodilation and skin atrophy present in DLE lesions, the vascular network that surrounds hair follicles becomes visible and is perceived as FRD through trichoscopy.[16] The presence of such a vascular network suggests that the follicular structure is still viable and patients should be aggressively treated.

White dots are more easily perceived in patients with dark scalp. They represent follicular and eccrine gland openings and are known as pinpoint white dots.[17]

Perifollicular and Interfollicular Patterns

The differential diagnosis between scalp DLE and lichen planopilaris (LPP) is a good example of how characterization of trichoscopic features such as having a perifollicular versus interfollicular pattern of distribution may help the clinician when using trichoscopy. Lichenoid inflammation in LPP is mainly folliculocentric and this will result in perifollicular inflammatory signs, like scaling. On the other hand, the diffuse lichenoid inflammation typical of DLE means that the interfollicular area also will be affected, and patients will present with diffuse scaling.[18] Likewise, pigment incontinence also will have distinct patterns. In LPP, pigment incontinence will be perceived as blue-gray dots in a target pattern (surrounding hair follicles), whereas in DLE blue-gray dots are diffusely spread, arranged in a speckled pattern.[19]

Vascular Structures

Thin arborizing vessels are a normal finding in the scalp and frequently seen in the temporal and occipital regions (**Fig. 8**). Simple red loops may also be seen in the normal scalp.[10] On the other hand, some vascular structures may be indicative of a scalp disorder. Thick arborizing vessels, for example, are typically present in connective tissue diseases such as DLE and dermatomyositis[20] or as a side-effect in areas of steroid-induced atrophy.[21]

AM I FACING A SCARRING CONDITION?

As a general rule, alopecias may be divided into nonscarring, a group in which patients retain the possibility of presenting hair regrowth; and scarring, when hair loss is irreversible. The trichoscopic hallmark of scarring alopecias is loss of follicular openings (**Fig. 9**). Therefore, when first approaching a patient with hair loss, clinicians should look for this variable to start considering possible differential diagnoses. Pitfalls do exist, as seen in patients with long-standing AA. In these cases, follicular openings may not be clearly visible, misleading one's diagnosis. Another clue for potentially scarring conditions is the presence of inflammatory signs, such as erythema and scaling or the presence of exudative lesions.[18,22] Even though this is not a strict rule, overt inflammation is usually part of the trichoscopic picture of potentially scarring conditions, whereas nonscarring conditions, such as AGA, AA, and telogen effluvium do not present obvious inflammatory features.

MY PATIENT HAS A RECEDING HAIRLINE: HOW TRICHOSCOPY MAY HELP?

The list of possible diagnoses of patients presenting a receding hair line includes AGA, AA in a *sisaipho* pattern, traction alopecia, and FFA. Differential diagnosis between them may not be trivial, particularly in early cases or in nonactive disease, in which typical

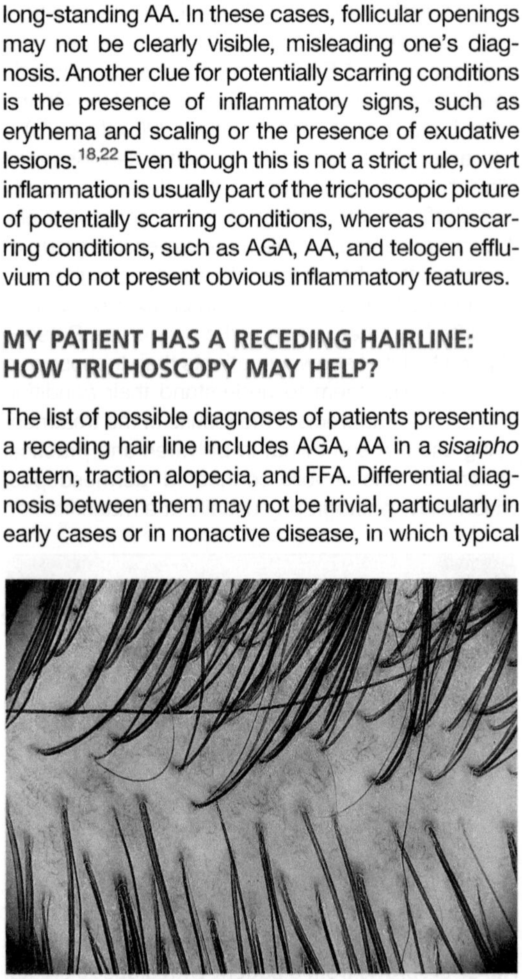

Fig. 8. Arborizing vessels.

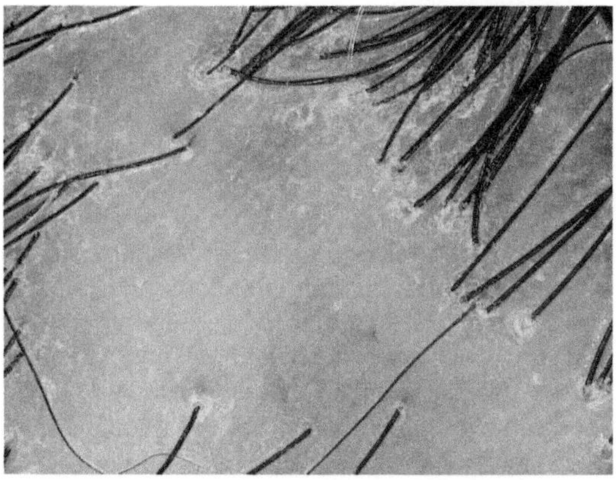

Fig. 9. Lichen planopilaris: absence of follicular openings; also note peripilar casts around hair shaft emergence.

clinical features may not be present. A useful clue is to check for the presence of vellus hairs in the hairline. In the normal hairline, there is a progressive "transition" from very thin vellus hairs present in the forehead to the thick terminal hairs of the scalp. In FFA, this "transition" is affected: the loss of vellus hairs in the hairline is a typical sign of the disease (see Fig. 2).[23] For such, when approaching a patient with a receding hairline, clinicians should bear in mind this decisive trichoscopic feature. When patients have active ongoing conditions, other trichoscopic features may help the diagnosis, such as the presence of exclamation marks and coudability hairs in AA,[24] perifollicular erythema, and scaling in FFA or hair casts in traction alopecia.[25]

DON'T FORGET THE BIGGER PICTURE

When clinicians and students are first introduced to trichoscopy, attempting to memorize lists of trichoscopic features for each disease is a common (but deceptive) reaction. Trichoscopy is a recent diagnostic tool and, as expected, new trichoscopic features are being continuously described. But, to understand trichoscopy, it is important to make correlation with disease pathogenesis. Many different trichoscopic features represent, in fact, the same pathogenic process. A good example of that is trichotillomania. In this compulsive disorder, we may find, among others, flame hairs, tulip hairs, hair powder, or the v-sign, but all these findings result from a common cause: hair shafts that were broken by the patient by traumatic pulling. Depending on the shape shafts assume after breakage, they receive a different name. To establish diagnosis, more important than knowing all these names, is to understand that they represent broken hair shafts.

In trichoscopy, it is also important to analyze the context in which a trichoscopic feature is present: what other trichoscopic features are also there? What is the patient history? What is the clinical picture? These are simple questions that should always be in the clinician's mind. Black dots, for example, may be found in a number of conditions.[26] Weakening and breakage of hair shafts forming black dots may result from either the cytotoxic insult of chemotherapeutic agents,[13,27] inflammation in AA, hypoxemia in pressure-induced alopecia,[13] or even traumatic pulling in trichotillomania. Focusing on a single trichoscopic feature, instead of looking at the bigger picture, may lead the clinician to the wrong diagnosis.

FEATURES UNIQUE TO THE DARK SCALP

Early articles discussing trichoscopy reported features mainly in the context of light-skinned patients. Only a few years ago publications started to focus on the particularities of the dark scalp, and this field still remains to be fully explored.[10,19,28]

A remarkable normal finding of the dark scalp is the visualization of a pigmented network (Fig. 10). This feature is present in the dark scalp due to the greater amount of pigment in the skin and reflects normal cutaneous architecture with rete ridges forming the darker network, whereas the thinner epidermis overlying the dermal papilla forms the lighter areas in-between. Assessing this pattern is particularly useful in the differential diagnosis of some forms of scarring alopecia. Although the pigmented network remains unaffected in folliculocentric conditions such as LPP, DLE presents with a lichenoid dermatitis that affects the whole dermal-epidermal junction in addition to hair follicles. For such, in DLE, the skin architecture is affected and loss of the pigmented network pattern is an expected trichoscopic feature of the disease in dark-skinned patient. Damage to the basal layer leads to pigment incontinence, which in turn results in the visualization of blue-gray dots in trichoscopy.

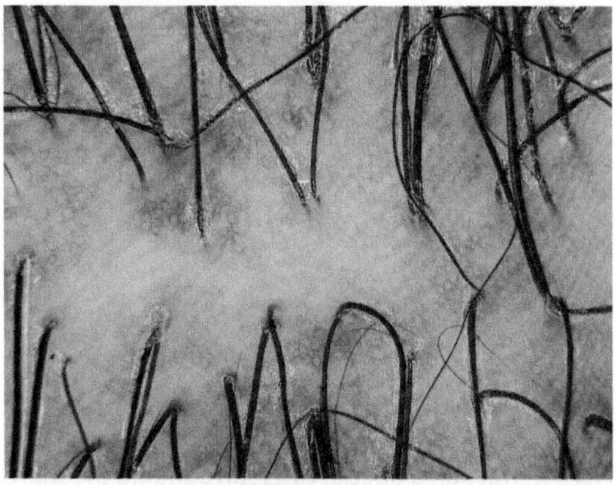

Fig. 10. Pigmented network.

Blue-gray dots, either in a target or speckled pattern as previously discussed, are also more commonly seen in patients with darker skin types.

When facing a potentially inflammatory condition of the scalp, clinicians should be aware that the severity of the process may be underestimated in one's evaluation, for the visualization of erythema may be hampered by the overlying intensely pigmented skin.

A trichoscopic feature described in the same population is the "starry sky" pattern, the presence of multiple pinpoint white dots on the darker skin background. This is a normal finding caused by the visualization of the eccrine grand openings.

Peripilar white gray halos have been described in the trichoscopy of central centrifugal cicatricial alopecia,[29] the most common cause of scarring alopecia in African American women.[30] They correspond on pathology to the lamellar fibrosis surrounding the outer root sheath. In our experience, they also may be seen in dark-skinned patients with other forms of folliculocentric scarring alopecias, such as FFA.

Traumatic hair styling makes some populations and ethnicities, such as Africans and African descendants particularly prone to traction alopecia. Hair casts are a useful trichoscopic sign of ongoing traction. On trichoscopy, hair casts appear as white to brown cylindrical structures that encircle the proximal hair shafts (**Fig. 11**). Traction-induced hair casts consist of the pulled out inner and/or outer root sheath and are not characterized by prominent parakeratosis.[25]

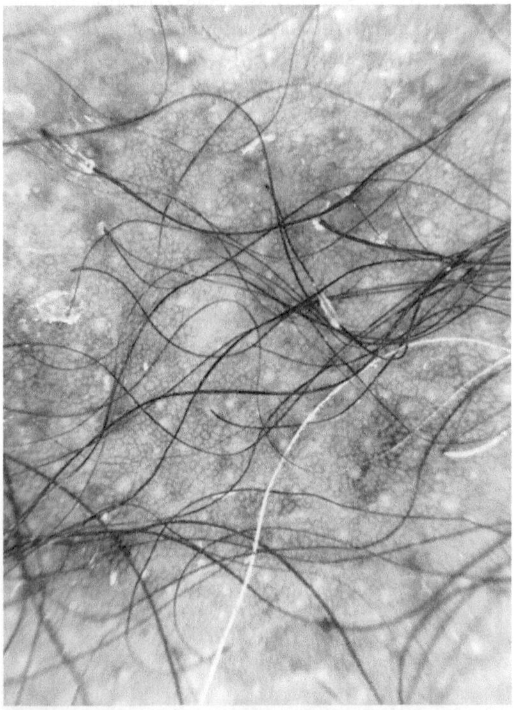

Fig. 11. Traction alopecia: casts surrounding the shafts at the margins of the patch indicate ongoing traction.

CHILDREN! WHAT TO EXPECT IN TRICHOSCOPY?

A variety of conditions are more frequently seen in children, ranging from infections and infestations to hair shaft formation disorders. The fact that trichoscopy is noninvasive and painless makes this diagnostic method particularly interesting in the evaluation of hair and scalp disorders in children.[31] Even so, few studies regarding the use of trichoscopy have been done exclusively in children and much of the current knowledge derives from studies in adults. However, some features that are inherent to this group should be observed.

In our experience, follicular units in children usually consist of 1 or 2 hairs and often have shafts of different diameters, which may mislead to the diagnosis of AGA by an unwary clinician.

A normal trichoscopic feature commonly seen in children is dirty dots. Dirty dots appear as brown, black, and occasionally red, yellow, and blue particulate dots and loose fibers and likely represent environmental particles.[32] This finding possibly results from the inability of the scalp to repel particulate debris from exogenous environmental sources due to low activity of the sebaceous glands in patients of early age. The involution of sebaceous glands with age may also explain the presence of dirty dots in the elderly.[33]

The low activity of sebaceous glands is also responsible for the lower incidence of yellow dots in children. Clinicians should keep this information in mind. Long-standing patches of AA may not reveal yellow dots, and visualization of follicular openings may be hampered. For this reason, cases of AA may end up being misdiagnosed as scarring alopecia, which in reality is quite uncommon in children.

PITFALLS IN TRICHOSCOPY: BE AWARE!

Pitfalls in trichoscopy are artifacts that may simulate hair disorders. It is important to identify such artifacts to avoid misdiagnosing a hair condition. The most important pitfalls are secondary to scalp deposits, scalp staining, and hair shaft deposits.

Scalp Deposits

Scalp deposits may be either due to deposition of environmental particles, like dust, or camouflage products. Environmental particles are the previously discussed "dirty dots." To the untrained eye, dirty dots may simulate a few trichoscopic features, depending on the shape and color of the particle. Some deposits are commonly misinterpreted as black dots, a sign of ongoing hair follicle damage observed in a few conditions, such as AA. Importantly, dirty dots can be completely removed after intense shampooing.

Another type of scalp deposit is camouflage products used by patients to conceal areas of decreased hair density. They can be present as a powder on the scalp surface or, more commonly, as fibers. In this later case, it is important not to confuse them with broken hair shafts.

Scalp Staining

Common causes of scalp staining include hair dye, topical medication, such as anthralin, or scalp tattoos, which is an increasingly popular method to camouflage decreased hair density.

Hair dye may be present on the scalp surface and within follicular openings simulating both interfollicular hyperpigmentation and dots (**Fig. 12**).[34] Anthralin also may stain follicular openings and resemble black dots. Because anthralin is used in the treatment of alopecia areata, identification of this pitfall is essential to not misclassify your patients as having active AA. Finally, ink deposition in scalp tattoos may have a blue hue and simulate a few trichoscopic features, such as blue-gray dots or even a blue nevus, depending on the pattern of distribution.

Hair Shaft Deposits

Another common pitfall is hair shaft deposits. They may be secondary to the use of dry shampoos, hair sprays, or other hair-styling products. These products may form concretions around hair shafts and mimic hair casts, as seen in LPP and traction alopecia, or even nits, simulating infestation by pediculosis (**Fig. 13**).[35,36]

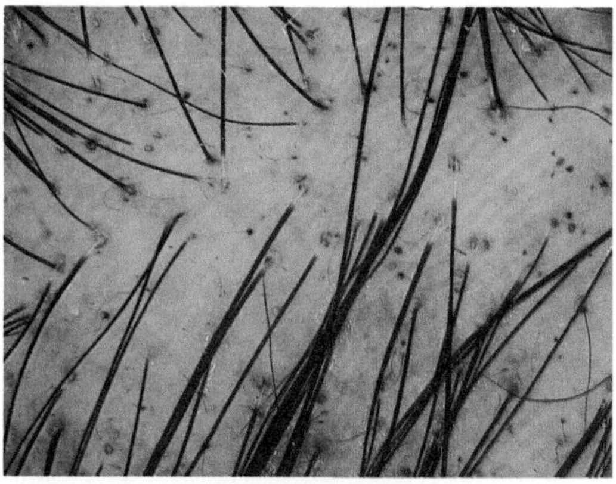

Fig. 12. Permanent hair dye staining.

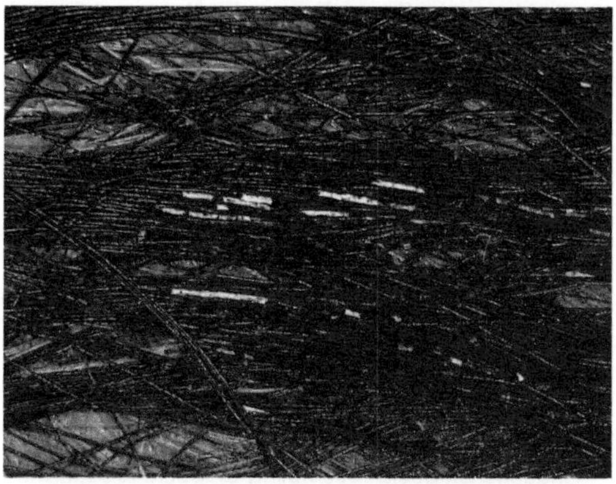

Fig. 13. Pseudocasts due to hair spray.

SUMMARY

The aim of this article was to bring selected information from the literature and our clinical experience that may help dermatologists to use trichoscopy in their everyday practice. Clinicians should keep in mind that trichoscopy is a recently described and evolving technique; many new concepts are constantly arising and constant update is required.

REFERENCES

1. Miteva M, Tosti A. Hair and scalp dermatoscopy. J Am Acad Dermatol 2012;67(5):1040–8.
2. Olszewska M, Rudnicka L, Rakowska A, et al. Trichoscopy. Arch Dermatol 2008;144(8):1007.
3. Lacarrubba F, Micali G, Tosti A. Scalp dermoscopy or trichoscopy. Curr Probl Dermatol 2015;47:21–32.
4. Vicenzi C, Tosti A. Instruments for scalp dermoscopy. In: Tosti A, editor. Dermoscopy of the hair and nails. 2nd edition. Boca Raton (FL): CRC Press; 2016. p. 25–8.
5. Rudnicka L, Rakowska A, Kerzeja M, et al. Hair shafts in trichoscopy: clues for diagnosis of hair and scalp diseases. Dermatol Clin 2013;31(4):695–708.
6. Pirmez R, Del Rei M. Cover image: a dashed hair. Br J Dermatol 2016;174(3):697–8.
7. Anzai A, Donati A, Valente NY, et al. Isolated eyebrow loss in frontal fibrosing alopecia: relevance of early diagnosis and treatment. Br J Dermatol 2016;175(5):1099–101.
8. Rudnicka L, Rusek M, Borkowska B. Introduction. In: Rudnicka L, Olszewska M, Rakowska A, editors. Atlas of trichoscopy–Dermoscopy in hair and scalp disease. 1st edition. London: Springer-Verlag; 2012. p. 3–8.
9. Verzì AE, Lacarrubba F, Micali G. Use of low-cost videomicroscopy versus standard videodermatoscopy in trichoscopy: a controlled, blinded noninferiority trial. Skin Appendage Disord 2016;1(4):172–4.

10. de Moura LH, Duque-Estrada B, Abraham LS, et al. Dermoscopy findings of alopecia areata in an African-American patient. J Dermatol Case Rep 2008;2(4):52–4.
11. Ross EK, Vincenzi C, Tosti A. Videodermoscopy in the evaluation of hair and scalp disorders. J Am Acad Dermatol 2006;55(5):799–806.
12. Pirmez R, Piñeiro-Maceira J, Sodré CT. Exclamation marks and other trichoscopic signs of chemotherapy-induced alopecia. Australas J Dermatol 2013;54(2): 129–32.
13. Papaiordanou F, da Silveira BR, Piñeiro-Maceira J, et al. Trichoscopy of noncicatricial pressure-induced alopecia resembling alopecia areata. Int J Trichology 2016;8(2):89–90.
14. Rudnicka L, Olszewska M, Rakowska A, et al. Trichoscopy update 2011. J Dermatol Case Rep 2011;5(4):82–8.
15. Tosti A, Torres F, Misciali C, et al. Follicular red dots: a novel dermoscopic pattern observed in scalp discoid lupus erythematosus. Arch Dermatol 2009; 145(12):1406–9.
16. Pirmez R, Piñeiro-Maceira J, Almeida BC, et al. Follicular red dots: a normal trichoscopy feature in patients with pigmentary disorders? An Bras Dermatol 2013;88(3):459–61.
17. Abraham LS, Piñeiro-Maceira J, Duque-Estrada B, et al. Pinpoint white dots in the scalp: dermoscopic and histopathologic correlation. J Am Acad Dermatol 2010;63(4):721–2.
18. Ramos-e-Silva M, Pirmez R. Red face revisited: disorders of hair growth and pilosebaceous unit. Clin Dermatol 2014;32:784–99.
19. Duque-Estrada B, Tamler C, Sodré CT, et al. Dermoscopy patterns of cicatricial alopecia resulting from discoid lupus erythematosus and lichen planopilaris. An Bras Dermatol 2010;85(2):179–83.
20. Vicenzi C, Tosti A. Trichoscopy patterns. In: Tosti A, editor. Dermoscopy of the hair and nails. 2nd edition. Boca Raton (FL): CRC Press; 2016. p. 1–20.
21. Pirmez R, Abraham LS, Duque-Estrada B, et al. Trichoscopy of steroid-induced atrophy. Skin Appendage Disord 2017;3:171–4.
22. Vendramini DL, Silveira BR, Duque-Estrada B, et al. Isolated body hair loss: an unusual presentation of lichen planopilaris. Skin Appendage Disord 2017; 2(3–4):97–9.
23. Lacarrubba F, Micali G, Tosti A. Absence of vellus hair in the hairline: a videodermatoscopic feature of frontal fibrosing alopecia. Br J Dermatol 2013; 169(2):473–4.
24. Pirmez R. Revisiting coudability hairs in alopecia areata: the story behind the name. Skin Appendage Disord 2016;2(1–2):76–8.
25. Tosti A, Miteva M, Torres F, et al. Hair casts are a dermoscopic clue for the diagnosis of traction alopecia. Br J Dermatol 2010;163(6):1353–5.
26. Kowalska-Oledzka E, Slowinska M, Rakowska A, et al. 'Black dots' seen under trichoscopy are not specific for alopecia areata. Clin Exp Dermatol 2012;37(6):615–9.
27. Pirmez R, Piñeiro-Maceira J, Gonzalez CG, et al. Loose anchoring of anagen hairs and pili torti due to erlotinib. Int J Trichology 2016;8(4):186–7.
28. Pirmez R, Duque-Estrada B, Donati A, et al. Clinical and dermoscopic features of lichen planus pigmentosus in 37 patients with frontal fibrosing alopecia. Br J Dermatol 2016;175(6):1387–90.
29. Miteva M, Tosti A. Dermatoscopic features of central centrifugal cicatricial alopecia. J Am Acad Dermatol 2014;71(3):443–9.
30. Olsen EA, Callender V, Sperling L, et al. Central scalp alopecia photographic scale in African American women. Dermatol Ther 2008;21:264–7.
31. Lencastre A, Tosti A. Role of trichoscopy in children's scalp and hair disorders. Pediatr Dermatol 2013;30(6):674–82.
32. Fu JM, Starace M, Tosti A. A new dermoscopic finding in healthy children. Arch Dermatol 2009; 145(5):596–7.
33. Miteva M, Lima M, Tosti A. Dirty dots as a normal trichoscopic finding in the elderly scalp. JAMA Dermatol 2016;152(4):474–6.
34. Angra K, LaSenna CE, Nichols AJ, et al. Hair dye: a trichoscopy pitfall. J Am Acad Dermatol 2015;72(4): e101–2.
35. Doche I, Vincenzi C, Tosti A. Casts and pseudocasts. J Am Acad Dermatol 2016;75(4):e147–8.
36. Pirmez R. Acantholytic hair casts: a dermoscopic sign of pemphigus vulgaris of the scalp. Int J Trichology 2012;4(3):172–3.

Trichoscopy in Hair Shaft Disorders

Lidia Rudnicka, MD, PhD[a], Małgorzata Olszewska, MD, PhD[b,*], Anna Waśkiel, MD[b], Adriana Rakowska, MD, PhD[b]

KEYWORDS

• Trichoscopy • Dermoscopy • Dermatoscopy • Alopecia • Hair shaft • Ectodermal dysplasia • Classification • Hair fragility

KEY POINTS

- Trichoscopy allows the practitioner to analyze the structure and size of growing hairs without the need to pull hair for examination.
- Trichoscopy allows establishing the diagnosis of most of the known hair shaft disorders.
- Some structures are only visible with dry trichoscopy, whereas other may require an immersion fluid.
- In patients suspected of trichothiodystrophy, a polarized dermoscope should be used.

INTRODUCTION

Trichoscopy (hair and scalp dermoscopy) has been successfully applied in practical dermatology in recent years.[1,2] One of the major fields of progress is the use of trichoscopy for evaluation of hair shaft diseases in children.[3,4] This noninvasive technique replaced light microscopy, which required pulling of multiple hairs for investigation. This was in particular burdensome for patients with hairs prone to fracturing and in diseases, where only few hairs might be affected, but the examination is crucial for establishing a diagnosis. A best example is Netherton syndrome, which occasionally required pulling a few hundred hair shafts to establish a diagnosis. In 2007 and 2008, a Polish group first described the application of trichoscopy in hair shaft disorders.[5,6] Now trichoscopy may be successfully applied in most of the inherited and acquired hair shaft disorders.

NORMAL HAIRS

Normal hair shafts are uniform in thickness and color throughout their length.[7,8] Terminal hairs may have a medulla, which is continuous, interrupted, fragmented, or absent.[9] Up to 10% of normal human scalp hairs are vellus hairs.[7,8] These are hairs that are less than 3-mm long and less than 30-μm thick.

CLASSIFICATION OF HAIR SHAFT ABNORMALITIES IN TRICHOSCOPY

A classification of hair shaft abnormalities in trichoscopy was proposed by Rudnicka and colleagues.[18] It distinguishes the following groups of hair shaft features observed by trichoscopy: (1) hair shafts with fractures, (2) hair narrowings, (3) hairs with nodelike structures, (4) curls and twists, (5) bands, and (6) short hairs. A short hair is defined as a hair in which an entire hair shaft is visible in 1 field of view of a dermoscope (10-fold to 20-fold magnification). These hairs are usually less than 10-mm long.

HAIR SHAFT DISEASES

Monilethrix and Monilethrix-Like Hairs

Monilethrix is characterized by regular, periodic thinning of hair shafts and a tendency to fracture

Disclosure Statement: No conflicts of interest.
[a] Department of Neuropeptides, Mossakowski Medical Research Centre Polish Academy of Sciences, Warsaw, Poland; [b] Department of Dermatology, Medical University of Warsaw, Pawinskiego 5, 02-106, Warszawa, Poland
* Corresponding author. Department of Dermatology, Medical University of Warsaw, Koszykowa 82A, 02-008, Warsaw, Poland.
E-mail addresses: malgorzata.olszewska@wum.edu.pl; malgorzataolszewska@yahoo.com

Dermatol Clin 36 (2018) 421–430
https://doi.org/10.1016/j.det.2018.05.009

at constricted points. Nodosities correspond to the normal hair caliber, whereas the defect is in the constricted sections.[10]

Monilethrix is a hereditary disorder, typically caused by autosomal dominant mutations in type II hair keratin genes KRT 81, KRT 83, and KRT 86.[11] Mutations in the desmoglein 4 (DSG4) gene are associated with autosomal recessive monilethrix and monilethrix-like congenital hypotrichosis, which differ from classic monilethrix by barely visible internodes, which do not show constant periodicity.[12]

From early childhood, patients with monilethrix present with short and fragile hairs that never grow long enough to require a haircut. Noninvolved hairs are seldom longer than 5 cm to 8 cm. Other hairy areas, such as eyebrows; eyelashes; or axillary, pubic, and body hair, may also be involved.[13] The disease tends to improve with age.

The hair shaft fragility is associated with perifollicular abnormalities, which range from subtle perifollicular erythema to large hyperkeratotic follicular papules. Other, rare, ectodermal symptoms in these patients may include koilonychia, brittle nails, syndactyly, juvenile cataract, decreased visual field, and dental abnormalities.[13]

Several studies have investigated the application of trichoscopy in diagnosing monilethrix. The first study by Rakowska and colleagues[6] showed that trichoscopy allows visualizing abnormalities in both terminal and vellus hairs of the scalp. Hair shafts show uniform elliptical nodosities and intermittent constrictions causing variation in hair shaft thickness (**Fig. 1**). Hairs are bended regularly at multiple locations and have a tendency to fracture at constriction sites.[5,6] The term, *regularly bended ribbon sign*, was suggested to differentiate trichoscopy features of monilethrix from pseudomonilethrix and other causes of hair loss.[6] Horny follicular papules appear as big yellow dots, when evaluated in trichoscopy with immersion fluid, while perifollicular scaling and keratotic follicular plugs may be observed in dry trichoscopy.

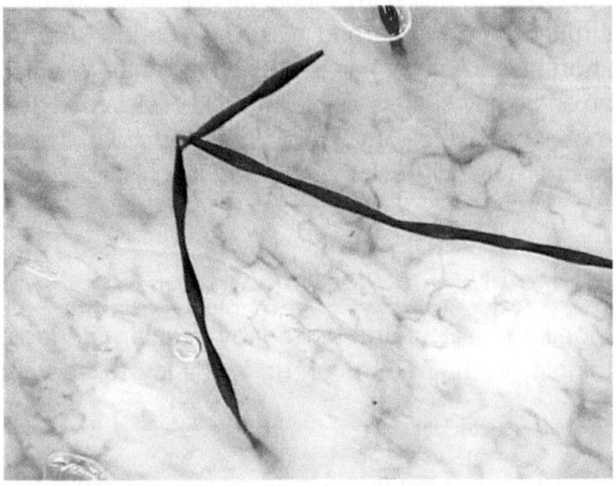

Fig. 1. Monilethrix. Trichoscopy shows hair shafts with regularly distributed nodes (correspond to normal hair shaft thickness) and internodes (correspond to narrowing of hair shaft). If only small proportion of hair shafts is affected, this abnormality is more likely to found in occipital area (×70).

A later report showed that beaded hairs arise from the keratotic papules on neck.[14] Typical trichoscopy findings were also observed in the affected body hairs of the forearms.

Not all hairs are affected by monilethrix. Probably the best areas for searching for typical abnormalities are the temporal and occipital areas, where most hair shafts show features of the disease. In rare cases, however, other locations are predominantly affected. The development of hair loss mimicking androgenetic alopecia with typical monilethrix hairs in the androgen-dependent areas of the scalp was reported.[15]

The term, *pseudomonilethrix*, was used to describe irregular, square-shaped, flattening of hair shafts. It remains controversial whether pseudomonilethrix is a true disease[16] or an artifact produced by either procedure of preparing hairs for microscopic examination or by excessive use of cosmetic hair care products.[17] There was no reported case of pseudomonilethrix on trichoscopy despite massive use of this diagnostic method in recent years. This may be an indirect confirmation that pseudomonilethrix is an artifact, which may be visible in light microscopy but is easy to identify as excessive use of hair cosmetics in the trichoscopic evaluation.

A pseudomonilethrix effect may be observed in patients who use hair styling gels.[6] Thus, patients should be advised not to use these products between hair washing and trichoscopy. Also, ultrasound gel used as immersion fluid can make hair shafts appear irregularly flattened.[6]

Pseudomonilethrix has to be distinguished from monilethrix-like hairs, which show the same type of ovoid constrictions as in monilethrix but with no regularity characteristic for true monilethrix. These constrictions have been also called Pohl-Pinkus constrictions. Monilethrix-like hair shafts may be observed in diseases with variable course, such as alopecia areata and lichen planopilaris, or in patients undergoing chemotherapy (**Box 1**).[18–20]

Trichorrhexis Nodosa

Trichorrhexis nodosa is a condition in which the shaft splits longitudinally into numerous small fibers within a restricted area of the shaft. The outer fibers bulge out, what causes a segmental increase in hair diameter. Macroscopically this may resemble nodules located along the hair

Box 1
Monilethrix-like hair shafts in trichoscopy

- Monilethrix
- Monilethrix-like congenital hypotrichosis
- Alopecia areata with variable activity in the course of disease
- Primary cicatricial alopecia (border of fibrotic area)
- Chemotherapy-induced alopecia
- Monilethrix-like effect from hair styling gel
- Monilethrix-like effect from immersion gel

shaft. Hairs eventually break at these points leaving brush-like ends.[21]

The condition may be inherited or acquired. The inherited form is usually associated with multisymptom syndromes. Trichorrhexis nodosa as a sole finding, not associated with other clinical symptoms, is observed in only 5.6% of children with this condition.[22] Conditions associated with trichorrhexis nodosa are listed in **Box 2**. It has been shown that trichorrhexis nodosa may be induced by mechanical trauma, such as scratching in scalp diesthesia.[23]

In patients with trichorrhexis nodosa, hair appears clinically dry and brittle with a tendency to break at different lengths. The uncut hair is usually longer compared with patients with monilethrix but usually breaks before it grows very long.

Trichoscopy may give slightly different images depending on magnification. At low magnification, trichorrhexis nodosa may not be visible. Hairs bending at sharp angles, but with rounded edges, may be indicative of the abnormality (**Fig. 2**). Trichoscopy may show nodular thickenings along the hair shaft, which appear light in the darker hair shaft. The hair shaft thickness is approximately 25% larger at the site of the nodule. When a hair shaft breaks at the site of the nodule, it leaves a slightly thickened, rounded hair shaft end, which may appear darker compared with light-colored hair shaft. In dry trichoscopy of dark hairs, these ends tend to appear lighter compared with the remaining hair shafts. At higher magnification, trichoscopy allows appreciating numerous small fibers, which produce a picture resembling 2 brooms or brushes aligned in opposition. Broken hairs leave brush-like ends with numerous small fibers at the distal end of the hair shafts.

Trichorrhexis Invaginata and Netherton Syndrome

Netherton syndrome is an autosomal recessive disorder in the wide spectrum of atopic dermatitis, characterized clinically by the triad of ichthyosis (most commonly ichthyosis linearis circumflexa), atopic diathesis, and trichorrhexis invaginata. The neonatal period is commonly complicated by congenital ichthyosiform erythroderma of variable expression.[24]

Ichthyosis linearis circumflexa, which consists of erythematous migratory polycyclic patches surrounded by serpiginous double-edged scales, is variable and episodic evolving with recurrent acute attacks lasting a few weeks.[25] Other associated manifestations of Netherton syndrome may include

Box 2
Diseases associated with trichorrhexis nodosa

- Physical trauma[71,72]
- Chemical trauma[73]
- Thermal trauma[74]
- Scalp pruritus[75]
- Scalp dysethesia[23]
- Mental retardation (for example Pollitt syndrome)[76]
- Diarrhea (for example trichohepatoenteric syndrome)[77]
- Argininosuccinic aciduria[78]
- Kabuki syndrome[79]
- Menkes disease[80]
- Ectodermal dysplasias[69,81]
- Biotin deficiency[21]
- Monilethrix-like congenital hypotrichosis[12]
- Hypovitaminosis A[a,82]
- Seborrheic dermatitis[75]
- Netherton syndrome (as additional, nonspecific finding)[21]
- Mutation in the XPD gene[83]
- Laron syndrome[84]
- Congenital disorder of glycosylation[b,85]
- Zinc deficiency[b,86,87]
- Hypotrichosis, hair structure defects, hypercysteine hair and glucosuria syndrome[a,88]
- Bazex-Dupré-Christol syndrome[a,89]
- Hypothyroidism[a,90]
- Congenital trichorrhexis nodosa without coexisting defects[21]

[a] One case published, according to the authors' literature search.
[b] Three cases published, according to the authors' literature search.

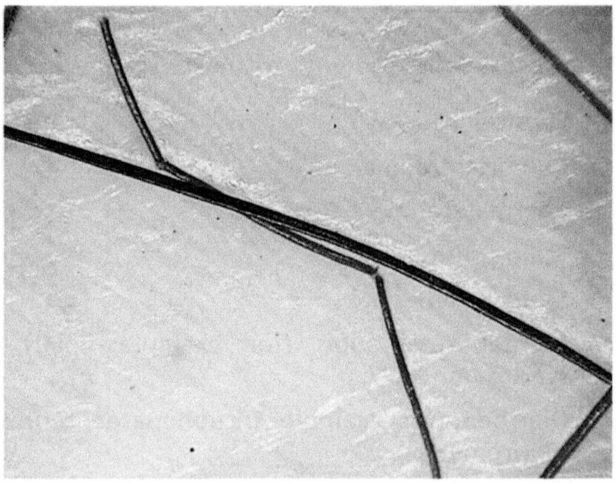

Fig. 2. Trichorrhexis nodosa. Trichoscopy reveals nodules along hair shafts, which are random areas where hair shaft splits longitudinally into numerous small fibers. The hair shafts have tendency to bend and break at these sites (×70).

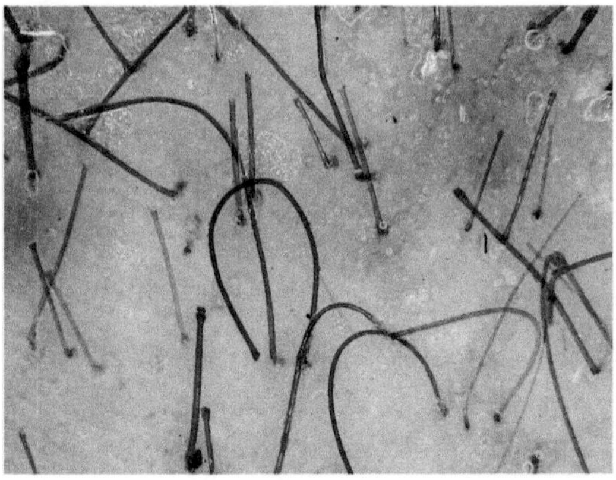

Fig. 3. Trichorrhexis invaginata and golf tee hairs. These 2 hair shafts abnormalities are pathognomonic for Netherton syndrome. Trichorrhexis invaginata is a term used to describe invagination of the distal portion of hair shaft into its proximal portion. Usually this abnormality is observed at several points along hair shaft, creating a bamboo-like appearance. Fractured bamboo hairs have cupped proximal end and are known as golf tee hairs (×20).

aminoaciduria, failure to thrive, mental and neurologic retardation, and immune abnormalities.

The disease is caused by loss-of-function mutations in the *SPINK5* gene, which encodes lymphoepithelial kasal-type inhibitor (LEKTI), a serine protease inhibitor with antitrypsin activity. LEKTI is normally expressed in epithelial and lymphoid tissues and may play an important role in anti-inflammatory and antimicrobial effects.[26] Mutations in the filaggrin gene (*FLG*) also have been described.[27]

Patients with Netherton syndrome have sparse hair, which is dry, short, spiky, and brittle. A diagnosis of Netherton syndrome may be established by identifying at least 1 hair shaft with trichorrhexis invaginata.[25]

Trichorrhexis invaginata, also called bamboo hair, is an abnormality of the hair in which the hair shaft telescopes in on itself (invaginates) at several points along the shaft. In low-magnification trichoscopy, this appears as multiple small nodules spaced along the shaft at irregular intervals (**Fig. 3**). High-magnification trichoscopy shows an invagination of the distal portion of the hair shaft into its proximal portion forming a ball-in-cup appearance, which is considered pathognomonic of Netherton syndrome. Occasionally, ragged, cupped proximal hair ends may be seen, where the distal end has fractured. This abnormality is often referred to as golf tee hairs.[28] Recently, matchstick hairs were described in a patient with Netherton syndrome.[29] They are visible by a handheld dermoscope as short hair shafts with a bulging tip and are equivalent to golf tee hairs.

Several investigators indicate that trichorrhexis invaginata (bamboo hairs) and golf tee hairs are easiest to find by trichoscopy of the eyebrow area,[28] because their density (the number of lesions per millimeter of hair shaft) is 10 times higher in the eyebrow area compared with the scalp in patients with Netherton syndrome.[30] Eyelashes may also exhibit trichoscopy features of trichorrhexis invaginata.[31]

Other hair anomalies, such as pili torti, trichorrhexis nodosa, and helical hairs, can be found in patients with Netherton syndrome, but they are not specific for the disease.[32]

Pili Torti

The term, *pili torti*, refers to twisted hair.[33] In pili torti sections of a hair shaft are flattened at irregular intervals and then rotated by 180° around its long axis.[32] Pili torti may be either inherited or acquired (**Table 1**).

The condition affects mainly scalp hair, but eyebrows, eyelashes, and axillary hair may show features of pili torti. Hairs are brittle and dry and may break before they grow long.[33] The abnormality is probably caused by alterations in the inner root sheath. The genetic background of most inherited diseases associated with pili torti is not known. The diversity of inherited syndromes associated with the disease may indicate that there also is a diversity in genes responsible for this abnormality.

Two types of the inherited variant of pili torti are distinguished: (1) the early-onset, classic type (Ronchese type), and (2) late onset (Beare type).

In the classic form (Ronchese type), the abnormality is observed since early childhood. Disease

Table 1
Conditions associated with pili torti

Congenital	Acquired
• Pili torti (Ronchese type) • Pili torti (Beare type) • Autosomal recessive ichthyosis with hypotrichosis • Bazex syndrome • Beare syndrome • Björnstad syndrome • Congenital disorder of glycosylation, type Ia • Crandall syndrome • Hipohidrotic ectodermal dysplasia • Hypotrichosis-osteolysis-periodontitis-palmoplantar keratoderma syndrome • Menkes syndrome • Rapp-Hodgkin syndrome • Trichodysplasia-xeroderma • Trichothiodystrophy (photosensitive) • Schöpf-Schulz-Passarge syndrome	• Alopecia areata • Cicatricial alopecia • Hair transplantation • Repetitive trauma • Retinoid treatment • Systemic sclerosis

onset is between third month and third year of life. The disease typically occurs in girls with blond hairs. Foci of alopecia are located predominantly in the temporal and occipital area, what is associated with increased friction in these areas. This type of pili torti may coexist with leukonychia, keratosis pilaris, dystrophic nails, ichthyosis, and dental abnormalities (in ectodermal syndromes). Inheritance is autosomal dominant or recessive.[1]

The second, late-onset type occurs after puberty (Beare type) and is more frequently associated with dark hair. Inheritance is autosomal dominant.[33]

The term, *Björnstad syndrome*, is used for describing coexistence of pili torti with sensorineural hearing loss. The disease is associated with mutations in the gene BCS1L.[34]

Pili torti may be also associated with several other, rare, inherited diseases and syndromes.[35]

Acquired forms of pili torti may result from repetitive trauma, oral retinoid treatment,[36] hair follicle changes in cicatricial alopecia,[37] and systemic sclerosis.

Light microscopy shows twists at irregular intervals along the shaft. Only part of hairs in a sample and only part of the hair length is affected.

Trichoscopy of pili torti shows twists of hair shafts along the long axis. Images taken at a low magnification may demonstrate the hair shafts bent at different angles at irregular intervals (**Fig. 4**). The abnormality is best observed in dry trichoscopy and at high magnification.[5]

Pili Annulati

Pili annulati means "ring hair." The term refers to an autosomal dominant disorder, which is characterized by hair shafts with alternating white and dark bands (rings).[38] A locus for pili annulati was mapped to chromosome 12q24.32-24.33,[39] but it remains unknown which gene is responsible for the disease. One case of pili annulati associated with Rothmund-Thomson syndrome with a mutation in RECQL4 was reported.[40]

There is no consensus on the origin of the white bands. Most authors indicate that the bands are due to air-filled gaps in the cortex.[41,42]

Pili annulati appears at birth or during infancy. The characteristic bands can be visible on clinical examination. Hair often appears shiny but is otherwise normal. The hairs are not excessively fragile. In some patients, however, increased sensitivity to weathering may occur in light the bands.[43,44] The abnormality is usually limited to scalp hair, but axillary, beard hair, and pubic hair may be affected.[38] Pili annulati is easier detected in blonde hair, because the banding pattern tends to be masked the additional pigment in dark colored hair.[38] There is no association between pili annulati and other hair or systemic abnormalities. Cases of pili

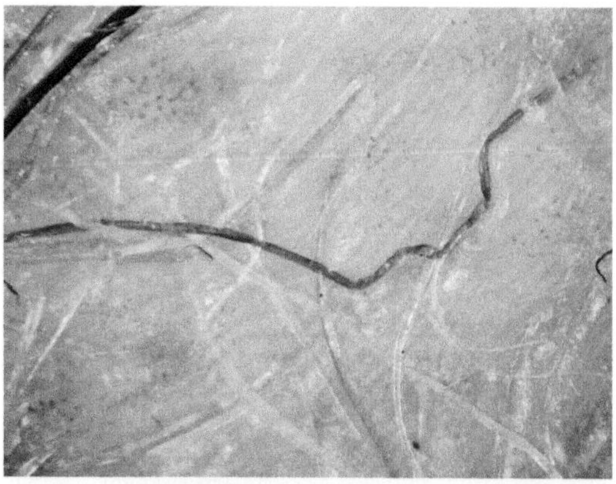

Fig. 4. Pili torti. Sections of hair shafts are flattened and rotated 180° around its long axis at irregular intervals. In trichoscopy, it is best visible in higher magnifications and without immersion fluid. The hair shafts are bended irregularly (×70).

annulati associated with alopecia areata were reported. Most probably this is a coincidental concomitant manifestation with a common disease than true pathogenetic association.[45]

In light microscopy, hair shafts show alternating light and dark bands. Bands that appear white macroscopically and in trichoscopy look dark in light microscopy, because light does not pass through the air-filled gaps in the cortex.

Trichoscopy demonstrates hair shafts with alternating white and dark bands in both, with dark and blond hairs (**Fig. 5**).[5] Approximately 20% to 80% of hairs are affected in individuals with pili annulati and the number of white bands is reduced distally.[3,45] It is unclear why the bands tend to disappear as the hair grows. It may be due to either a weathering process resulting in collapse of the cavities or damage to the cuticle, allowing penetration of the immersion fluid into the cavities.

In trichoscopy, pili annulati has to be differentiated from fragmented or intermittent medulla in healthy individuals. Intermittent medulla is visible in trichoscopy as a longitudinal, white-colored structure, which covers less than 50% of the hair shaft width. In pili annulati, which is an abnormality of the cortex, the light-colored bands cover 50% to 100% of the hair shaft thickness.[1]

A differential diagnosis is pseudopili annulati,[46] in which the banded clinical appearance of hairs is an optical effect resulting from the partial twisting of the hair shaft in an oscillating manner. In such cases, trichoscopy show no white bands but only twisted hairs.

A pitfall may be hairs, which are nonuniformly colorized, mainly in the case of low-pigment hairs dyed dark.[1]

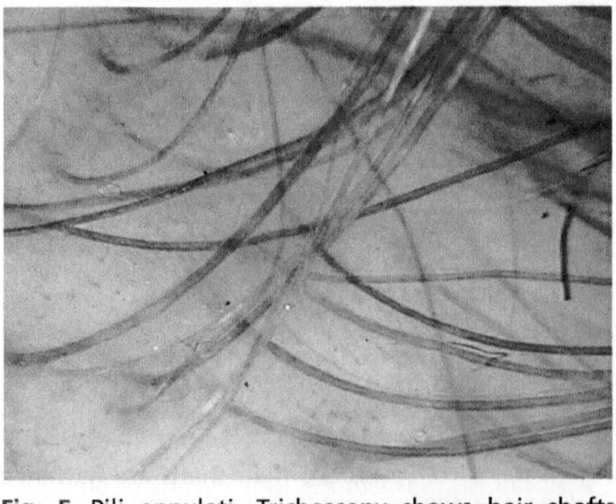

Fig. 5. Pili annulati. Trichoscopy shows hair shafts with alternating white and dark bands. White bands cover more than 50% of hair shaft thickness and have no clear-cut borders (×70).

Woolly Hair

The term, *woolly hair*, refers to an abnormal variant of fine, tightly curled hair with 180° longitudinal twisting and increased tendency to fracture. Transverse sections of hair shafts show varying, ovoid shapes of different morphology.[47,48] Hair may be sparse and hypopigmented.[46] Trichorrhexis nodosa and pili annulati may coexist.[47]

Hutchinson and colleagues[49] classified the condition into 3 variants: (1) woolly hair nevus, (2) autosomal dominant woolly hair (hereditary woolly hair), and (3) autosomal recessive woolly hair (familial woolly hair).

The nonsyndromic autosomal recessive inherited form is associated with mutations within genes: P2RY5, LIPH, LPA, KRT25, and mPA-PLA1.[50–55] In the autosomal dominant type, a mutation within the helix initiation motif of the keratin 74 (KRT74) was described.[56] Depending on type of genetic background clinical appearance of the disease is variable from hair curling to hypotrichosis or total alopecia.

Woolly hair nevus is a distinct, nongenetically determined condition. It presents clinically as localized area with well-circumscribed border. The hair in this area is tightly curled, sometimes hypopigmented. First manifestation is at birth or during first 2 years of life.[57]

In woolly hair, trichoscopy demonstrates intensely wavy hair with a crawling snake appearance and broken hair shafts. Trichoscopy is not decisive for diagnosis, but the typical wavy appearance of hairs may indicate the need for detailed clinical evaluation.[5]

Trichothiodystrophy

Trichothiodystrophy (sulfur-deficient brittle hair) is associated with a group of neuroectodermal disorders.[58] Multiple symptoms may be associated with trichothiodystrophy. A recent systematic review of 112 published cases identified individuals at the age from 12 weeks to 47 years. In these patients, hair abnormalities were associated with developmental delay/intellectual impairment (86%), short stature (73%), ichthyosis (65%), abnormal characteristics at birth (55%), ocular abnormalities (51%), infections (46%), photosensitivity (42%), maternal pregnancy complications (28%), and defective DNA repair (37%). The spectrum of clinical features varied from mild disease with only hair involvement to severe disease with profound developmental defects, recurrent infections, and a high mortality at a young age.[59]

A new clinicogenetic classification of trichothiodystrophy distinguishes 3 types of disease: (1) the photosensitive type with mutations in genes encoding transcription/repair factor IIH (TFIIH) subunits (XPD, XPB, and TTDA), (2) the nonphotosensitive type, with TTDN1 mutation, and (3) the nonphotosensitive type, with no mutation in the gene encoding TTDN1 with no identified genetic basis.[60,61]

Clinical symptoms of trichothiodystrophy vary widely in type and severity. The single common feature in all patients is fragile hair.[62] In addition, hair loss may occur with periodic cyclicity. Increased hair loss during infections was observed.[63] Scalp hair, eyebrows, and eyelashes are brittle, unruly, and of variable lengths. Some investigators indicate that eyelashes may be long in trichothiodystrophy.[61]

Light microscopy shows hair shafts with an irregular, undulating contour and clean transverse fractures through the hair shaft (trichoschisis).[64]

The basis for diagnosis is examination of hair shafts in polarized light microscopy. Under polarized light, hair shafts show alternating bright and dark bands, often called tiger tail banding.[58] The diagnosis of trichothiodystrophy in polarized light microscopy should not be made on the basis of few hairs that appear to have alternating bright and dark bands. Rather, all hair should show the tiger tail pattern.[58]

Polarized light microscopy may be replaced by polarized transilluminating trichoscopy performed with a polarized handheld dermoscope.[65]

Nonpolarized trichoscopy has limited value in identifying trichothiodystrophy. It is not possible to demonstrate the characteristic phenomena, which are observed under polarized light microscopy (tiger tail). Trichoscopy examination can only suggest the necessity for further diagnosis of trichothiodystrophy, when hair shafts assessed at a high magnification have a nonhomogenous structure resembling grains of sand and their contour is very slightly wavy (**Fig. 6**).[5] Trichoschisis may be observed in trichoscopy, but distinction between trichoschisis and trichoclasis is rarely possible.[5]

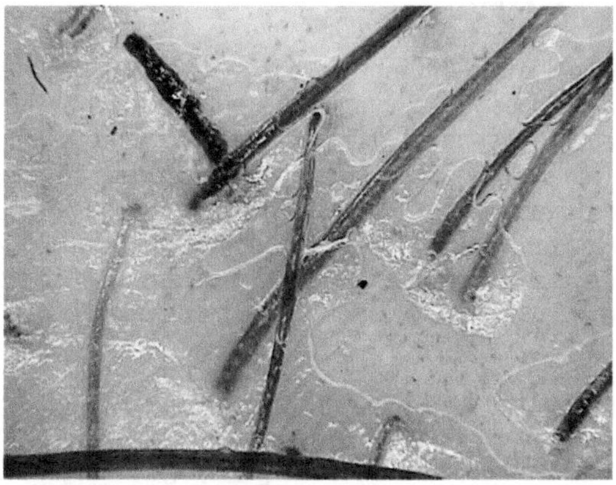

Fig. 6. Trichothiodystrophy. Trichoscopy in these cases does not reveal characteristic tiger tail hair shafts, which can be only detected in polarized light microscopy. It only can suggest the need for further diagnosis of trichothiodystrophy. In this image, short hair with transverse fracture, nonhomogenous structure, and wavy contour can be noticed (×70).

ECTODERMAL DYSPLASIAS

Hair shaft abnormalities are the main dermatological features of ectodermal dysplasias. Ectodermal dysplasias are a group of more than 200 genetic disorders caused by more than 50 different mutations in different genes, most commonly in the ectodysplasin A (*EDA*) 1, *EDA* receptor, and *EDA* receptor–associated death domain genes, which encode a ligand, a receptor, and an intracellular signal mediator of a single linear pathway.[66,67]

Ectodermal dysplasias are characterized by dysplasia of 2 or more tissues of ectodermal origin. These include abnormalities affecting hair, teeth, nails, sweat glands, and other tissues of ectodermal origin. In patients with ectodermal dysplasias, scalp hair is often sparse, light-pigmented, thin, dry, brittle, and curly.[68,69] In most patients, the number of hairs is significantly decreased.[70]

Trichoscopy shows hair abnormalities in most if not all patients with ectodermal dysplasias.[70] The most consistent findings are: increased percentage of follicular units with only 1 hair and heterogeneity in hair shaft pigmentation.[1,70] Patients have multiple hypopigmented (gray) hairs, regardless of age.[70] Various hair shaft structure abnormalities may be observed. These include pili torti, trichoschisis, and pili canaliculi. Trichorrhexis nodosa or monilethrix-like hairs may be present.[70] Occasionally, high-magnification trichoscopy reveals hair shafts with nonhomogenous, grainy structure, and a slightly wavy contour, which may be indicative of trichothiodystrophy. Cicatricial alopecia is extremely rare but may be present. In such cases trichoscopy shows homogenous ivory-white areas lacking follicular openings.[70]

Trichoscopy of eyebrows and eyelashes may show shows empty follicular openings, which appear as brown-gray, but in many cases commonly no abnormalities are observed.[70]

It is advisable to perform both, dry trichoscopy and trichoscopy with immersion fluid in patients suspected of hair abnormalities in the course of ectodermal dysplasias. Dry trichoscopy allows better visualization of hair shaft structure abnormalities, especially in patients with light-colored hair. Trichoscopy with immersion fluid allows to better evaluate the inner structure of hair shafts and skin surface abnormalities.

SUMMARY

A major field of progress in recent years is the use of trichoscopy, a noninvasive technique, for evaluation of hair shaft diseases in children and adults. Trichoscopy replaced light microscopy, which required pulling of multiple hairs for investigation. Now trichoscopy may be successfully applied in all known inherited and acquired hair shaft disorders.

REFERENCES

1. Rudnicka L, Olszewska M, Rakowska A. Atlas of trichoscopy: dermoscopy in hair and scalp disease. London: Springer; 2012.
2. Rudnicka L, Olszewska M, Rakowska A, et al. Trichoscopy: a new method for diagnosing hair loss. J Drugs Dermatol 2008;7:651–4.
3. Rudnicka L, Olszewska M, Slowinska M. Trichoscopy update 2011. J Dermatol Case Rep 2011;5:82–8.
4. Olszewska M, Rudnicka L, Rakowska A, et al. Trichoscopy. Arch Dermatol 2008;144:1007.
5. Rakowska A, Slowinska M, Kowalska-Oledzka E, et al. Trichoscopy in genetic hair shaft abnormalities. J Dermatol Case Rep 2008;2:14–20.
6. Rakowska A, Slowinska M, Czuwara J, et al. Dermoscopy as a tool for rapid diagnosis of monilethrix. J Drugs Dermatol 2007;6:222–4.
7. Rakowska A. Trichoscopy (hair and scalp videodermoscopy) in the healthy female. Method standardization and norms for measurable parameters. J Dermatol Case Rep 2009;3:14–9.
8. Vogt A, MK, Blume-Peytavi U. Biology of the hair follicle. In: Blume-Peytavi U, Tosti A, Whiting D, et al, editors. Hair; from basic science to clinical application. Berlin: Springer-Verlag; 2008. p. 1–22. ISBN: 3540469087.
9. Wagner R, Joekes I. Hair medulla morphology and mechanical properties. J Cosmet Sci 2007;58: 359–68.
10. Neila Iglesias J, Rodriguez Pichardo A, Garcia Bravo B, et al. Masquerading of trichotillomania in a family with monilethrix. Eur J Dermatol 2011; 21:133.
11. Nedoszytko B, Lewicka-Potocka Z, Szczerkowska-Dobosz A, et al. Monilethrix in monozygotic twins with very rare mutation in KRT 86 gene. J Eur Acad Dermatol Venereol 2017;31:e409–10.
12. Zlotogorski A, Marek D, Horev L, et al. An autosomal recessive form of monilethrix is caused by mutations in DSG4: clinical overlap with localized autosomal recessive hypotrichosis. J Invest Dermatol 2006; 126:1292–6.
13. Mirmirani P, Huang KP, Price VH. A practical, algorithmic approach to diagnosing hair shaft disorders. Int J Dermatol 2011;50:1–12.
14. Sharma VK, Chiramel MJ, Rao A. Dermoscopy: a rapid bedside tool to assess monilethrix. Indian J Dermatol Venereol Leprol 2016;82:73–4.
15. Jain N, Khopkar U. Monilethrix in pattern distribution in siblings: diagnosis by trichoscopy. Int J Trichology 2010;2:56–9.
16. Zitelli JA. Pseudomonilethrix. An artifact. Arch Dermatol 1986;122:688–90.
17. Itin PH, Schiller P, Mathys D, et al. Cosmetically induced hair beads. J Am Acad Dermatol 1997;36: 260–1.
18. Rudnicka L, Rakowska A, Kerzeja M, et al. Hair shafts in trichoscopy: clues for diagnosis of hair and scalp diseases. Dermatol Clin 2013;31:695–708, x.
19. Rudnicka L, Rakowska A, Olszewska M. Trichoscopy: how it may help the clinician. Dermatol Clin 2013;31:29–41.
20. Pirmez R, Pineiro-Maceira J, Sodre CT. Exclamation marks and other trichoscopic signs of chemotherapy-induced alopecia. Australas J Dermatol 2013;54(2):129–32.
21. Bartels NGB-PU. Hair loss in children. In: Blume-Peytavi U, Tosti A, Whiting D, et al, editors. Hair growth and disorders. Leipzig (Germany): Springer; 2008. p. 293–4.
22. Smith VV, Anderson G, Malone M, et al. Light microscopic examination of scalp hair samples as an aid in the diagnosis of paediatric disorders: retrospective review of more than 300 cases from a single centre. J Clin Pathol 2005;58:1294–8.
23. Rakowska A, Olszewska M, Rudnicka L. Trichoscopy of scalp dysesthesia. Postepy Dermatol Alergol 2017;34:245–7.
24. Singh G, Miteva M. Prognosis and management of congenital hair shaft disorders with fragility-Part I. Pediatr Dermatol 2016;33:473–80.
25. Boussofara L, Ghannouchi N, Ghariani N, et al. Netherton's syndrome: the importance of eyebrow hair. Dermatol Online J 2007;13:21.
26. Sarri CA, Roussaki-Schulze A, Vasilopoulos Y, et al. Netherton syndrome: a genotype-phenotype review. Mol Diagn Ther 2017;21:137–52.
27. Shi ZR, Xu M, Tan GZ, et al. A case of Netherton syndrome with mutation in SPINK5 and FLG. Eur J Dermatol 2017;27:536–7.
28. Rakowska A, Kowalska-Oledzka E, Slowinska M, et al. Hair shaft videodermoscopy in netherton syndrome. Pediatr Dermatol 2009;26:320–2.
29. Goujon E, Beer F, Fraitag S, et al. 'Matchstick' eyebrow hairs: a dermoscopic clue to the diagnosis of Netherton syndrome. J Eur Acad Dermatol Venereol 2010;24:740–1.
30. Powell J. Increasing the likelihood of early diagnosis of Netherton syndrome by simple examination of eyebrow hairs. Arch Dermatol 2000;136: 423–4.

31. Neri I, Balestri R, Starace M, et al. Videodermoscopy of eyelashes in Netherton syndrome. J Eur Acad Dermatol Venereol 2011;25(11):1360–1.
32. Whiting DA, Dy LC. Office diagnosis of hair shaft defects. Semin Cutan Med Surg 2006;25:24–34.
33. Mirmirani P, Samimi SS, Mostow E. Pili torti: clinical findings, associated disorders, and new insights into mechanisms of hair twisting. Cutis 2009;84: 143–7.
34. Shigematsu Y, Hayashi R, Yoshida K, et al. Novel heterozygous deletion mutation c.821delC in the AAA domain of BCS1L underlies Bjornstad syndrome. J Dermatol 2017;44:e111–2.
35. Sikorska MS-DA, Purzycka-Bohdan D, Nowicki R. Pili torti and multiple facial milia as an expression of ectodermal dysplasia in monozygotic twins. Przegl Dermatol 2014;101:35–9.
36. Hays SB, Camisa C. Acquired pili torti in two patients treated with synthetic retinoids. Cutis 1985; 35:466–8.
37. Sakamoto F, Ito M, Saito R. Ultrastructural study of acquired pili torti-like hair defects accompanying pseudopelade. J Dermatol 2002;29:197–201.
38. Cheng AS, Bayliss SJ. The genetics of hair shaft disorders. J Am Acad Dermatol 2008;59:1–22 [quiz: 3–6].
39. Giehl KA, Rogers MA, Radivojkov M, et al. Pili annulati: refinement of the locus on chromosome 12q24.33 to a 2.9-Mb interval and candidate gene analysis. Br J Dermatol 2009;160:527–33.
40. Bhoyrul B, Lindsay H, Robinson R, et al. Pili annulati in a case of Rothmund-Thomson syndrome with a novel frameshift mutation in RECQL4. J Eur Acad Dermatol Venereol 2018;32(6):e221–3.
41. Streck AP, Moncores M, Sarmento DF, et al. Study of nanomechanical properties of human hair shaft in a case of pili annulati by atomic force microscopy. J Eur Acad Dermatol Venereol 2007;21:1109–10.
42. Giehl KA, Schmuth M, Tosti A, et al. Concomitant manifestation of pili annulati and alopecia areata: coincidental rather than true association. Acta Derm Venereol 2011;91:459–62.
43. Feldmann KA, Dawber RP, Pittelkow MR, et al. Newly described weathering pattern in pili annulati hair shafts: a scanning electron microscopic study. J Am Acad Dermatol 2001;45:625–7.
44. Nam CH, Park M, Choi MS, et al. Pili annulati with multiple fragile hairs. Ann Dermatol 2017; 29:254–6.
45. Giehl KA, Ferguson DJ, Dawber RP, et al. Update on detection, morphology and fragility in pili annulati in three kindreds. J Eur Acad Dermatol Venereol 2004; 18:654–8.
46. Lee SS, Lee YS, Giam YC. Pseudopili annulati in a dark-haired individual: a light and electron microscopic study. Pediatr Dermatol 2001;18(1): 27–30.
47. Chien AJ, Valentine MC, Sybert VP. Hereditary woolly hair and keratosis pilaris. J Am Acad Dermatol 2006;54(2 Suppl):S35–9.
48. Jimenez-Sanchez MD, Garcia-Hernandez MJ, Camacho FM. Woolly hair with alopecia areata in a Caucasian girl. Eur J Dermatol 2010;20:245–6.
49. Hutchinson PE, Cairns RJ, Wells RS. Woolly hair. Clinical and general aspects. Trans St Johns Hosp Dermatol Soc 1974;60:160–77.
50. Horev L, Tosti A, Rosen I, et al. Mutations in lipase H cause autosomal recessive hypotrichosis simplex with woolly hair. J Am Acad Dermatol 2009;61: 813–8.
51. Horev L, Babay S, Ramot Y, et al. Mutations in two genes on chromosome 13 resulting in a complex hair and skin phenotype due to two rare genodermatoses: KLICK and autosomal recessive woolly hair/ hypotrichosis simplex. Br J Dermatol 2011;164: 1113–6.
52. Horev L, Saad-Edin B, Ingber A, et al. A novel deletion mutation in P2RY5/LPA(6) gene cause autosomal recessive woolly hair with hypotrichosis. J Eur Acad Dermatol Venereol 2010;24:858–9.
53. Shimomura Y, Wajid M, Ishii Y, et al. Disruption of P2RY5, an orphan G protein-coupled receptor, underlies autosomal recessive woolly hair. Nat Genet 2008;40:335–9.
54. Shimomura Y, Ito M, Christiano AM. Mutations in the LIPH gene in three Japanese families with autosomal recessive woolly hair/hypotrichosis. J Dermatol Sci 2009;56:205–7.
55. Yu X, Chen F, Ni C, et al. A missense mutation within the helix termination motif of KRT25 causes autosomal dominant woolly hair/hypotrichosis. J Invest Dermatol 2018;138:230–3.
56. Shimomura Y, Wajid M, Petukhova L, et al. Autosomal-dominant woolly hair resulting from disruption of keratin 74 (KRT74), a potential determinant of human hair texture. Am J Hum Genet 2010;86:632–8.
57. Kumaran S, Dogra S, Handa S, et al. Woolly hair nevus. Pediatr Dermatol 2004;21:609–10.
58. Itin PH, Sarasin A, Pittelkow MR. Trichothiodystrophy: update on the sulfur-deficient brittle hair syndromes. J Am Acad Dermatol 2001;44:891–920 [quiz: 1–4].
59. Arseni L, Lanzafame M, Compe E, et al. TFIIH-dependent MMP-1 overexpression in trichothiodystrophy leads to extracellular matrix alterations in patient skin. Proc Natl Acad Sci U S A 2015;112: 1499–504.
60. Morice-Picard F, Cario-Andre M, Rezvani H, et al. New clinico-genetic classification of trichothiodystrophy. Am J Med Genet A 2009;149A:2020–30.
61. Zhou X, Khan SG, Tamura D, et al. Brittle hair, developmental delay, neurologic abnormalities, and photosensitivity in a 4-year-old girl. J Am Acad Dermatol 2010;63:323–8.

62. Itin PH, Fistarol SK. Hair shaft abnormalities–clues to diagnosis and treatment. Dermatology 2005;211: 63–71.
63. Liang C, Kraemer KH, Morris A, et al. Characterization of tiger-tail banding and hair shaft abnormalities in trichothiodystrophy. J Am Acad Dermatol 2005; 52:224–32.
64. Forslind B, Andersson MK, Alsterborg E. Hereditary hair changes revealed by analysis of single hair fibres by scanning electron microscopy. Scanning Microsc 1991;5:867–74 [discussion: 74–5].
65. Yang YW, Yarbrough K, Mitkov M, et al. Polarized transilluminating dermoscopy: bedside trichoscopic diagnosis of trichothiodystrophy. Pediatr Dermatol 2018;35:147–9.
66. Cluzeau C, Hadj-Rabia S, Jambou M, et al. Only four genes (EDA1, EDAR, EDARADD, and WNT10A) account for 90% of hypohidrotic/anhidrotic ectodermal dysplasia cases. Hum Mutat 2011;32:70–2.
67. Mikkola ML. Molecular aspects of hypohidrotic ectodermal dysplasia. Am J Med Genet A 2009;149A: 2031–6.
68. Mehta U, Brunworth J, Fete TJ, et al. Head and neck manifestations and quality of life of patients with ectodermal dysplasia. Otolaryngol Head Neck Surg 2007;136:843–7.
69. Rouse C, Siegfried E, Breer W, et al. Hair and sweat glands in families with hypohidrotic ectodermal dysplasia: further characterization. Arch Dermatol 2004;140:850–5.
70. Rakowska A, Gorska R, Rudnicka L, et al. Trichoscopic hair evaluation in patients with ectodermal dysplasia. J Pediatr 2015;167:193–5.
71. Martin AM, Sugathan P. Localised acquired trichorrhexis nodosa of the scalp hair induced by a specific comb and combing habit - a report of three cases. Int J Trichology 2011;3:34–7.
72. Mirmirani P. Ceramic flat irons: improper use leading to acquired trichorrhexis nodosa. J Am Acad Dermatol 2010;62:145–7.
73. Burkhart CG, Burkhart CN. Trichorrhexis nodosa revisited. Skinmed 2007;6:57–8.
74. Callender VD, McMichael AJ, Cohen GF. Medical and surgical therapies for alopecias in black women. Dermatol Ther 2004;17:164–76.
75. Chernosky ME, Owens DW. Trichorrhexis nodosa. Clinical and investigative studies. Arch Dermatol 1966;94:577–85.
76. Pollitt RJ, Jenner FA, Davies M. Sibs with mental and physical retardation and trichorrhexis nodosa with abnormal amino acid composition of the hair. Arch Dis Child 1968;43:211–6.
77. Fabre A, Andre N, Breton A, et al. Intractable diarrhea with "phenotypic anomalies" and tricho-hepato-enteric syndrome: two names for the same disorder. Am J Med Genet A 2007;143:584–8.
78. Erez A, Nagamani SC, Lee B. Argininosuccinate lyase deficiency-argininosuccinic aciduria and beyond. Am J Med Genet C Semin Med Genet 2011;157:45–53.
79. Abdel-Salam GM, Afifi HH, Eid MM, et al. Ectodermal abnormalities in patients with kabuki syndrome. Pediatr Dermatol 2011;28(5):507–11.
80. Wang XH, Lu JL, Zhang LP, et al. Clinical and laboratory features of the Menkes disease. Zhonghua Er Ke Za Zhi 2009;47:604–7 [in Chinese].
81. Kelly SC, Ratajczak P, Keller M, et al. A novel GJA 1 mutation in oculo-dento-digital dysplasia with curly hair and hyperkeratosis. Eur J Dermatol 2006;16: 241–5.
82. Colomb D, Cretin J, Vibert J, et al. Trichorrhexis nodosa in a hypothrepsic child with hypovitaminosis A. Lyon Med 1970;223:337–8 [in French].
83. Botta E, Nardo T, Broughton BC, et al. Analysis of mutations in the XPD gene in Italian patients with trichothiodystrophy: site of mutation correlates with repair deficiency, but gene dosage appears to determine clinical severity. Am J Hum Genet 1998; 63:1036–48.
84. Lurie R, Ben-Amitai D, Laron Z. Laron syndrome (primary growth hormone insensitivity): a unique model to explore the effect of insulin-like growth factor 1 deficiency on human hair. Dermatology 2004;208:314–8.
85. Silengo M, Valenzise M, Pagliardini S, et al. Hair changes in congenital disorders of glycosylation (CDG type 1). Eur J Pediatr 2003;162:114–5.
86. Traupe H, Happle R, Grobe H, et al. Polarization microscopy of hair in acrodermatitis enteropathica. Pediatr Dermatol 1986;3:300–3.
87. Slonim AE, Sadick N, Pugliese M, et al. Clinical response of alopecia, trichorrhexis nodosa, and dry, scaly skin to zinc supplementation. J Pediatr 1992;121:890–5.
88. Blume-Peytavi U, Fohles J, Schulz R, et al. Hypotrichosis, hair structure defects, hypercysteine hair and glucosuria: a new genetic syndrome? Br J Dermatol 1996;134:319–24.
89. Colomb D, Ducros B, Boussuge N. Bazex, Dupre and Christol syndrome. Apropos of a case with prolymphocytic leukemia. Ann Dermatol Venereol 1989; 116:381–7 [in French].
90. Lurie R, Hodak E, Ginzburg A, et al. Trichorrhexis nodosa: a manifestation of hypothyroidism. Cutis 1996;57:358–9.

Onychoscopy
Dermoscopy of the Nails

Bianca Maria Piraccini, MD, PhD*, Aurora Alessandrini, MD[1], Michela Starace, MD, PhD[1]

KEYWORDS

• Onychoscopy • Nail dermoscopy • Onycholysis • Nail infection • Subungual mass • Melanonychia
• Subungual hematoma • Traumatic onycholysis

KEY POINTS

- In recent years, onychoscopy has become increasingly appreciated as an effective tool to facilitate the clinical assessment of nail diseases.
- In daily practice, onychoscopy may confirm the clinical diagnosis and guide the management of nail diseases and treatments by permitting a better visualization of signs.
- The 2 main lesions for which nail onychoscopy are crucial are pigmented lesions and onycholysis, with or without subungual hyperkeratosis.
- Pigmented nail lesions are common and can be challenging for clinicians, especially in making a differential diagnosis.
- Onycholysis is not specific of any disease but it is often associated with the more frequent nail diseases.

INTRODUCTION

Nail disorders are often a diagnostic challenge for dermatologists in daily practice and the introduction of dermoscopy during the routine evaluation helps to better manage nail alterations. Currently, nail dermoscopy, or onychoscopy, is sometimes used by nail experts only to magnify the clinical features of nail diseases that are not well visualized with naked eye; whereas, other times, it is helpful for a more accurate diagnosis and to avoid invasive methods. The use of onychoscopy is expanding from the managing of nail melanocytic lesions to all types of nail alterations. It has been shown to decrease the number of unnecessary excisions of benign lesions. In daily practice, onychoscopy may be a useful tool with which to elucidate common findings about specific diseases, to reinforce presumptive clinical diagnoses, as well as to guide the management and prognosis of different nail diseases. The use of onychoscopy can be applied to all visible parts of the nail unit; however, it is also possible to observe the nail matrix, the only nonvisible part, in conjunction with intraoperative methods. The dermatoscope may be used dry in evaluation of the nail plate surface or matrix diseases or with ultrasound gel in cases of nail pigmentation, onycholysis, and for the evaluation of the distal nail margin. For the examination of the nail apparatus, the authors recommend the use of a gel, such as ultrasound gel, as an immersion medium because the decreased viscosity permits it to stay on the nail plate and fill any concavities without rolling off. The recommended procedure is to start with initial dry observation, followed by application of an interface medium. For the evaluation of nail diseases and to appreciate the thin signs within the nail plate, it is useful to vary the focus of the device during the

Conflict of Interest: None.
Department of Specialised Experimental and Diagnostic Medicine, Dermatology, Alma Mater Studiorum, Università di Bologna, Bologna, Italy
[1] Present address: Via Massarenti 1, Bologna 40138, Italy.
* Corresponding author. Dermatology Unit, Via Massarenti 1, Bologna 40138, Italy.
E-mail address: Biancamaria.piraccini@unibo.it

Dermatol Clin 36 (2018) 431–438
https://doi.org/10.1016/j.det.2018.05.010

examination. Another suggestion is to start with low magnification (10 times), at which it is possible to observe the nail as a whole, and to then move to higher magnifications, depending of the onychoscopic features, up to 70 times.

This article summarizes cases in which onychoscopy is useful in daily practice. In particular, the 2 main lesions for which the role of nail dermoscopy is crucial are pigmented lesions and onycholysis, with or without subungual hyperkeratosis.

Pigmented Nail Lesions

According to the patterns found, nail experts agree that onychoscopy is useful to distinguish melanic from nonmelanic pigmentation, such as blood or exogenous substances.[1] Melanonychia refers to a black-brown-grey pigmentation of the nail plate. It usually appears as a longitudinal band, which starts from the proximal margin and extends to the distal margin of the nail, following the growth of the nail. Three steps have been identified for evaluating cases of melanonychia[2]:

1. Establish whether the pigment is melanic
2. If it is melanic, determine if the pigmentation is due to activation or proliferation of nail matrix melanocytes
3. If it is a proliferation, determine whether it is benign or malignant.

Generally, a melanic pigmentation is brown-black in color, located within the nail plate, and the shape is a longitudinal band (but transversal or total aspects have been detected); whereas exogenous pigmentations include different substances that adhere to or are below the nail plate and do not usually have a longitudinal appearance but are located near the nail folds or in the center of the nail plate with homogenous distribution. Common causes of nonmelanic pigmentations are subungual hematoma, *Pseudomonas* infection (green nails), or fungal melanonychia.

In subungual hematoma, which is among the most frequent causes of a brown-black nail pigmentation, onychoscopy is diagnostic because it shows typical features: the pigmentation appears as a red-purple-brown round structure with homogeneous color and it has a globular pattern in the proximal edge and a linear distribution in the distal edge, with peripheral fading. A higher onychoscopy magnification permits the differentiation of acute hematoma from chronic hematoma. Typical of the acute phase are well-circumscribed reddish dots or streaks, or a filamentous pattern, at the distal edge, together with the red-purple to black color of the lesion, whereas the red-brown color associated with splinter hemorrhages and a linear pattern indicates a chronic or minor trauma[3] (**Fig. 1**). However, any subungual hematoma that does not grow out with the nail and that is not continuously being transferred toward the distal edge but persists at the same place requires a further examination to exclude other diagnoses.[4]

In green nails, the pigmentation is characterized by a green or black discoloration and is due to colonization by *Pseudomonas aeruginosa* that produces a pigment named pyocyanin, which adheres to the irregular nail plate surface or is located under an onycholytic nail plate.[5] The exogenous deposition above the nail plate may clinically resemble a band of melanonychia when it has a longitudinal arrangement along the lateral side of the nail plate. Onychoscopy typically shows a bright green color that fades to yellow at the periphery. Onychoscopy also allows recognition of dark pigmentation due to pyocyanin presence under the nail plate from melanonychia because it shows a convex proximal shape of the pigmentation, which does not start from the matrix (**Fig. 2**). In this case, clipping away the detached nail plate is advised to observe the deposition of the pigment, which can be gently scraped away with gauze with antiseptic solution until it reveals a normal nail bed.[2]

A longitudinal black band of the nail can be also due to fungal melanonychia, a rare variant of onychomycosis caused by *Trichophyton rubrum var melanoides* or by other fungi. In fungal melanonychia, onychoscopy shows a multicolored pigmentation that is wider in the distal end and ranges in color from yellow to brown to gray and/or black or red (when hemorrhages are present). The main pattern

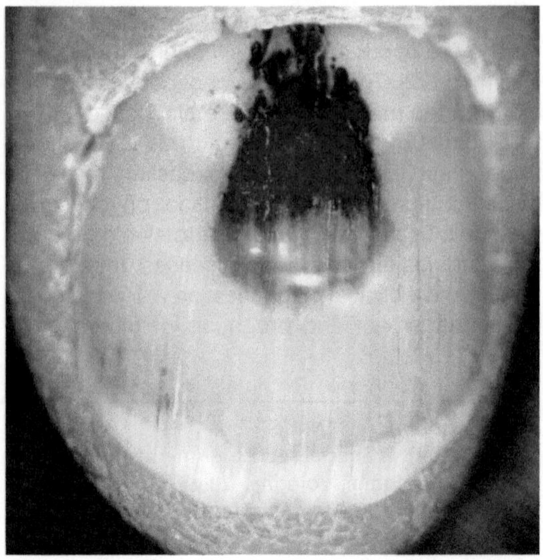

Fig. 1. Onychoscopy of subungual hematoma of a fingernail.

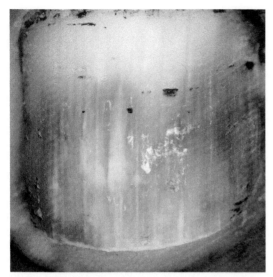

Fig. 2. Onychoscopy of *Pseudomonas aeruginosa* infection, seen after removing nail polish.

is homogeneous, occasionally with black pigment aggregates 0.1 mm or greater in size, which are either coarse granules or pigmented clumps.[6] Onychoscopy of the distal margin shows a thick subungual hyperkeratosis with yellow and brown-black scales that correspond to the accumulation of fungal colonies[7] (**Fig. 3**). Other main onychoscopic alterations are a matte black nail plate pigmentation, seen as lines, and a disrupted black linear pigmentation with a blurred appearance.[6]

After an exogenous deposition of the pigmentation has been excluded, as in cases of a longitudinal melanonychia, the second step is the distinction between a benign activation of melanocytes and a true melanocytic proliferation. Unfortunately, the examination of longitudinal melanonychia is limited to the inspection of the pigment that was deposited in the nail plate weeks to months earlier[8]; however, onychoscopy is essential for the first evaluation of the pigmentation. Before observing a melanonychia with a dermatoscope to distinguish the origin of the pigment, some clinical features must be noted, including (1) modality of onset of the band: time and course; (2) number of digits involved; and (3) history of the patient: age, race, personal and pathologic history, drugs, and hobbies. Next, the dermoscope can be used to observe the distal margin of the nail plate. If the pigmentation is located on the lower part of the nail plate, the lesion is likely to start in the distal matrix; on the other hand, if the pigmentation is found in the dorsum of the nail plate, it indicates a more proximal origin of the pigment.[9] This information can be used to better target the biopsy and to avoid a visible definitive nail dystrophy if the surgery is limited to the distal matrix. Onychoscopy then provides useful additional information that can be added to the clinical details to help the clinician to decide if a nail biopsy is required, including

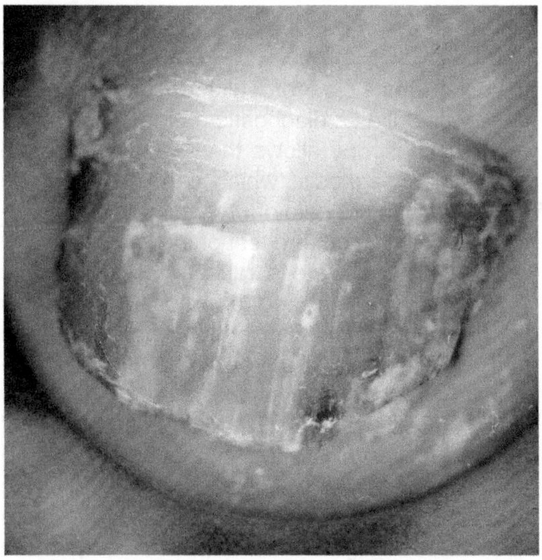

Fig. 3. Onychoscopy of fungal melanonychia: black pigmentation with yellow and brown scales.

1. The background of the band is brown to black and the color can be more or less pronounced and homogeneous
2. The borders can be well-defined or less sharp
3. The width can range from a few millimeters to the entire nail plate
4. The longitudinal lines of the band can be regular or irregular in thickness along their length, continuous or interrupted, and parallel to each other or not.

The collection of this information permits classification of the band of longitudinal melanonychia[4,10]:

Melanocyte activation

- The bands are often polydactylic, monochromic, stable in size and shape, or may have a well-defined cause (eg, drugs, repetitive trauma, dermatologic condition, inducing periungual inflammation, systemic factors, predisposing ethnic origin)
- Adults and children can be affected
- Onychoscopy shows a homogeneous gray background with thin, longitudinal, gray lines and regular borders (**Fig. 4**).

Benign melanocyte proliferation (lentigo or nevus of the nail matrix)

- The band is monodactyl and polychromic, with changes in width and color over time
- Adults and children can be affected

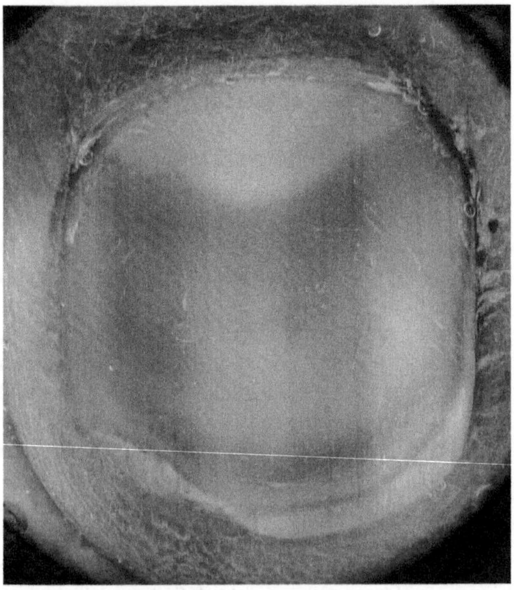

Fig. 4. Onychoscopy of longitudinal melanonychia due melanocytic activation: homogeneous coloration of the background with thin, longitudinal, gray lines.

- Onychoscopy in adults shows a brown background associated with regular parallel lines of identical color and width
- Onychoscopy in children shows a brown background with longitudinal lines that may have different color and irregular width.

Malignant melanocyte proliferation (nail matrix melanoma)

- The band is monodactyl, multicolor, and rapidly enlarging
- Adults are affected
- Onychoscopy shows a brown background associated with longitudinal lines that are irregular in color, width, spacing, and parallelism (**Fig. 5**).

According to the literature,[11] the use of onychoscopy in cases of suspected nail melanoma is useful particularly in 2 situations: (1) when nail melanoma presents as an ulcerated nodule of the nail bed (amelanotic melanoma), onychoscopy can sometimes show the presence of the so-called micro-Hutchinson sign, a periungual melanic pigmentation due to tumor spread that is not visible by naked-eye observation; and (2) when nail melanoma presents as a band of longitudinal melanonychia, not associated with periungual pigmentation and/or nail plate changes. In these cases, observation of an irregular pattern of lines and borders should suggest a nail matrix biopsy.

The following algorithm has been created to indicate, step by step, the correct procedure to

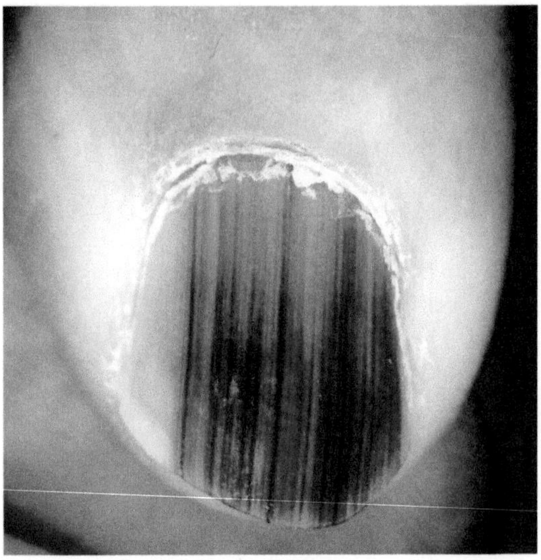

Fig. 5. Onychoscopy of a melanoma in situ of fifth fingernail: longitudinal lines irregular in color, width, spacing, and parallelism.

follow in the case of an adult patient with suspected nail apparatus melanoma. Look first at the nail plate and the periungual tissue to find any pigmentation visible by the naked eye and then look with a dermoscope. If there is periungual pigmentation, the diagnosis of melanoma is highly suggested and biopsy is mandatory. In cases of a nail bed nodule with ulceration, its association with Hutchinson sign is diagnostic for invasive nail melanoma. The use of a dermatoscope may detect micro-Hutchinson sign and irregular vascular structures with atypical vessels. All cases should indeed be biopsied.

Onycholysis

The second nail sign for which onychoscopy can be very useful as a diagnostic method is onycholysis. Onychoscopy allows the examiner to make the correct diagnosis, which can eventually be confirmed with the help of other diagnostic instruments, such as a culture test or nail biopsy and/or avulsion. The nail plate is transparent and, when it is attached to the nail bed, has a pink color that is due to nail bed vascularization. When separated from the nail bed, in onycholysis, the nail plate appears white due to the presence of air underneath.[12] Bacterial colonization or presence of exogenous particles may change the color to yellow-green-black. Onycholysis starts with the disruption of the distal onychocorneal band, which is the site of the greatest adhesion of nail plate to nail bed. This is not specific to any diseases but it is frequently associated with the most common nail diseases when combined with other onychoscopic signs that often allow differential diagnosis.

In case of onycholysis, it is important to assess some clinical parameters:

- Modality of onset: acute or chronic, time, duration
- Pain associated with development
- Clinical signs: color, shape of the border of detachment, presence of hyperkeratosis
- Onychoscopy signs: specific for any type of onycholysis.

Based on these alterations, onycholysis can be distinguished in traumatic onycholysis:

- Bilateral and symmetric detachment of nail plate with a chronic modality of onset over time
- It is painless
- The line of detachment of the plate from the bed is linear, regular, and smooth, and surrounded by a normally pale pink-bed, without hyperkeratosis.

The subungual space is usually whitish to yellow and, frequently, black drops or lines corresponding to hemorrhages due to traumas can be observed. A pathway resembling atrial fibrillation to the distal margin is a traumatic sign (**Fig. 6**).

Onycholysis due to distal subungual onychomycosis[13]

- Usually affects 1 or both great toenails with a stable onycholysis
- Is painless
- The 4 important dermoscopic patterns are a jagged edge of the proximal margin of the onycholytic area, with sharp structures (spikes) directed toward the proximal fold; white-yellow longitudinal striae in the onycholytic nail plate; an overall appearance of the affected nail plate in parallel bands of different colors, resembling the aurora borealis and, in fact, named Aurora borealis pattern; and ruined appearance of the subungual yellow hyperkeratosis due to the accumulation of dermal debris of fungal invasion, more visible with frontal dermoscopy[14] (**Fig. 7**).

Other types pf onychomycosis for which onychoscopy can be useful include white superficial onychomycosis (WSO), proximal subungual onychomycosis (PSO), and dermatophytoma. In WSO, fungi invade the dorsal nail plate, forming white opaque formations, which are easily scraped away. The dermoscopic pattern of WSO is a nail plate with several small white opaque and friable patches (**Fig. 8**). For a better result of the image, performing dry dermoscopy is recommended because the use of a gel for an interface induces a partial disappearance of the white discoloration that includes the scales irregularly spread on the nail surface. Onychoscopy helps in the differential diagnosis with superficial nail fragility due to prolonged wearing of nail polish and transverse toenail leukonychia due to trauma. In PSO, fungi reach the ventral part of the proximal nail plate via proximal nail fold, so they are located under the proximal part of the nail. PSO due to

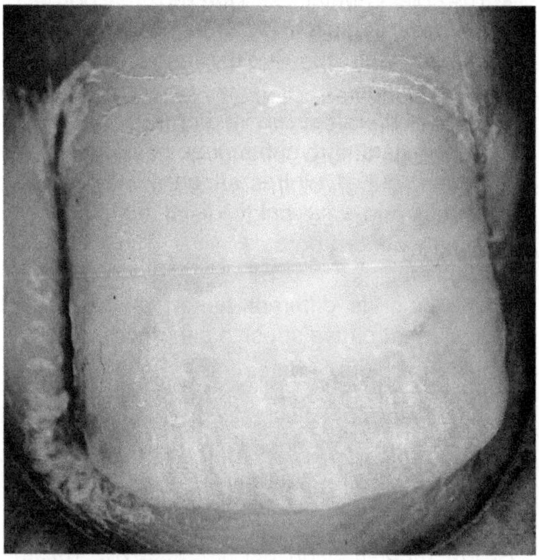

Fig. 6. Onychoscopy of traumatic onycholysis, characterized by a linear, regular, and smooth line of detachment of nail plate from nail bed, surrounded by a normally pale pink-bed, without hyperkeratosis.

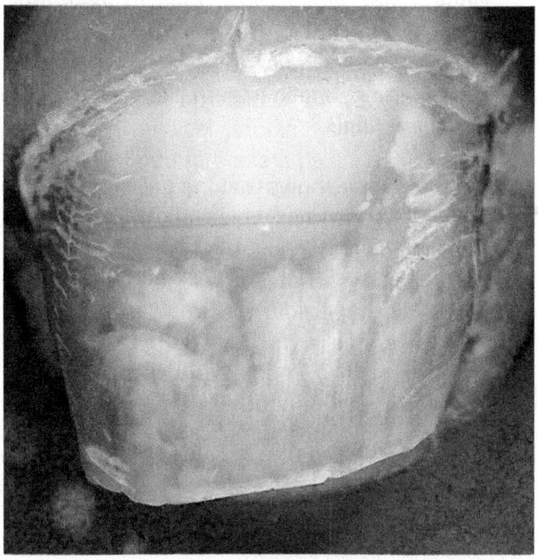

Fig. 7. Onychoscopy of distal subungual onychomycosis: white-yellow longitudinal striae in the onycholytic nail plate.

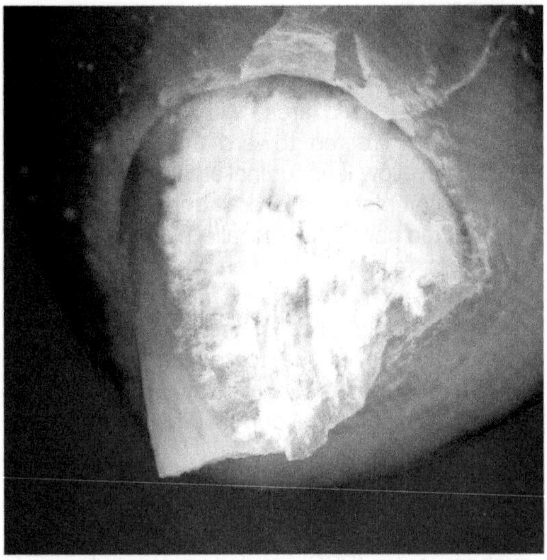

Fig. 8. Onychoscopy of white superficial onychomycosis of the fifth toenail.

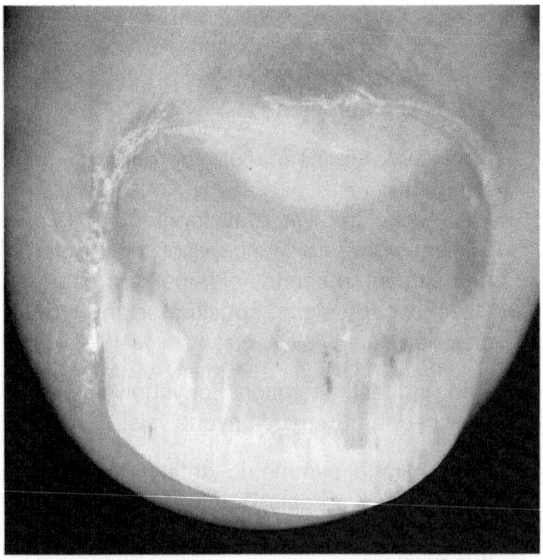

Fig. 9. Onychoscopy of onycholysis due to nail psoriasis: an erythematous border surrounding the distal edge of the detachment. Splinter hemorrhages are also visible.

dermatophytes is very rare and is characterized by a white area under the proximal nail plate, in the lunula area, better visualized by a dermatoscope. Dermatophytoma is a subungual accumulation of hyphae and scales, which appears as yellow-orange round areas under the nail plate, connected distally with a longitudinal band of onycholysis. Dermoscopy shows an irregular subungual accumulation with a round shape, yellow-orange in color, connected by a thin narrow channel to the distal edge of the nail plate.

Onycholysis due to nail psoriasis

- Can involve the matrix or the bed and the signs differ accordingly but an extremely wide spectrum of symptoms may be present, which vary in severity and type
- Is typical in psoriatic fingernails, greater in the dominant hand
- Is painless
- Onychoscopy shows that the proximal margin of the onycholysis, which clinically appears red-pink is color, is bright yellow-orange, and is associated with a slightly dented margin (Fig. 9).

Dermoscopy of the hyponychium is also very helpful to confirm the diagnosis of psoriasis in patients with simple onycholysis or mild nail bed hyperkeratosis showing irregularly distributed, dilated, tortuous, and elongated capillaries, similar to those seen in skin psoriasis.[15] Capillary density is positively correlated with the disease severity and response to treatment. Capillaries are better visualized at 40 times magnification. With a hand-held dermatoscope, they appear as regular red dots[16] and may also be visible on the proximal nail fold in very marked inflamed diseases.

Idiopathic onycholysis

- Fingernails are usually affected as a result of cleaning underneath the nail with a sharp object, greater in the nondominant hand. The aspect is diffusely homogeneous; possible alteration of proximal nail folds can be present due to manipulation by the patient
- It is painless
- The color is whitish and the proximal border of onycholysis is usually straight or linear and regular with the typical aspect of roller-coaster type.
- No hyperkeratosis is present (Fig. 10).

Onycholysis due to subungual mass

- Usually only 1 digit is affected with irregular aspect and with bulgy distal margin and a slightly dented border
- Is painful
- The color is different based on subungual mass that cause specific alterations.

In cases of onychopapilloma, a filiform keratotic subungual mass or a fissure is present at the distal margin in correspondence with the streak. This is associated with a longitudinal red band, starting from the lunula and reaching to the distal margin, with splinter hemorrhages[17,18] (Fig. 11). In subungual exostosis, a benign bony proliferation of the distal phalanx occurring beneath the nail, onychoscopy shows onycholysis and subungual hyperkeratosis. The most common finding of vascular

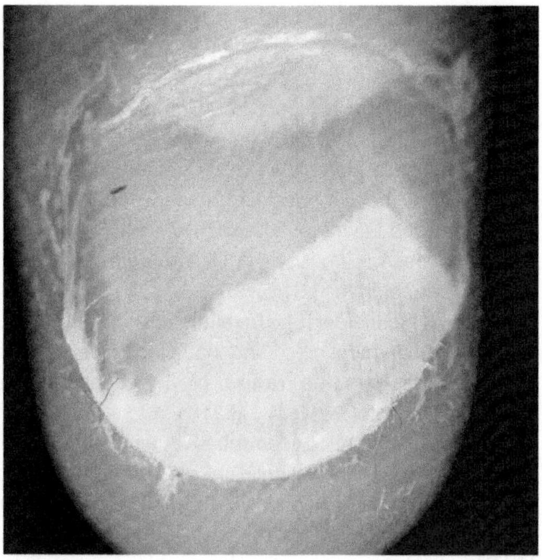

Fig. 10. Onychoscopy of idiopathic onycholysis, characterized by a whitish color and the proximal border of onycholysis with the typical aspect of roller-coaster type.

ectasia is probably due to neoangiogenesis associated with subungual mass.[19] A radiograph is necessary to confirm the suspected disease.

DISCUSSION

Oonychoscopy should be used routinely in the evaluation of nail diseases because it provides important information. Dermoscopic observation of the nail can be performed with a handheld dermoscope, which allows visualization of the entire nail simultaneously, or with a videodermoscope, which allows different magnifications. The main technical problem with onychoscopy comes from nail plate convexity and hardness, which makes it difficult to obtain complete apposition of the lens to the surface: a gel should be used as an interface medium.

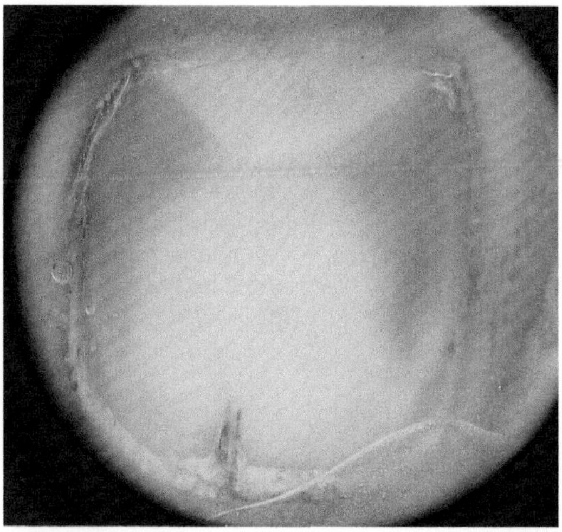

Fig. 11. Onycholysis due to the presence of filiform onychopapilloma.

Increasingly, onychoscopy-based diagnostic criteria for various nail diseases are being refined and evolved. Onychoscopy has come a long way from being an investigational fad to being a reliable diagnostic tool. It definitely permits better visualization of nail signs but also, for some diseases, it adds greatly to the clinical examination and reveals suggestive features not otherwise visible to the naked eye. Over the years, the clarity of dermoscopic characteristics for various nail disease has increased. Furthermore, newer indications and findings are being reported. Currently, the indications for onychoscopy include nail pigmentation, onychomycosis, nail psoriasis, nail lichen planus, traumatic nail abnormalities, and nail tumors such as onychomatricoma and glomus tumor. Pigmented nail lesions are common and can be challenging for clinicians, especially in making a differential diagnosis. Usually, the presence of a pigmented and/or dystrophic nail should raise the suspicion of melanoma and this should be excluded before considering other diagnoses. In onycholysis, onychoscopy can be very useful for observing, with high magnification, the space detached as a result of different causes, such as traumatic event, nail psoriasis, onychomycosis, and the presence of subungual mass.

REFERENCES

1. Di Chiacchio N, Hirata AH, Daniel R, et al. Consensus on melanonychia nail plate dermoscopy. An Bras Dermatol 2013;88:309–13.
2. Piraccini BM, Dika E, Fanti PA. Nail disorders: practical tips for diagnosis and treatment. Dermatol Clin 2015;33:185–95.
3. Sato T, Tanaka M. The reason for red streaks on dermoscopy in the distal part of a subungual hemorrhage. Dermatol Pract Concept 2014;4(2):83–5.
4. Braun RP, Baran R, Le Gal FA, et al. Diagnosis and management of nail pigmentation. J Am Acad Dermatol 2007;56(5):835–47.
5. Chiriac A, Brzezinski P, Foia L, et al. Chloronychia: green nail syndrome caused by *Pseudomonas aeruginosa* in elderly persons. Clin Interv Aging 2015; 14(10):265–7.
6. Kilinc Karaarslan I, Acar A, Aytmur D, et al. Dermoscopic features in fungal melanonychia. Clin Exp Dermatol 2015;40(3):271–8.
7. Wang YJ, Sun PL. Fungal melanonychia caused by Trichophyton rubrum and the value of dermoscopy. Cutis 2014;94(3):E5–6.

8. Hirata SH, Yamada S, Almeida FA, et al. Dermoscopy of the nail bed and matrix to assess melanonychia striata. J Am Acad Dermatol 2005;53(5):884–6.
9. Braun RP, Baran R, Saurat JH, et al. Surgical pearl: dermoscopy of the free edge of the nail to determine the level of nail plate pigmentation and the location of the probable origin in the proximal or distal nail matrix. J Am Acad Dermatol 2006;55:512–3.
10. Thomas L, Dalle S. Dermoscopy provides useful information for the management of melanonychia striata. Dermatol Ther 2007;20:3–10.
11. Starace M, Dika E, Fanti PA, et al. Nail apparatus melanoma: dermoscopic and histopathologic correlations on a series of 23 patients from a single centre. J Eur Acad Dermatol Venereol 2018;32(1):164–73.
12. Daniel CR 3rd, Iorizzo M, Piraccini BM, et al. Simple onycholysis. Cutis 2011;87(5):226–8.
13. Piraccini BM, Balestri R, Starace M, et al. Nail digital dermoscopy (onychoscopy) in the diagnosis of onychomycosis. J Eur Acad Dermatol Venereol 2013;27(4):509–13.
14. De Crignis G, Valgas N, Rezende P, et al. Dermatoscopy of onychomycosis. Int J Dermatol 2014;53(2):e97–9.
15. Iorizzo M, Dahdah M, Vincenzi C, et al. Videodermoscopy of the hyponychium in nail bed psoriasis. J Am Acad Dermatol 2008;58(4):714–5.
16. Lencastre A, Lamas A, Sà D, et al. Onychoscopy. Clin Dermatol 2013;31(5):587–93.
17. Tosti A, Schneider SL, Ramirez-Quizon MN, et al. Clinical, dermoscopic, and pathologic features of onychopapilloma: a review of 47 cases. J Am Acad Dermatol 2016;74(3):521–6.
18. Micali G, Verzì AE, Lacarrubba F. Alternative uses of dermatoscopy in daily clinical practice: an update. J Am Acad Dermatol 2018 [pii:S0190-9622(18)32143-1] [Epub ahead of print].
19. Piccolo V, Argenziano G, Alessandrini A, et al. Dermoscopy of subungual exostosis: a retrospective study of 10 patients. Dermatology 2017;233:80–5.

Dermoscopy for the Diagnosis of Conjunctival Lesions

Elisa Cinotti, MD, PhD[a,*], Anna La Rocca, MD[a], Bruno Labeille, MD[b], Damien Grivet, MD[c,d], Linda Tognetti, MD[a], Victor Lambert, MD[c,d], Mathilde Kaspi, MD[c,d], Niccolò Nami, MD[a], Michele Fimiani, MD[a], Jean Luc Perrot, MD, PhD[b], Pietro Rubegni, MD, PhD[a]

KEYWORDS

• Dermoscopy • Eye • Conjunctiva • Lesion • Melanoma • Squamous cell carcinoma • Nevus • Tumor

KEY POINTS

- Dermoscopy is not only valuable for the skin but can also be used for the diagnosis of conjunctival lesions.
- The anatomy of the conjunctiva is different from the skin; therefore, dermoscopic features of conjunctival tumors are different from the respective tumors of the skin.
- Conjunctival melanoma is characterized by irregularly distributed dots and a higher prevalence of gray color compared with nevi.
- Squamous cell carcinoma of the conjunctiva is characterized by hairpin and glomerular vessels.

INTRODUCTION

Conjunctival lesions comprise a large and varied spectrum of conditions, including inflammatory lesions and benign and malignant epithelial, melanocytic, vascular, fibrous, and lymphoid tumors.[1,2] Clinical observation often fails to make the diagnosis, and complete excisional biopsy is carried out in order to perform a histologic examination with possible functional and aesthetic consequences in this sensitive area.[2]

Noninvasive imaging techniques are extremely important for helping clinicians in the diagnosis of conjunctival lesions. Ophthalmologists currently use the slit lamp for the observation of conjunctival lesions, a binocular microscope equipped with an optical system that only provides clinical images of the anterior segment of the eye at high magnifications. New noninvasive imaging techniques, such as reflectance confocal microscopy, optical coherence tomography, and high-frequency ultrasound biomicroscopy, are under development for the investigation of the conjunctiva; but they are expensive and are only available in highly specialized centers.[3–8]

Disclosures: None.

[a] Department of Medical, Surgical and Neurological Science, Dermatology Section, University of Siena, S. Maria Alle Scotte Hospital, Viale Bracci 16, Siena 53100, Italy; [b] Department of Dermatology, University Hospital of Saint-Etienne, Saint-Etienne Cedex 2 42055, France; [c] Department of Ophthalmology, University Hospital of Saint-Etienne, Saint-Etienne Cedex 2 42055, France; [d] Laboratory Biology, Engineering, and Imaging of Corneal Graft, Jean Monnet University, EA2512, Saint-Etienne 42000, France
* Corresponding author.
E-mail address: elisacinotti@gmail.com

Dermatol Clin 36 (2018) 439–449
https://doi.org/10.1016/j.det.2018.05.011

In dermatology, the dermoscope is currently used to aid the clinical diagnosis of many skin diseases; it increases the diagnostic accuracy of skin tumors with respect to the simple naked eye.[9] There are some studies of dermoscopy concerning the oral and genital mucosa,[10–12] whereas the conjunctiva is rarely evaluated.[8,13–16] The authors' study aims to evaluate the current literature about the use of dermoscopy for the conjunctiva and to analyze the dermoscopic features of a large series of conjunctival tumors.

METHODS

Patients and Setting

One hundred and twenty-seven consecutive patients (60 women, 67 men, mean age 47 years, standard deviation [SD] 22.1, range 7–94 years) presenting with 147 conjunctival lesions were recruited at the Dermatology Department of the University Hospital of Saint-Etienne, France, between September 1, 2013 and January 30, 2017 to exclude the presence of malignant tumors. Eyelid margin tumors were excluded. An institutional review board approval was obtained (institutional review board at the University Hospital of Saint-Etienne, France, number IORG0007394; study filed under reference number IRBN332014/CHUSTE). A patient-informed consent was always obtained orally during the first consultation and before the examination.

Examined Lesion Diagnosis

All lesions were evaluated by a team of 3 dermatologists and 3 ophthalmologists. A surgical excision and a histopathologic examination were performed in 38 cases suspicious for malignant tumors under clinical, slit lamp, dermoscopy, and/or in vivo reflectance confocal microscopy examination. Histopathology of the 38 excised lesions revealed 16 malignant tumors, including 8 squamous cell carcinomas (SCCs), 8 melanomas (3 local recurrences after surgery and 3 with an involvement of the eyelid) and 22 benign lesions (18 nevi and 4 primary acquired melanoses [PAMs]). In particular, nevi were all compound except for 2 that were limited to the stroma (dermal nevi).

The remaining 109 lesions were not excised because they were considered benign and did not show any changes following consecutive monitoring for at least 12 months. Their clinical diagnosis was of 51 nevi, 42 PAMs, 5 cases of pterygia, 5 cases of pinguecula, 3 cases of scleromalacia, 1 angioma, 1 dermoid cyst, and 1 lymphangiectasia. Scleromalacias were also included in the authors' study even if they were not of the conjunctiva but of the underlying sclera because they are in the differential diagnosis with conjunctival lesions.

Clinical Data

The following data were collected for each lesion: demographic information of patients, anatomic site (bulbar, tarsal, limbal para-limbal and caruncle), presence of brown or blue pigmentation, shape (macule, papule, nodule and plaque), and larger diameter.

Dermoscopic Examination

Dermoscopy was performed with the PowerShot G7 camera (Canon, Melville, NY) combined with the FotoFinder Systems (FotoFinder Systems GmbH, Bad Birnbach, Germany) at × 20 magnification. Before the examination, topical anesthesia was administered using oxybuprocaine hydrochloride (1.6 mg/0.4 mL) (oxybuprocaine Thea) and tetracaine hydrochloride 1% (tetracaine Thea) applied in the inferior conjunctival fornix of the eye, and a transparent ophthalmic gel of carbomer 974P (Gel larmes Thea) was applied to the ocular region to be examined. A disposable sterile transparent film (Visulin) was applied to the tip of the dermoscope for the first 50 patients. For the rest of the patients, the tip of the camera was disinfected by applying a layer of Tristel Duo foam and by using ethanol wipes (Cidalkan ethanol) before and after the application of the foam.

Analysis of Dermoscopic Images

Dermoscopic images were evaluated together by 3 experts in noninvasive skin imaging (P.R., E.C., and N.N.) blinded from the histologic diagnosis. Each lesion was scored using the dermoscopic patterns described by Blum and colleagues[10] for genital and oral mucosal lesions: dots, globules or clods, circles, lines (parallel, reticular, or curved lines), structureless pigmentation, and number of patterns that was present within a single lesion. All these patterns were referred only to the distribution of the pigmentation.

In addition to these criteria, the authors also studied the vascular pattern: linear thin, linear thick, comma, arborizing, hairpin, and glomerular vessels. Vessels were calculated only when absent in the surrounding conjunctiva or when they exhibited a different pattern from vessels of the surrounding conjunctiva.

With regard to color, the authors scored the presence of brown, black, blue, gray, red (excluded red color of the vessels), white, yellow, and pink and the number of colors in a lesion. In case of a brown color, the authors specified if it was light brown and/or dark brown.

Statistical Analysis

Data are described using mean and SD for quantitative variables and number and percentages for qualitative variables. Continuous data were compared using unpaired *t* tests. Fisher exact test was used for the comparison of proportions. A $P<.05$ indicated statistical significance.

RESULTS

Clinical Features

Clinical data are reported in **Table 1**. A slight male predominance was observed (52%). Patients with malignant lesions (MMs plus SCCs) were significantly older than patients with benign lesions (mean 67, SD 15.8; range 43–94 years vs mean 42; SD 21, range 7–94 years; t value = 3.3988, P = .0193). With regard to the anatomic site, most lesions were located on the bulbar conjunctiva (59%). Interestingly, SCCs were located at the limbus with an extension to the bulbar conjunctiva in all cases except one. The latter case corresponded to a patient who had 2 SCCs in the same eye, one located on the bulbar conjunctiva and another on the limbus. Tumors of the caruncle were only nevi and one angioma. Lesions were relatively small at the diagnosis (mean 4.9, SD 3.6, range 1–15 mm). Therefore, most of them were macules (68%) or papules (22%).

All lesions with histologic examination were clinically pigmented except for the 8 SCCs. The group

Table 1
Clinical features of the conjunctival tumors

	Lesions with Histologic Examination				Benign Lesions Without Histologic Examination			
	MM	SCC	Nevus	PAM	Nevus	PAM	Achromic Lesions[a]	Total
Number of Lesions	8	8	18	4	51	42	16	147
Sex of the patients n (%)								
Male	2 (25)	8 (100)	13 (72)	1 (25)	23 (45)	18 (43)	11 (69)	76(52)[b]
Female	6 (75)	0	5 (28)	3 (75)	28 (55)	24 (57)	5 (31)	71(48)[b]
Age of the patients (y)								
Mean age (y) (SD)	67 (18)	67 (18)	40 (23)	27 (4)	37 (20)	47 (17)	54 (26)	47.0 (22.1)
Age range (y)	43–94	44–86	83–9	24–33	7–74	16–83	15–94	7–94
Anatomic site n (%)								
Bulbar	2 (25)	1 (13)	11 (61)	3 (75)	29 (57)	29 (69)	11 (69)	86(59)
Tarsal	3 (38)	0	1 (6)	0	0	1 (2)	0	5 (3)
Paralimbal	3 (38)	0	4 (22)	1 (25)	5 (10)	9 (21)	3 (19)	25(17)
Caruncle	0	0	2 (11)	0	14 (27)	0	1 (6)	17 (12)
Limbal	0	7 (88)	0	0	3 (6)	3 (7)	1 (6)	14(10)
Shape n (%)								
Macule	4 (50)	0	11 (61)	4 (100)	36 (71)	42 (100)	3 (19)	100 (68)
Papule	2 (25)	4 (50)	6 (33)	0	15 (29)	0	5 (31)	32 (22)
Nodule	0	0	0	0	0	0	0	0
Plaque	2 (25)	4 (50)	1 (6)	0	0	0	8 (50)	15 (10)
Presence of pigmentation n (%)								
Brown	8 (100)	0	18 (100)	4 (100)	45 (88)	42 (100)	0	111 (76)
Blue	0	0	0	0	5 (10)	0	0	5 (3)
Lesion size mm (SD)								
Maximum diameter	5 (4)	8 (6)	4 (2)	5.0 (1.4)	4 (3)	5 (3)	7 (4)	4.9 (3.6)
Size range	2–15	2–20	1–8	3–6	1–15	1–12	2–5	1–15

[a] Pinguecula, pterygia, scleromalacia, lymphangectasia, angioma, and dermoid cyst.
[b] Some patients have more than one lesion.

without the histologic examination included 93 pigmented lesions (51 nevi and 42 PAMs) and 16 clinically achromic lesions (5 cases of pterygia, 5 cases of pinguecula, 3 cases of scleromalacia, 1 angioma, 1 dermoid cyst, and 1 lymphangiectasia).

Dermoscopic Features

Dermoscopic features of the tumors are reported in **Table 2**. Interestingly, parallel and reticular lines were never found and curved lines forming circles

Table 2
Dermoscopic features of the conjunctival tumors

	Lesions with Histologic Examination				Benign Lesions Without Histologic Examination			
	MM	SCC	Nevus	PAM	Nevus	PAM	Achromic Lesions[a]	Total
	n (%)	n (%)	n (%)	n (%)	n (%)	n (%)	n (%)	n (%)
Number of Lesions	8	8	18	4	51	42	16	147
Dermoscopic patterns								
Lines	0	0	0	0	0	0	0	0
Circles	0	0	1 (6)	0	2 (4)	0	0	3 (2)
Structureless	8 (100)	0	15 (83)	2 (50)	32 (63)	11 (26)	2 (12)	70 (48)
Globules	2 (25)	0	9 (50)	0	25 (49)	0	0	36 (24)
Dots	8 (100)	0	14 (78)	4 (100)	27 (53)	42 (100)	0	95 (65)
Number of patterns								
1	0	0	4 (22)	2 (50)	22 (43)	31 (74)	2 (12)	61 (41)
2	6 (75)	0	7 (39)	2 (50)	24 (47)	11 (26)	0	50 (34)
3	2 (25)	0	7 (39)	0	4 (8)	0	0	13 (9)
4	0	0	0	0	1 (2)	0	0	1 (0.6)
Type of vessels								
Linear thin	0	1 (13)	0	0	0	0	1 (6)	2 (1)
Linear thick	0	0	0	0	0	0	0	0
Comma	0	0	0	0	0	0	1 (6)	1.0 (0.6)
Arborizing	0	0	0	0	0	0	1 (6)	1.0 (0.6)
Hairpin	0	6 (75)	0	0	0	0	0	6 (4)
Glomerular	0	6 (75)	0	0	0	0	0	7 (4)
Color								
Brown	8 (100)	0	18 (100)	4 (100)	51 (100)	42 (100)	2 (12)	125 (85)
Light brown	8 (100)	0	17 (94)	4 (100)	42 (82)	41 (98)	2 (12)	114 (78)
Dark brown	7 (88)	0	13 (72)	2 (50)	33 (65)	6 (14)	0	61 (41)
Gray	5 (63)	7 (88)	1 (6)	0	7 (14)	2 (5)	5 (31)	27 (18)
Blue	0	0	1 (6)	0	5 (10)	0	5 (31)	11 (7)
Black	0	0	0	0	1 (2)	0	0	1 (0.6)
White	0	8 (100)	1 (6)	0	3 (6)	0	3 (19)	15 (10)
Yellow	0	0	0	0	0	1 (2)	8 (50)	9 (6)
Pink	0	5 (63)	0	0	0	0	0	5 (3)
Red	1 (13)	0	0	0	0	0	1 (6)	2 (1)
Number of colors								
1	2 (25)	0	15 (83)	4 (100)	40 (78)	39 (93)	9 (56)	109 (74)
2	6 (75)	4 (50)	3 (17)	0	6 (12)	3 (7)	6 (38)	28 (19)
3	0	4 (50)	0	0	5 (10)	0	1 (6)	10 (7)
>3	0	0	0	0	0	0	0	0

[a] Pinguecula, pterygia, scleromalacia, lymphangectasia, angioma, and dermoid cyst.

were found in only 3 nevi. All MMs were pigmented, and their pigmentation was arranged in dots and in a structureless pattern. In 2 cases, globules were also present. All MMs had more than one color. A light brown color was present in all cases, dark brown in 88%, and gray in 63%. A red structureless color was also observed in one case.

Nevi were all pigmented and their pigmentation was mainly structureless or distributed in dots and/or globules. In 3 cases the pigmentation formed circles. All nevi had a brown pigmentation; gray, blue, black and white colors were also visible in isolated cases. The comparison of the dermoscopic features of nevi with histologic examination and MMs showed more frequently a gray pigmentation in MMs than nevi ($P = .0045$).

All PAMs exhibited a brown pigmentation distributed in dots that could be confluent in a structureless pattern. In nearly all cases they were light brown, and in only a small proportion of cases they were dark brown. The latter cases were found in patients with photo-type VI.

SCCs were all whitish (100%) and greyish (88%) lesions and were characterized by hairpin and glomerular (75%) vessels. Interestingly, all MMs and SCCs presented neo-angiogenesis around and inside the tumors that have not been scored in **Table 2** when the vessels inside the lesions had the same pattern of the vessels in the peripheral conjunctiva.

The clinically achromic lesions did not show any brown pigmentation under dermoscopy except in 2 pinguecula that exhibited a structureless light brown pigmentation. All pinguecula had a yellowish color, and all pterygia were characterized by a light gray color. In 2 pterygia, gray color had light blue shadows; light blue color characterized 3 cases of scleromalacia. Only the dermoid cyst showed vessels, and they were thin arborizing at the periphery and thin linear and comma vessels in its central part.

DISCUSSION

To the authors' knowledge, this is the first study concerning the dermoscopic features of a series of conjunctival lesions. In the literature, there are no data on dermoscopic features of inflammatory conjunctival lesions and only 4 case reports about tumors that described a sebaceous carcinoma of the tarsal conjunctiva with polymorphous vessels and brilliant yellow background[13] and 3 MMs. The first MM involved the tarsal conjunctiva and showed atypical pigment network, irregular dots and globules, regression structure, and a blue-white veil[14]; the second MM involved the eyelid margin and showed structureless dark brown–gray pigmentation[8]; and the third MM was located on the para-limbal area and showed brown dots confluent in an homogeneous pigmentation.[16] Moreover, the authors' group previously performed a study on 39 conjunctival pigmented tumors that were imaged with a noncontact camera that provided digital images at 16 × and evaluated many dermoscopic parameters by a dedicated software (digital surface dermoscopy). MMs were found to be larger and darker and had more internal contrast than benign lesions.[15]

In the present study, malignant tumors were represented by SCCs and MMs, which are known to be the 2 most common malignant tumors of the conjunctiva,[1,17] whereas benign lesions mainly included nevi and PAMs. All MMs were characterized by a brown pigmentation organized in irregular distributed dots that were confluent in a structureless pattern (**Fig. 1**). In most cases the pigmentation was dark brown, and this fact helped both the clinical and dermoscopic diagnosis (see **Fig. 1**). Gray was observed in more than half of the cases (63%, see **Fig. 1**) and probably corresponded to a melanocytic invasion of the superficial part of the stroma. It should be noted that differently from cutaneous MM, conjunctival MM is by definition a proliferation of melanocytes that invade the stroma and could not be limited to the epithelium.[1] MM recurrences presented as small macules that were suspicious because of their location in the surgical scar and the irregular distribution of the pigmentation. Moreover, 2 cases had a multifocal extension suggestive of a diffuse spread of melanocytes.

All nevi were pigmented and exhibited a brown pigmentation at clinical examination except for 5 Ota nevi that were blue (**Fig. 2**). Under dermoscopy, gray, blue, black, and white were also visible in a small proportion of cases. The authors could not find any dermoscopic criteria that allowed the differential diagnosis with MM except for the higher presence of gray color in MM than nevi ($P = .0045$). However, in 40% of cases, clear cysts were visible inside the nevus suggesting epithelial cystic nevi (see **Fig. 2**), whereas in MM cysts were never observed in the authors' series and were reported in only 7% of MMs in a larger study.[18] Notably, dermoscopy helped to identify the cysts of minor size not visible under the naked eye. Differently from MMs and PAMs, nevi showed globules in half of the cases (see **Fig. 2**) in addition to dots and structureless pigmentation; this aspect could be related to the presence of well-defined roundish melanocytic nests. The normal caruncle is characterized by thin vessels and pinkish color. In case of light-brown nevi of the

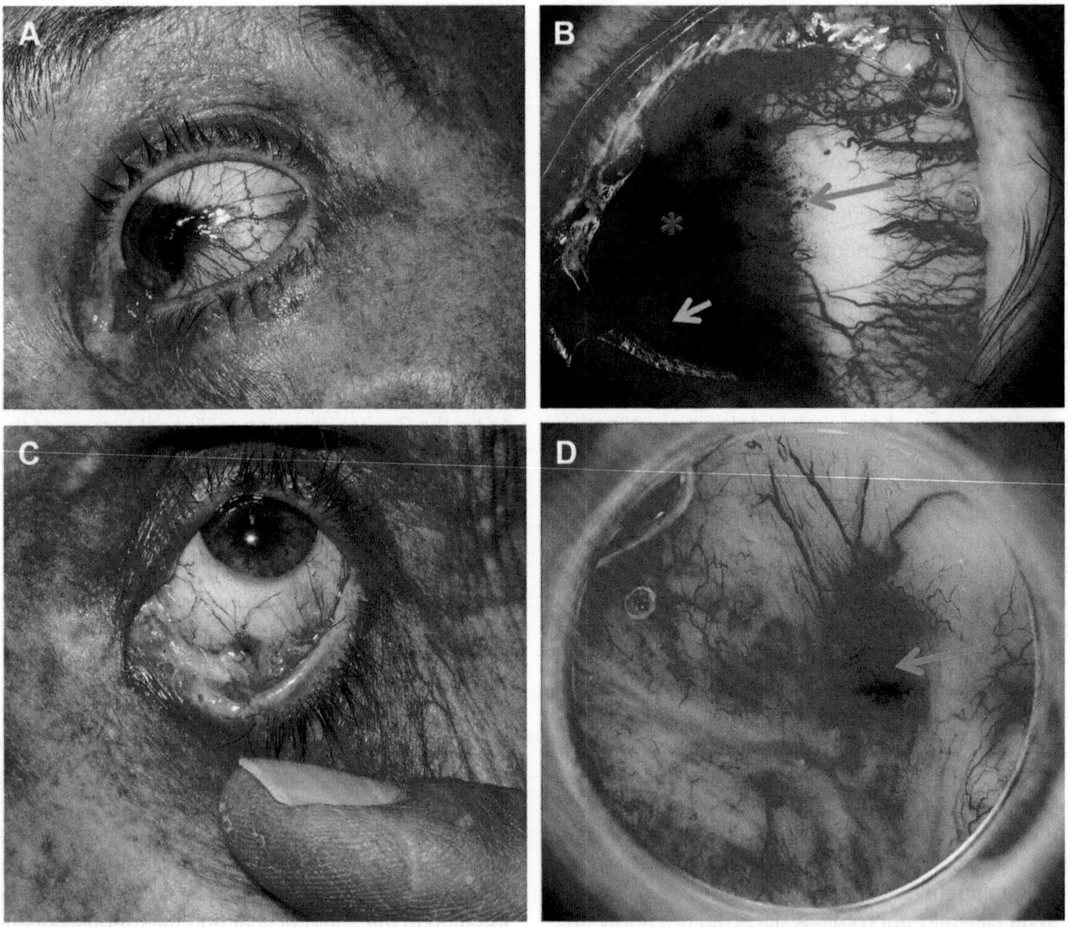

Fig. 1. Melanomas: clinical (*A, C*) and dermoscopic (*B, D*) aspect. Primary (*A, B*) and recurrent (*C, D*) melanomas are characterized by a dark-brown pigmentation organized in irregular distributed dots (*green arrow*) that are confluent in a structureless pattern (*red asterisk*). Gray color is also visible (*blue arrow*).

caruncle, these vessels were also visible in the background and contributed to enhance the pink color of this area.

The second largest group of benign melanocytic tumors in the authors' study was represented by PAMs. All lesions were flat and exhibited dots that were often confluent in a structureless pigmentation (**Fig. 3**). Different from MM, dots were regularly distributed all over the lesions. Moreover, different from MMs, PAMs were mainly light brown and were dark brown in a few cases that corresponded to racial melanosis. Histopathologically, PAM is characterized by the proliferation of melanocytes in the epithelium.[1] Notably, when the authors stretched the tip of the dermoscope onto one side of the conjunctiva containing the PAM, they could observe that the epithelium formed multiple pigmented folds (they called this *the flag sign*) and left a nonpigmented area behind (**Fig. 4**). This sign demonstrated that the pigmentation of PAM involved only the conjunctiva and not the episclera and sclera, different from what could be observed in MM.

All SCCs were raised tumors that originated on the limbus area with a subsequent extension onto the cornea surface as grayish lesions and onto the bulbar conjunctiva as whitish-pinkish plaques filled of characteristic hairpin vessels with glomerular extremities (**Fig. 5**). Dermoscopy allowed to precisely define the extension of SCCs that was not always possible to be identified by the naked eye. The grayish color of the tumor on the limbus could be induced by the overlap of the whitish proliferation of the SCC and the underlying iris. The pinkish color was more present in large-size lesions probably due to the greater neo-angiogenesis. In only 2 cases were the characteristic hairpin and glomerular vessels not present: one case corresponded to an initial small SCC and in the other case they were probably

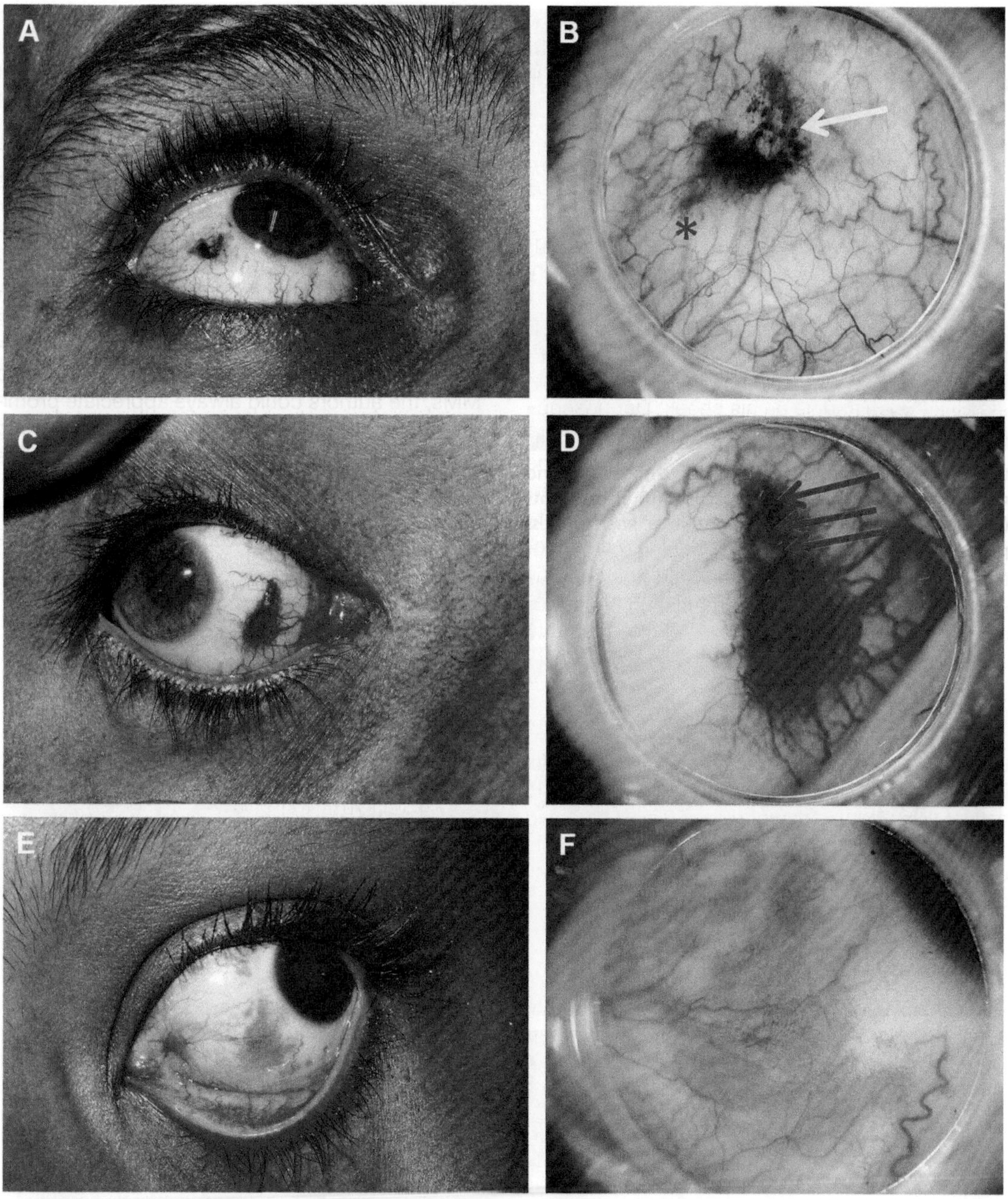

Fig. 2. Two compound nevi (*A–D*) and one nevus of Ota (*E, F*): clinical (*A, C, E*) and dermoscopic (*B, D, F*) aspect. Dermoscopy (*B, D*) shows some globules (*yellow arrow*) and some cysts (*pink arrows*) surrounded by curved pigmented lines.

masked by a hyperkeratotic whitish surface (see **Fig. 5**).

Pinguecula and pterygium are benign lesions in differential diagnoses with initial SCC. They corresponded to an elastotic degeneration of collagen associated with a fibrovascular proliferation covered by an overlying epithelium and appeared as plaques over the bulbar (pingueculum) or perilimbal (pterygium) conjunctiva. Pingueculum is limited to the bulbar conjunctiva and does not grow across the cornea differently from pterygium. Pinguecula were characterized by a yellowish homogeneous color that was never observed in SCC, and in 2 cases they also showed a structureless light-brown pigmentation that was probably induced by the overlap of the yellow color with the red blood vessels (**Fig. 6**). In the authors' series, pterygium could be recognized from SCC because it had a lighter gray color, which left the underlying retina partially visible (see **Fig. 6**). Notably, pingueculum and pterygium and all other clinically achromic lesions of this series did not show any hairpin or glomerular vessels.

In normal conjunctiva, vessels can often be seen and the interpretation of tumor vessels could be more difficult than in the skin. In the authors' study, they decided not to count the vessels of a lesion when the same type of vessel was also present in the surrounding nonlesional conjunctiva. Therefore, a large part of the tumor was scored as having no vessels even if vessels were seen. Interestingly, in the conjunctiva around all SCCs and MMs, the authors could always appreciate prominent feeder linear vessels that were directed into the lesions. Moreover, neo-angiogenesis was more evident for raised tumors. On the contrary, when visible in the surrounding conjunctiva of benign lesions, vessels were mainly thin. In case

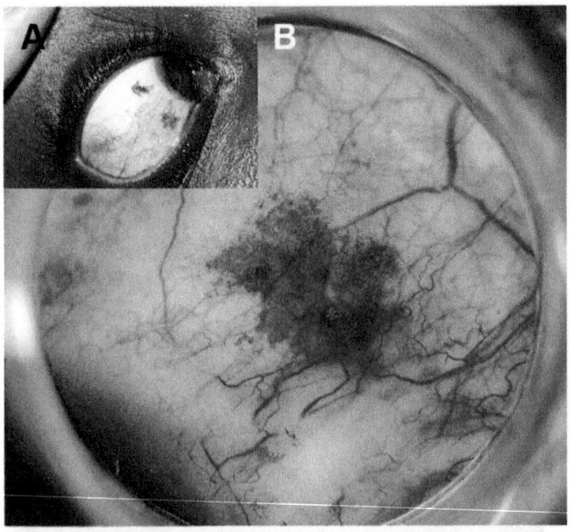

Fig. 3. Primary acquired melanosis: clinical (*A*) and dermoscopic (*B*) aspect. Dermoscopy (*B*) shows dots (*green arrow*) that are confluent in a structureless pattern (*red asterisk*).

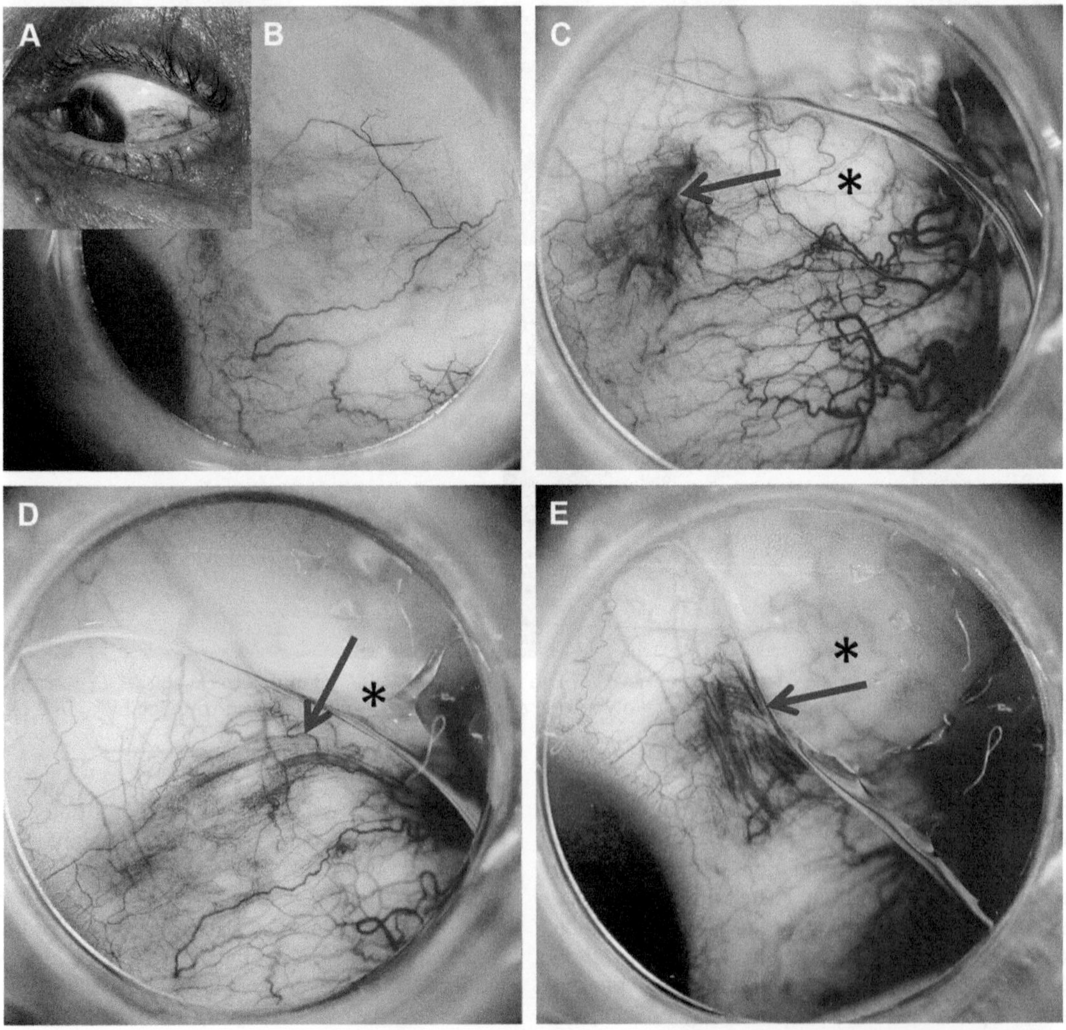

Fig. 4. Clinical (*A*) and dermoscopic (*B–E*) aspect of a PAM with the flag sign. The dermoscopic aspect of the PAM (*B*) is changed by stretching the conjunctiva onto one side (*C–E*). The conjunctiva forms multiple pigmented folds (*red arrows*) and leaves a nonpigmented area behind (*asterisk*).

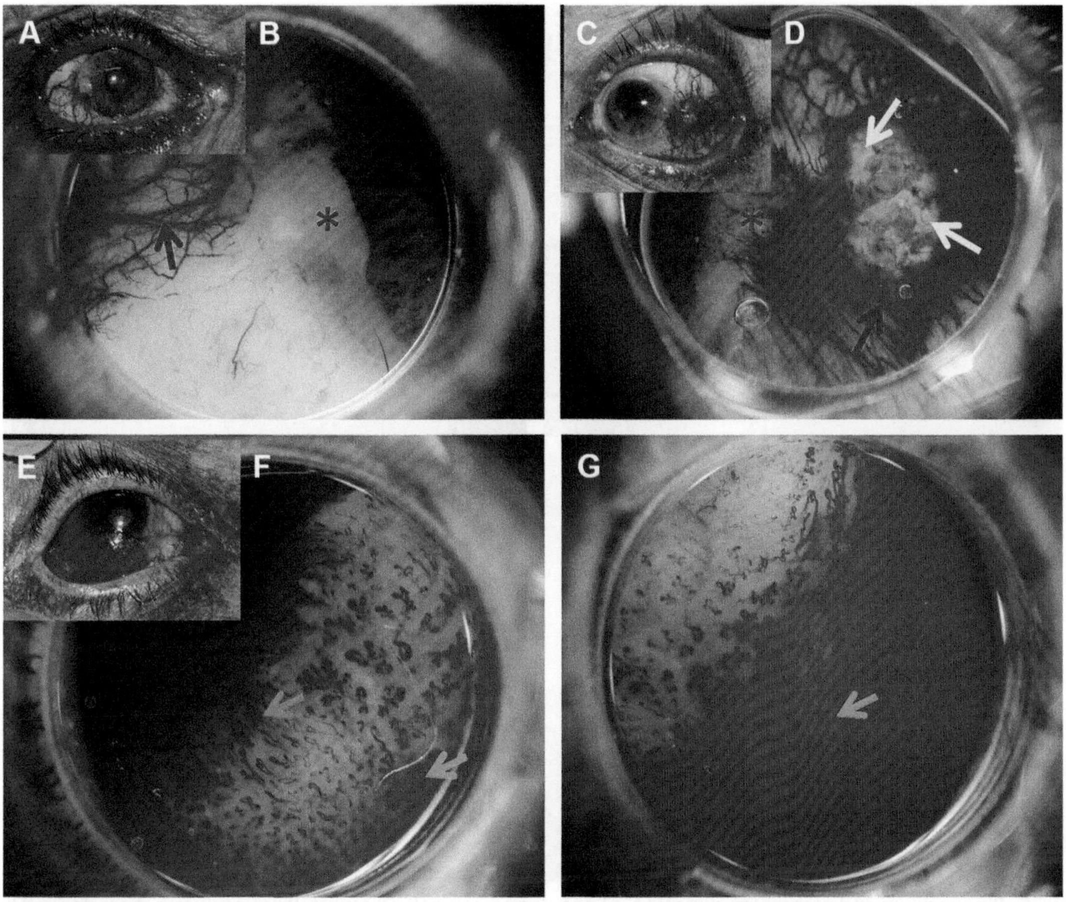

Fig. 5. Three cases of SCC: clinical (*A, C, E*) and dermoscopic (*B, D, F, G*) aspect. Dermoscopy shows a grayish structureless pigmentation on the cornea (*red asterisk*) and whitish-pinkish areas on the bulbar conjunctiva (*yellow arrows*). Characteristic hairpin vessels (*blue arrow*) with glomerular extremities (*green arrow*) are visible as well as elongated feeding vessels (*pink arrows*).

of benign lesions, vessels were also often visible in the surrounding conjunctiva but in most cases they were thin. In a large study on 601 MMs and 440 SCCs, feeder vessels were clinically observed in 48% and 58% of cases, whereas intrinsic vessels were observed in 33% and 69% of cases, respectively[18]; it is, therefore, possible that these percentages could have been more elevated by using dermoscopy.

Another significant difference compared with the skin concerns pigment distribution. Interestingly, in the authors' study, the pigmentation was never organized in parallel and reticular lines and was less frequently organized in globules than in the skin probably because, unlike the skin, the junction between the epithelium and the stroma is flat. Pigmentation was mainly organized in dots that corresponded to the proliferation of isolated melanocytes; in case of an increase melanocyte proliferation, the dots were confluent in a structureless pigmentation. Curved lines were observed in only 3 cases: in 2 cases the pigmentation surrounded the cysts associated with the nevus (see **Fig. 2**), and in the other case the pigmentation was probably in circles because of the extension onto the limbal area. Li and Xin[14] described the presence of a pigment network in their MM of the tarsal conjunctiva. The presence of the network could be related to this particular location. However, in the authors' series, the nevus and the 3 MMs of the tarsal conjunctiva did not show this pattern.

The authors' pilot study showed that dermoscopy can add important elements to the clinical diagnosis of the conjunctival lesions. These lesions have different aspects compared with cutaneous ones, and the authors found some features that seem to characterize the conjunctiva, such as the irregular dots and gray color in MMs and the presence of hairpin and glomerular vessels in

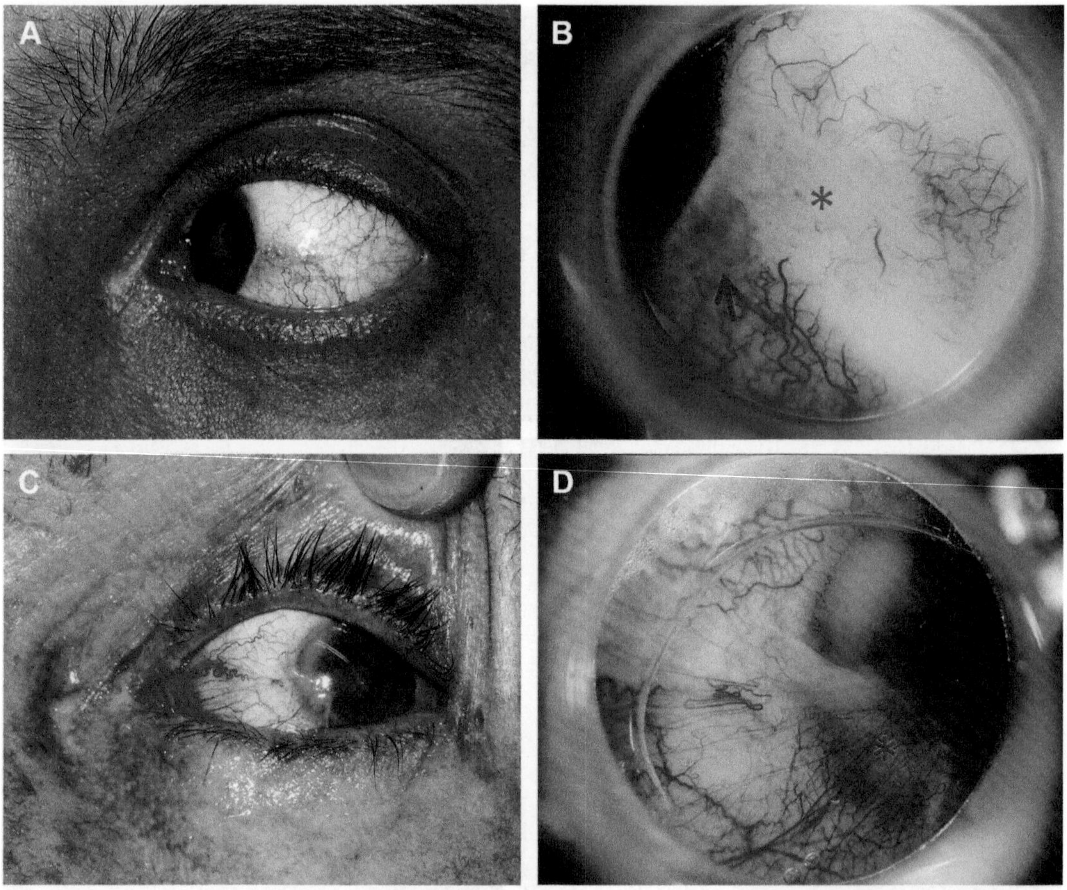

Fig. 6. Pingueculum and pterygium: clinical (*A, C*) and dermoscopic (*B, D*) aspect. Pingueculum is characterized by a yellowish homogeneous color (*blue asterisk*) with a focal structureless light-brown pigmentation (*violet arrow*), and pterygium shows a light-gray color, which leaves the underlying retina partially visible (*pink asterisk*).

SCCs. The authors' research could be a starting point for other studies that evaluate different dermoscopic criteria in order to help clinicians recognize benign and malignant conjunctival tumors.

REFERENCES

1. Shields CL, Shields JA. Tumors of the conjunctiva and cornea. Surv Ophthalmol 2004;49:3–24.
2. Maschi C, Caujolle J-P, Liolios I, et al. Benign conjunctival tumors. J Fr Ophtalmol 2013;36:796–802.
3. Cinotti E, Perrot JL, Campolmi N, et al. The role of in vivo confocal microscopy in the diagnosis of eyelid margin tumors: 47 cases. J Am Acad Dermatol 2014;71:912–918 e2.
4. Cinotti E, Perrot J-L, Labeille B, et al. Handheld reflectance confocal microscopy for the diagnosis of conjunctival tumors. Am J Ophthalmol 2015;159: 324–333 e1.
5. Cinotti E, Singer A, Labeille B, et al. Handheld In vivo reflectance confocal microscopy for the diagnosis of eyelid margin and conjunctival tumors. JAMA Ophthalmol 2017;135:845–51.
6. Cinotti E, Labeille B, Cambazard F, et al. Confocal microscopy for special sites and special uses. Dermatol Clin 2016;34:477–85.
7. Cinotti E, Perrot JL, Labeille B, et al. In vivo confocal microscopy for eyelids and ocular surface: a new horizon for dermatologists. G Ital Dermatol Venereol 2015;150:127–9.
8. Cinotti E, Haouas M, Grivet D, et al. In vivo and ex vivo confocal microscopy for the management of a melanoma of the eyelid margin. Dermatol Surg 2015;41:1437–40.
9. Vestergaard ME, Macaskill P, Holt PE, et al. Dermoscopy compared with naked eye examination for the diagnosis of primary melanoma: a meta-analysis of studies performed in a clinical setting. Br J Dermatol 2008;159:669–76.
10. Blum A, Simionescu O, Argenziano G, et al. Dermoscopy of pigmented lesions of the mucosa and the mucocutaneous junction: results of a multicenter

study by the International Dermoscopy Society (IDS). Arch Dermatol 2011;147:1181–7.
11. Ronger-Savle S, Julien V, Duru G, et al. Features of pigmented vulval lesions on dermoscopy. Br J Dermatol 2011;164:54–61.
12. Cinotti E, Couzan C, Perrot JL, et al. In vivo confocal microscopic substrate of grey colour in melanosis. J Eur Acad Dermatol Venereol 2015; 29:2458–62.
13. Satomura H, Ogata D, Arai E, et al. Dermoscopic features of ocular and extraocular sebaceous carcinomas. J Dermatol 2017;44:1313–6.
14. Li K, Xin L. Palpebral conjunctiva melanoma with dermoscopic and clinicopathological characteristics. J Am Acad Dermatol 2014;71:e35–7.
15. Tosi GM, Rubegni P, Schuerfeld K, et al. Digital surface microscopy analysis of conjunctival pigmented lesions: a preliminary study. Melanoma Res 2004;14: 375–80.
16. Volpini BMF, Maia M, Agi J, et al. Synchronous conjunctival melanoma and lentigo maligna melanoma. An Bras Dermatol 2017;92:565–7.
17. Shields CL, Demirci H, Karatza E, et al. Clinical survey of 1643 melanocytic and nonmelanocytic conjunctival tumors. Ophthalmology 2004;111: 1747–54.
18. Shields CL, Alset AE, Boal NS, et al. Conjunctival tumors in 5002 cases. comparative analysis of benign versus malignant counterparts. The 2016 James D. Allen Lecture. Am J Ophthalmol 2017;173:106–33.

Dermoscopy of Inflammatory Genital Diseases: Practical Insights

Alessandro Borghi, MD*, Annarosa Virgili, MD,
Monica Corazza, MD

KEYWORDS

• Dermoscopy • Inflammatory genital diseases • Lichen sclerosus • Lichen planus • Psoriasis
• Eczema • Plasma cell mucositis

KEY POINTS

- Genital inflammatory diseases may have similar appearances and represent a diagnostic challenge for clinicians.
- Genital inflammatory diseases may be confused with infectious and malignant conditions as well.
- Practical guidance for the use of dermoscopy in the assessment of the main inflammatory genital diseases is provided within this article, namely for lichen sclerosus, lichen planus, psoriasis, lichen simplex chronicus, and plasma cell mucositis.
- Dermoscopy potentially improves the differential diagnosis of genital inflammatory diseases by defining specific patterns.

INFLAMMATORY GENITAL DISORDERS: PRACTICAL PITFALLS

Dermoscopy was originally introduced as an integrative part in the clinical evaluation of pigmented lesions and skin tumors because it improves diagnostic accuracy.[1] Since then, the applicability of dermoscopy has been extended to numerous general dermatologic disorders, including nonpigmented tumors, inflammatory skin diseases,[2–4] hair and nail abnormalities,[5,6] skin infections, and infestations.[7]

Genital inflammatory disorders may represent a diagnostic challenge for both clinicians and pathologists.[8,9] In fact, an extraordinarily broad range of etiologies accounts for genital lesions, not only inflammatory in nature, but also cancerous and infectious conditions. The commonest inflammatory diseases that involve the genital sites are lichen sclerosus, lichen planus, lichen simplex chronicus, eczema, including atopic dermatitis and contact dermatitis, and psoriasis. Other less common disorders include plasma cell mucositis of Zoon and fixed drug eruption.

In many cases, these disorders, which are extremely heterogeneous for etiopathogenesis, course, and prognosis, may have similar appearances. In addition, the genital area is exposed to friction, maceration, physiologic occlusion, and mechanical and chemical irritation. Consequently, the normal features of these common dermatoses may be lost or modified in this region.

Because of their location, these dermatoses may be confused with sexually transmitted diseases. On the other hand, genital inflammatory disorders may coexist with contagious conditions and this can further make their diagnosis tricky.[10]

Cancer may develop in the context of some inflammatory conditions, without pathognomonic

Conflicts of Interest: None.
Department of Medical Sciences, Section of Dermatology and Infectious Diseases, University of Ferrara, Via L. Ariosto 35, Ferrara 44121, Italy
* Corresponding author.
E-mail address: alessandro.borghi@unife.it

Dermatol Clin 36 (2018) 451–461
https://doi.org/10.1016/j.det.2018.05.013

clinical changes, especially in the early phases.[11–13] Furthermore, a number of physiologic genital variants or lesions should be recognized and differentiated from inflammatory disorders, such as cysts, syringomas, seborrheic keratosis, pearly papules, Fordyce spots, and hyperpigmentation. Another important aspect is that because of their anatomic location, genital lesions, mostly vulvar lesions, are often noted incidentally, especially in asymptomatic cases. Thus, their onset, duration, and behavior may be unknown.

Although a histopathological examination may be necessary to shed light on this wide variety of differential diagnoses, dermoscopy could be included as a part of the clinical inspection of genital diseases.[14–16] Specific dermoscopic patterns and features have been described for several inflammatory genital disorders. As a consequence, in this field, too, dermoscopy could become a noninvasive diagnostic aid to support diagnosis and avoid unnecessary invasive investigation. Furthermore, by recording dermoscopic photographs, the course of inflammatory conditions can be monitored. This is of particular value for those disorders that can evolve toward cancer or lead to anatomic changes, like lichen sclerosus. Response to treatment can be objectively assessed, too.[17,18]

PRACTICAL TIPS FOR GENITAL DERMOSCOPY

During assessment of genital sites by dermoscopy, to prevent microbiological contamination of the probes and the subsequent potential transmission of infections between patients, previous studies have evaluated the possibility of covering the glass plate of the dermoscopic instrument with a disposable, polyvinyl chloride (PVC) food wrap (Domopak; Comital Cofresco SpA, Volpiano [Torino], Italy) with the interposition of mineral oil.[19,20] The use of PVC film during dermoscopic examination of mucosal surfaces was shown to act as a safe barrier for virologic contamination and to permit an unmodified view of the pigmented lesions.

DERMOSCOPY OF INFLAMMATORY GENITAL DISEASES

The chief objective of this article was to provide practical guidance for the use of dermoscopy in the assessment of inflammatory genital diseases. The main dermoscopic clues described so far for this group of disorders are summarized as follows and in **Table 1**.

Lichen Sclerosus

Genital lichen sclerosus (GLS) is a chronic inflammatory, immune-mediated disease that affects the anogenital areas.[21] GLS primary lesions are flat, ivory-colored spots that may coalesce into thin crinkly patches. Ecchymosis and itching-related excoriations are common, especially in female patients,[22] and occasionally hyperkeratosis is a prominent feature. Postinflammatory scarring may cause destruction of anogenital architecture. In female patients, this may lead to progressive labial fusion, tearing of tissue, introital stenosis, and burying of the clitoris. Phimosis, adhesions of the foreskin to the glans, and meatal stenosis are typical sequelae in male patients. An increased risk of genital cancer is also recognized.[23,24] GLS is a very distressing disease, in fact most patients complain of the symptoms, mainly itching, burning, and sexual dysfunction.[25–27]

In the early stages of the disease the diagnosis can be difficult. The main differential diagnoses are lichen planus (LP), lichen simplex chronicus, vitiligo, immunobullous disorders such as mucous membrane pemphigoid, and vulvar or penile intraepithelial neoplasia.[21,28]

To date, only a few studies have specifically addressed the dermoscopic features of GLS, with quite similar findings.[29,30] A whitish background together with patchy structureless areas, varying in color from white to white-yellowish to milky-pinkish, represent the prevalent dermoscopic feature of GLS (**Fig. 1**). These dermoscopic clues may be observable also in the case of absence of pallor at the clinical evaluation. They correspond to sclerosis and hyalinization, which are the main pathologic changes in lichen sclerosus (LS).[29] A marked decrease in vessel concentration in the context of GLS lesions when compared with unaffected surfaces is the other dermoscopic hallmark of this disease. Vessels are polymorphic in shape, without any specific arrangement. The correlation between dermoscopic vascular pattern and disease duration is controversial; Larre Borges and colleagues[29] did not find any association, whereas Borghi and colleagues[30] have observed that dotted vessels occur mostly in the early stage of GLS.

Gray-blue dots arranged in a typical peppering pattern can frequently be observed in GLS. Melanophages displaced in both the upper dermis and the perifollicular site are the histologic counterpart of this dermoscopic peppering, which is a consequence of the inflammatory process. Because of this, it is observed in other chronic, genital inflammatory diseases as well.[31] Postinflammatory hyperpigmentation may be so marked that in a few male patients it is reported to clinically and dermoscopically mimic melanoma.[32,33] In a case of pigmented postinflammatory penile LS, Sollena and colleagues[33] described a dermoscopic pattern

Table 1
Dermoscopic criteria of inflammatory genital diseases

	Dermoscopic Criteria	
Genital Disease	Vascular Findings	Nonvascular Findings
Lichen sclerosus	1. Marked decrease in vessel concentration 2. Vessels polymorphic in shape (linear and dotted) 3. No specific arrangement 4. Red purpuric dots, globules, or blotches	1. Whitish background 2. Patchy, structureless whitish areas 3. Gray-blue dots/globules with peppering pattern 4. Comedo-like openings 5. Scales
Lichen planus	1. Thick linear, irregular vessels, including hairpin vessels 2. No dotted vessels 3. Diffuse arrangement throughout lesions 4. Radial or parallel arrangement at the periphery of lesions 5. Sea-anemone pattern	1. Wickham striae, with the following configuration: Reticular Homogeneous Rounded-globular Annular Radial streaming Dots/"starry sky" Gray-white and/or blue-white veil 2. Dull or intense red background 3. Blue-gray dots/globules 4. Peppering pigment 5. Comedo-like openings
Psoriasis	1. Dotted vessels 2. Tortuous capillaries, with a "bushy" homogeneous aspect 3. Uniform and regular arrangement	1. No scales 2. Light red background
Lichen simplex chronicus	1. Rich vascularization, linear, serpentine, and dotted in shape 2. Diffuse arrangement	1. White-grayish background
Plasma cell mucositis	1. Prominent curved vessels with different width (serpentine, convoluted, and chalice-shaped vessels)	1. Focal/diffuse red-yellowish to orange-brownish structureless areas

characterized by linear and curved streaks associated with a cobblestone-like pattern and brown globules. The investigators underlined that the absence of irregular dots/globules, polymorphous vessels, and blue-whitish veil helped in the differential diagnosis from melanoma.

Red to purpuric, structureless, well-circumscribed dots, globules, or blotches, which correspond to blood spots, are common findings in GLS, especially in female cases.[15,30,34]

Both scales and yellow comedo-like openings, the latter correlating on histology with dilated infundibula with follicular cornified plugging, are additional findings that can be observed in some cases of GLS, as well as in extragenital sites.[35,36]

Lichen Planus

LP is a chronic muco-cutaneous inflammatory disease of unknown origin.[37] It is considered a prototypic skin disease in the category of "lichenoid tissue reaction/interface dermatitis", in which cytotoxic lymphocytes attack basal keratinocytes leading to apoptosis.[38] Various potential triggers, for example, viral or bacterial antigens, metal ions, drugs or physical factors, could initiate this autoimmune process.[39,40]

The skin and oral mucosa are the most frequently involved areas, but genital manifestations can occur.[37,41] In female patients, LP affecting the mucosal side of the vulva is a distinct clinical variant.[42] It typically involves the inner surface of the labia minora and consists of a glazed erythema that may easily bleed on touching[43]; erosions may frequently develop.[44] In a typical case of vulvar LP the erythema is surrounded by a lacy, hyperkeratotic white border, with or without Wickham striae (WS) in the surrounding skin. Vaginal inflammation is a supportive clinical feature.[45] Patients mainly complain of burning and pain and treatment may be extremely difficult.[41,43,44] Vulvar LP (VLP) may clinically resemble other inflammatory or tumoral

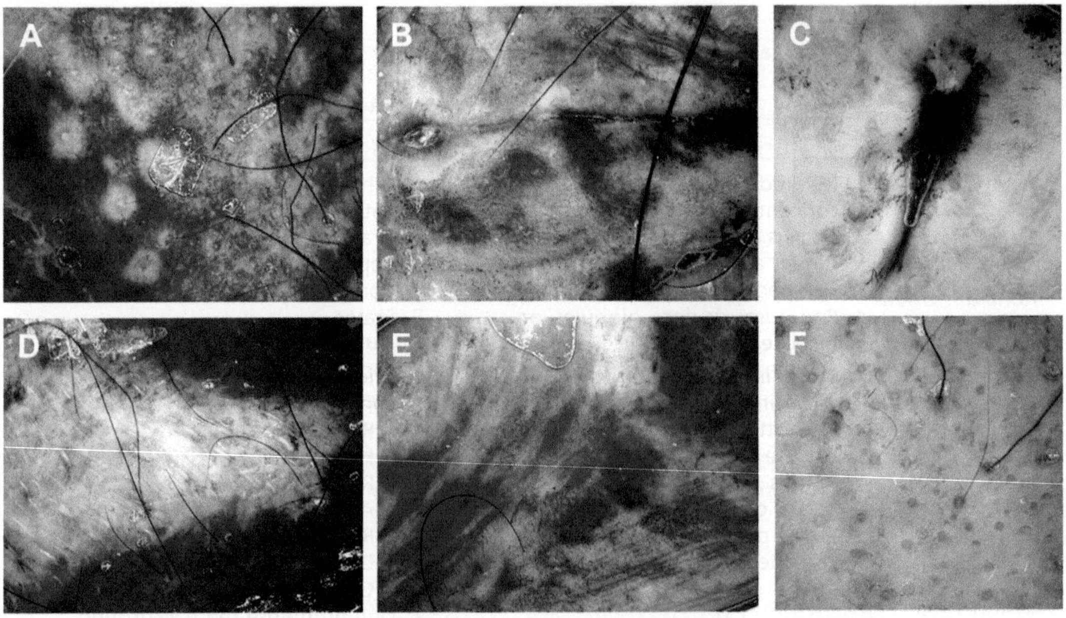

Fig. 1. (*A*) Dermoscopic features of vulvar white spot disease. (*B*) Patchy structureless whitish areas in a vulvar lichen sclerosus; gray/brownish peppering is visible. (*C*) Whitish background in a penile lichen sclerosus, with red purpuric blotches and globules corresponding to ecchymosis, adjacent to the urethral orifice and brown pigmentation. (*D*) Whitish background with vascular "desertification" in a female case. (*E*) White and milky-pinkish structureless areas with abundant peripheral peppering (vulva). (*F*) Numerous comedo-like openings on a white background (labia majora).

vulvar diseases, like plasma cell vulvitis, LS, vulvar intraepithelial neoplasia, contact dermatitis, and candidosis vulvitis.[46] In male patients, LP typically presents on the glans penis and may have an annular pattern. Erosive, hypertrophic, or papulosquamous LP are less common variants.[39]

To date, only 1 article has described the dermoscopic features of VLP in a series of 10 women.[31] A rather characteristic dermoscopic pattern was reported. It mainly combines (1) thick linear, irregular vessels, including hairpin and spermatozoa-like vessels, arranged diffusely throughout LP lesions (it is noteworthy that dotted vessels were not seen in any patient); (2) peripheral WS exhibiting different morphologic patterns, even combined; and (3) an intense red background (**Fig. 2**).

WS represent the dermoscopic hallmark of VLP, even though in the reported case series they were not a constant feature, like in cutaneous LP.[47,48] WS appeared mainly as deep pearly whitish structures, arranged in different patterns similar to those described in skin LP, namely reticular, annular, dotted/"starry sky" and rounded/globular configuration. Peripheral thin projections giving a comb-like appearance also were observed, usually intermingled with parallel vessels. On the other hand, WS mimicking leaf venation or the crystal structure of snow were not seen in vulvar cases, thus suggesting that WS morphologic patterns may be influenced by the location of the disease. In more than half of the study patients, WS also presented as a structureless, blue-white or gray-white area, similar to a veil.[31,49] White homogeneous areas were observed at the sinuous, hyperkeratotic border of the lesions, probably corresponding to the typical, macerate border surrounding the erosive areas in VLP. Although in most cases WS were clinically observable, dermoscopy ensured a far clearer visibility of the WS than was possible with the naked eye.

The gray-blue dots with a characteristic peppered arrangement may represent additional diagnostic clues, although observed in vulvar LS as well.[30] A gray pigmentation with a sea-anemonelike pattern around linear vessels was also described as a peculiar feature of the genital site.

Psoriasis

Psoriasis is a chronic, inflammatory skin disease with a prevalence in the general population of approximately 2% to 3%.[50] Based on data from the literature, involvement of the genital skin occurs in 30% to 60% of patients with psoriasis.[51] Most often, genital psoriasis is part of either a more generalized plaque psoriasis or inverse

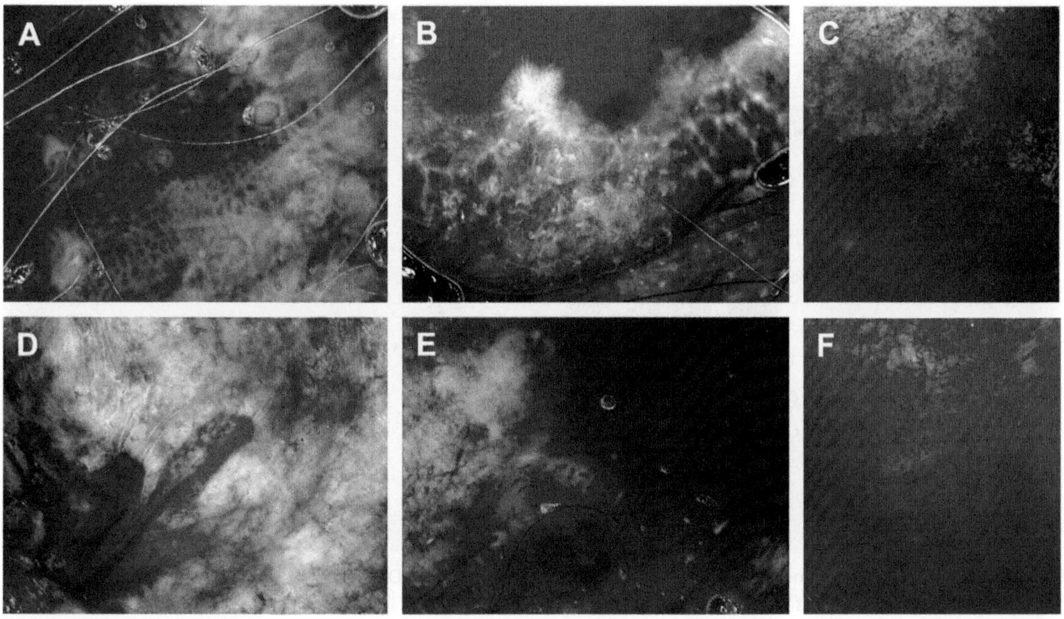

Fig. 2. Representative dermoscopic features of vulvar lichen planus: (*A*) annular/reticular WS; yellow comedo-like openings are also observed; (*B*) reticular WS at the periphery of an intense red surface; (*C*) typical thick linear, irregular vessels diffusely arranged over a red background; a blue-white veil, that corresponds to WS, is visible; (*D*) sinuous white homogeneous border surrounding an erosive bright red area; (*E*) peripheral WS appearing as a white area with parallel vessels (comblike pattern); (*F*) typical vascularization over an intense red background.

psoriasis, although isolated presentation of psoriasis on the external genitalia can occur in 2% to 5% of psoriatic patients.[52] Psoriasis affecting genital skin may be associated with considerable psychosexual morbidity, discomfort, and embarrassment, and may considerably impair quality of life.[51,53,54] However, in clinical practice, as well as in the available trials, psoriatic genital involvement and its burden are issues scarcely addressed.

Psoriasis on the genital skin often presents as well-demarcated, brightly erythematous, thin plaques and usually lacks the typical scaling, due to maceration and friction. This can lead to misidentification by both patients and health care providers. The appearance of vulvar psoriasis is often symmetric and can range from silvery, scaling patches adjoining the external faces of the labia majora to moist greyish plaques or glossy red plaques without scaling in the skin folds.[51,52] In male patients, well-defined, nonscaling erythematous plaques most commonly affect the glans penis, but scrotal and penile skin may be involved too. In addition to plaque-type genital psoriasis, the genital area also can be involved with pustular psoriasis. Due to the Koebner phenomenon, genital psoriasis may be worsened by irritation from urine and feces, tightfitting clothes, tampons, sanitary pads, shaving, and sexual intercourse.[54]

Even though several articles have described the dermoscopic features of different types and locations of psoriasis,[55,56] surprisingly enough only 2 studies assessed them at genital level.[57,58] In these reports, all the investigated psoriatic lesions showed a uniform pattern. It consists of either dilated and tortuous capillaries, with a typical "bushy" homogeneous aspect or dotted vessels, depending on magnification, regularly distributed over a light red background. This pattern, which was not observed in other nonpsoriatic dermatitis of the genitalia, histologically corresponds to dilated, elongated, and tortuous capillary loops in the papillary dermis. On dermoscopic observation, genital lesions usually lack scaling as well, as at clinical presentation.

In our experience, as well (AB, AV and MC, 2018, unpublished data), dotted vessels with uniform and regular distribution over a pale red background represent the stereotypical aspect of genital psoriasis (**Fig. 3**). Therefore, this typical combination of vascular morphology and arrangement is the main dermoscopic criterion in the differential diagnosis of genital psoriasis.

Lichen Simplex Chronicus

Anogenital lichen simplex chronicus (LSC) is a benign, chronic, itching, and extremely

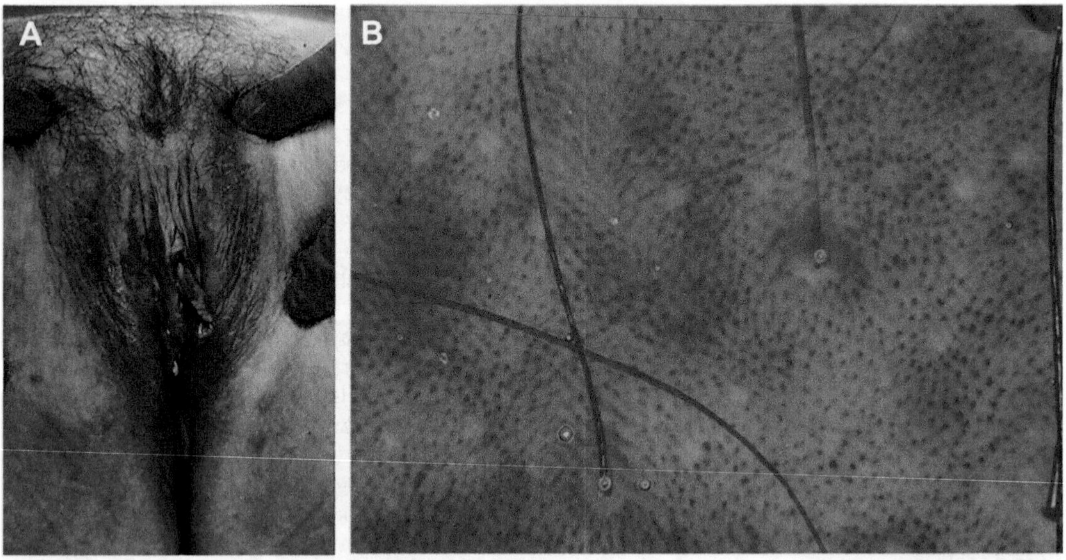

Fig. 3. Clinical (*A*) and dermoscopic (*B*) features of vulvar psoriasis. Dermoscopy (*B*) shows dotted vessels uniformly arranged over a light red background.

uncomfortable disorder characterized by lichenification, with varying degrees of excoriations caused by scratching and rubbing. LSC develops predominantly in mid to late adult life; it is a common condition, especially in women, but its incidence and prevalence are not established.[59]

Anogenital LSC can occur de novo on healthy, mucocutaneous tissue (primary or idiopathic LSC) or as a consequence of preexisting, underlying itching dermatitis, such as psoriasis, LS, and contact dermatitis (secondary LSC).[59] Both types of LSC are an expression of the same basic process in which the itch-scratch cycle preponderates in perpetuating the disease. The skin responds by thickening progressively with more prominent skin markings, turning slightly grayish-brown, and becoming coarse and rough (lichenification) with abrasions and fissures.

In our experience (AB, AV an MC, 2018, unpublished data), on dermoscopy anogenital LSC shows a whitish-grayish background, which presumably corresponds to the characteristic orthokeratotic epidermal hyperplasia found on histopathological examination. However, unlike LS, here the whitish background is characterized by a rich vascularization, mainly composed of linear, serpentine vessels, but also by dotted vessels, arranged diffusely within the affected surfaces (**Fig. 4**). This distinctive

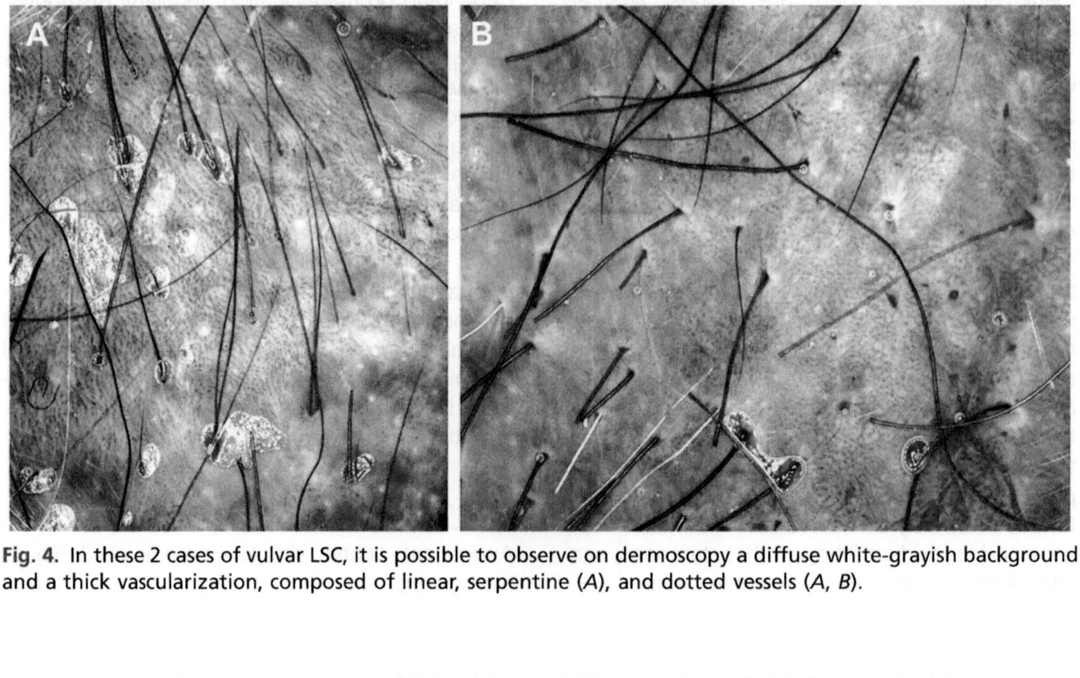

Fig. 4. In these 2 cases of vulvar LSC, it is possible to observe on dermoscopy a diffuse white-grayish background and a thick vascularization, composed of linear, serpentine (*A*), and dotted vessels (*A*, *B*).

dermoscopic picture, which combines the grayish-white background with the dense vascularization, is typical of long-lasting forms of LSC, in which a noticeable lichenification is clinically present.

Plasma Cell Mucositis

Plasma cell mucositis (PCM) is an uncommon chronic, inflammatory disease that owes its name to the characteristic dermal plasma cell infiltrate.[60] PCM has been described at several anatomic sites. The first cases described by Zoon[61] involved the glans penis and prepuce and 2 years later the vulvar counterpart was reported.[62] Analogous lesions have also been reported to occur on airways, oral cavity, and digestive tract, and recently the generic, unifying, and morphologically descriptive term of "idiopathic lymphoplasmacellular mucositis-dermatitis" has been suggested.[63] The incidence and etiopathogenesis of PCM are unknown, although a variety of triggering factors have been hypothesized.[63]

It is an entirely benign disorder, but it can cause local discomfort and render differential diagnosis with other genital disorders difficult. Both the delay in diagnosis observed and the inappropriate treatments often received by patients seem to indicate frequent misdiagnosis or nondiagnosis, especially by physicians unfamiliar with this condition.[64] Biopsy is usually necessary to rule out other conditions that are considered in the differential diagnosis, such as fixed drug eruptions, LP, LS, cicatricial pemphigoid, erythroplasia of Queyrat, invasive squamous cell carcinoma, Kaposi sarcoma, contact dermatitis, or psoriasis.

PCM is clinically characterized by well-circumscribed, shiny, erythematous flat, but barely palpable, patches that involve the glans, prepuce, or both, in men[65] and different sites at the vulvar level, mainly the introitus, inner face of labia minora, and periurethral area in women.[64]

Dermoscopy of plasma cell balanitis (PCB) has been recently described.[66,67] The main features on dermoscopic observation are peculiar focal/diffuse orange-yellowish structureless areas and fairly focused curved vessels. The former, also described as irregular pigmentations varying in color from yellowish to orange-brownish with a "rusty," spatter-like pattern, correspond to hemosiderin deposition. They tend to persist even after a successful treatment, inducing a remarkable

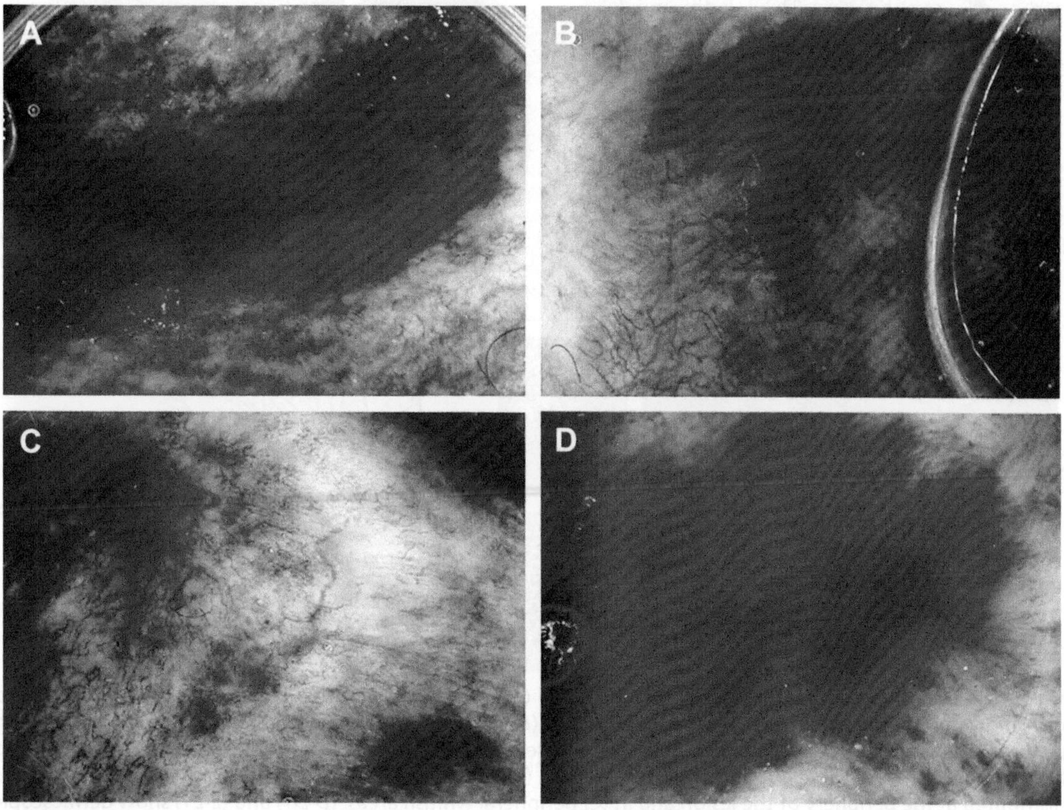

Fig. 5. Dermoscopic features of 4 cases of plasma cell vulvitis. In all cases (*A-D*), both prominent curved vessels and focal/diffuse reddish to orange-yellowish structureless areas are present. In (*C*), a "rusty," spatterlike pattern is observable.

improvement of the disease in terms of both erythema and lesion size.[66] The presence of prominent curved vessels with different width, such as serpentine, spermatozoa-like, convoluted, and chalice-shaped vessels, is a constant feature of PCB dermoscopy. The combination of these dermoscopic features may be of support in the differential diagnosis. Plasma cell vulvitis shares the same dermoscopic features described in male cases, as reported in **Fig. 5**.

Differential Diagnoses: Neoplastic Disorders

Intraepithelial neoplasia of genitalia may constitute a diagnostic challenge, as its onset is insidious and it can mimic different dermatologic genital disorders, including inflammatory and infectious diseases. Therefore, a brief reference to the dermoscopy of the condition may be useful in this context.

Regardless of the numerous changes proposed across the years in the classification and terminology of intraepithelial neoplasia of genitalia,[68] penile intraepithelial neoplasia (PeIN) and vulvar intraepithelial neoplasia (VIN) share quite similar etiopathogenesis. In particular, 2 different pathways underlie both conditions, namely human papillomavirus (HPV)-dependent and HPV-independent pathomecanisms.[69,70] The non-HPV pathway is usually associated with chronic inflammatory diseases, mainly LS.

At dermoscopic examination, intraepithelial neoplasia of genitalia presents as irregular plaques with asymmetry of structure and color.[71–73] In particular, they can present different colors, usually combined, ranging from dull pink to bright red, with whitish areas. Focal structureless gray-blue/brownish areas, as well as brown/brown-gray dots arranged in linear fashion may be observed, mainly located at the periphery of the lesion. Intraepithelial neoplasia presents thick vascularization, dotted, glomerular, and linear in shape with variable size and irregular and patchy distribution over the lesion surface. Papillary structures with fissures and ridges, leading to a focal cerebriform appearance, may be observed within the lesion (**Fig. 6**A–C).

Extramammary Paget disease (EMPD) can constitute a diagnostic challenge, as it can mimic several dermatologic disorders, mainly

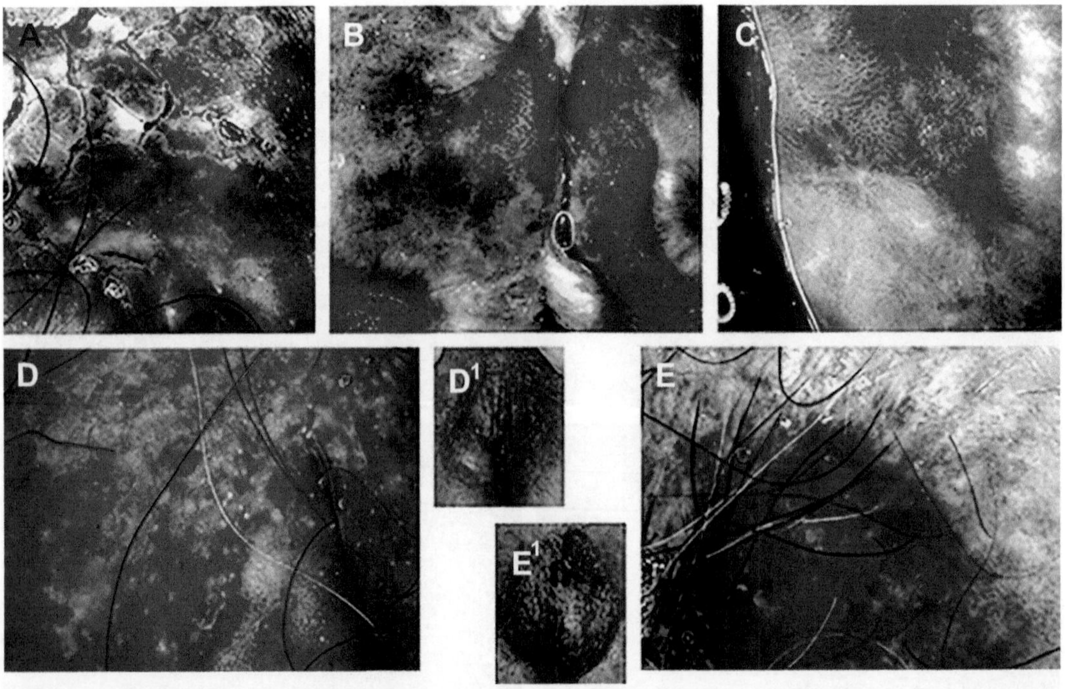

Fig. 6. (*A–C*) Dermoscopic features of 2 cases of VIN. In (*A*), papillary structures varying in color from whitish to brown-gray are visible within a red, vascularized lesion. (*B, C*) Dermoscopic images from the same patient. In both pictures, abundant dotted, glomerular, and linear vessels irregularly distributed over a dull pink to bright red background are observable. Dermoscopy revealed in (*B*) structureless gray-blue/brownish and whitish areas distributed at the periphery of the lesion and in (*C*) peripheral whitish areas. (*D-D1*) and (*E-E1*) show dermoscopic and clinical pictures, respectively, of 2 cases of vulvar Paget disease. In both cases, dermoscopy reveals thick polymorphic vessels arranged diffusely throughout pink-reddish background; milky-red areas, either isolated or coalescing, are present as well.

inflammatory diseases.[74] Its diagnosis is often delayed and is usually made on the histologic examination performed in the presence of a chronic dermatosis not responding to local treatments. The first report of dermoscopy in EMPD backs to 2011 and regards a pigmented vulvar PD (VPD) described as "dermoscopic equivocal."[75] All reported experiences on dermoscopic appearance of pigmented mammary and extramammary Paget disease have defined dermoscopy not diriment for diagnosis because it often reveals heterogeneous patterns mimicking other conditions, especially melanoma.[76–78] Recently, Mun and colleagues[79] assessed the dermoscopic patterns of 35 cases of EMPD, including genital forms. The investigators found several dermoscopic variables significantly associated with EMPD, namely dotted and glomerular vessels as well as milky-red areas, which may improve the diagnostic accuracy of this rare tumor. In our experience (AB, AV, and MC, 2018), in cases of VPD we have observed similar findings to those reported by Mun and colleagues,[79] as shown in **Fig. 6**D, E.

SUMMARY

Based on the summarized data, the recognition of specific dermoscopic patterns may enhance diagnostic accuracy and improve differential diagnosis in the field of genital inflammatory diseases, especially in the early phases or in the case of clinical doubts. Both the vessels, in terms of vascular morphology and arrangement, and the colors observed within the lesions, as well as their combination, are the major criteria to be considered in the dermoscopic assessment of genital conditions. As with any other condition in any other area of the body, these dermoscopic findings must be interpreted within the overall history and clinical features of the genital disorder.

REFERENCES

1. Argenziano G, Soyer HP, Chimenti S, et al. Dermoscopy of pigmented skin lesions: results of a consensus meeting via the Internet. J Am Acad Dermatol 2003;48:679–93.
2. Zalaudek I, Argenziano G, Di Stefani A, et al. Dermoscopy in general dermatology. Dermatology 2006; 212:7–18.
3. Lallas A, Zalaudek I, Argenziano G, et al. Dermoscopy in general dermatology. Dermatol Clin 2013; 31:679–94.
4. Lacarrubba F, Verzì AE, Dinotta F, et al. Dermatoscopy in inflammatory and infectious skin disorders. G Ital Dermatol Venereol 2015;150:521–31.
5. Miteva M, Tosti A. Hair and scalp dermatoscopy. J Am Acad Dermatol 2012;67:1040–8.
6. Lencastre A, Lamas A, Sá D, et al. Onychoscopy. Clin Dermatol 2013;31:587–93.
7. Micali G, Lacarrubba F, Massimino D, et al. Dermatoscopy: alternative uses in daily clinical practice. J Am Acad Dermatol 2011;64:1135–46.
8. Andreassi L, Bilenchi R. Non-infectious inflammatory genital lesions. Clin Dermatol 2014;32:307–14.
9. van der Meijden WI, Boffa MJ, Ter Harmsel WA, et al. 2016 European guideline for the management of vulval conditions. J Eur Acad Dermatol Venereol 2017;31:925–41.
10. Stamm AW, Kobashi KC, Stefanovic KB. Urologic dermatology: a review. Curr Urol Rep 2017;18:62.
11. Hoang LN, Park KJ, Soslow RA, et al. Squamous precursor lesions of the vulva: current classification and diagnostic challenges. Pathology 2016;48:291–302.
12. Schlosser BJ, Mirowski GW. Lichen sclerosus and lichen planus in women and girls. Clin Obstet Gynecol 2015;58:125–42.
13. Morris BJ, Krieger JN. Penile inflammatory skin disorders and the preventive role of circumcision. Int J Prev Med 2017;8:32.
14. Paštar Z, Lipozenčić J. Significance of dermatoscopy in genital dermatoses. Clin Dermatol 2014;32:315–8.
15. Oakley A. Dermatoscopic features of vulval lesions in 97 women. Australas J Dermatol 2016;57:48–53.
16. Micali G, Lacarrubba F. Augmented diagnostic capability using videodermatoscopy on selected infectious and non-infectious penile growths. Int J Dermatol 2011;50:1501–5.
17. Borghi A, Corazza M, Minghetti S, et al. Clinical and dermoscopic changes of vulvar lichen sclerosus after topical corticosteroid treatment. J Dermatol 2016;43:1078–82.
18. Lacarrubba F, D'Amico V, Nasca MR, et al. Use of dermatoscopy and videodermatoscopy in therapeutic follow-up: a review. Int J Dermatol 2010;49:866–73.
19. Zampino MR, Borghi A, Corazza M, et al. A preliminary evaluation of polyvinyl chloride film use in dermoscopic analysis of mucosal areas. Arch Dermatol 2005;141:1044–5.
20. Zampino MR, Borghi A, Caselli E, et al. Virologic safety of polyvinyl chloride film in dermoscopic analysis of mucosal areas. Arch Dermatol 2007;143:945–6.
21. Fistarol SK, Itin PH. Diagnosis and treatment of lichen sclerosus: an update. Am J Clin Dermatol 2013;14:27–47.
22. Virgili A, Borghi A, Cazzaniga S, et al. Gender differences in genital lichen sclerosus. Data from a multicentre Italian study on 729 consecutive cases. G Ital Dermatol Venereol 2018. https://doi.org/10.23736/S0392-0488.17.05819-9.
23. Cooper SM, Gao XH, Powell JJ, et al. Does treatment of vulvar lichen sclerosus influence its prognosis? Arch Dermatol 2004;140:702–6.

24. Kravvas G, Shim TN, Doiron PR, et al. The diagnosis and management of male genital lichen sclerosus: a retrospective review of 301 patients. J Eur Acad Dermatol Venereol 2018;32(1):91–5.
25. Virgili A, Borghi A, Toni G, et al. Prospective clinical and epidemiologic study of vulvar lichen sclerosus: analysis of prevalence and severity of clinical features, together with historical and demographic associations. Dermatology 2014;228:145–51.
26. Lansdorp CA, van den Hondel KE, Korfage IJ, et al. Quality of life in Dutch women with lichen sclerosus. Br J Dermatol 2013;168:787–93.
27. Edmonds EV, Hunt S, Hawkins D, et al. Clinical parameters in male genital lichen sclerosus: a case series of 329 patients. J Eur Acad Dermatol Venereol 2012;26:730–7.
28. Murphy R. Lichen sclerosus. Dermatol Clin 2010;28: 707–15.
29. Larre Borges A, Tiodorovic-Zivkovic D, Lallas A, et al. Clinical, dermoscopic and histopathologic features of genital and extragenital lichen sclerosus. J Eur Acad Dermatol Venereol 2013;27: 1433–9.
30. Borghi A, Corazza M, Minghetti S, et al. Dermoscopic features of vulvar lichen sclerosus in the setting of a prospective cohort of patients: new observations. Dermatology 2016;232:71–7.
31. Borghi A, Corazza M, Minghetti S, et al. Preliminary study on dermoscopic features of vulvar lichen planus: new insights for diagnosis. J Eur Acad Dermatol Venereol 2016;30:1063–5.
32. Tchernev G, Chokoeva AA, Mangarov H. Penile melanosis associated with lichen sclerosus et atrophicus: first description in the medical literature. Open Access Maced J Med Sci 2017;5:692–3.
33. Sollena P, Caldarola G, Di Stefani A, et al. Lichen sclerosus of the glans simulating melanoma. J Am Acad Dermatol 2017;76:S49–51.
34. Lacarrubba F, Dinotta F, Nasca MR, et al. Localized vascular lesions of the glans in patients with lichen sclerosus diagnosed by dermatoscopy. G Ital Dermatol Venereol 2012;147:510–1.
35. Micali G, Verzì AE, Lacarrubba F. Alternative uses of dermatoscopy in daily clinical practice: an update. J Am Acad Dermatol 2018 Jun 16. pii: S0190-9622(18)32143-1. [Epub ahead of print].
36. Lacarrubba F, Pellacani G, Verzì AE, et al. Extragenital lichen sclerosus: clinical, dermoscopic, confocal microscopy and histologic correlations. J Am Acad Dermatol 2015;72:S50–2.
37. Le Cleach L, Chosidow O. Clinical practice. Lichen planus. N Engl J Med 2012;366:723–32.
38. Sontheimer RD. Lichenoid tissue reaction/interface dermatitis: clinical and histological perspectives. J Invest Dermatol 2009;129:1088–99.
39. Lehman JS, Tollefson MM, Gibson LE. Lichen planus. Int J Dermatol 2009;48:682–94.
40. Lodi G, Pellicano R, Carrozzo M. Hepatitis C virus infection and lichen planus: a systematic review with meta-analysis. Oral Dis 2010;16:601–12.
41. Fahy CMR, Torgerson RR, Davis MDP. Lichen planus affecting the female genitalia: a retrospective review of patients at Mayo Clinic. J Am Acad Dermatol 2017;77:1053–9.
42. Belfiore P, Di Fede O, Cabibi D, et al. Prevalence of vulval lichen planus in a cohort of women with oral lichen planus: an interdisciplinary study. Br J Dermatol 2006;155:994–8.
43. Micheletti L, Preti M, Bogliatto E, et al. Vulva lichen planus in the practice of a vulval clinic. Br J Dermatol 2000;143:1349–50.
44. Lewis FM, Bogliatto F. Erosive vulval lichen planus–a diagnosis not to be missed: a clinical review. Eur J Obstet Gynecol Reprod Biol 2013;171:214–9.
45. Helgesen AL, Gjersvik P, Jebsen P, et al. Vaginal involvement in genital erosive lichen planus. Acta Obstet Gynecol Scand 2010;89:966–70.
46. Niamh L, Naveen S, Hazel B. Diagnosis of vulval inflammatory dermatoses: a pathological study with clinical correlation. Int J Gynecol Pathol 2009;28: 554–8.
47. Vázquez-López F, Manjón-Haces JA, Maldonado-Seral C, et al. Dermoscopic features of plaque psoriasis and lichen planus: new observations. Dermatology 2003;207:151–6.
48. Vázquez-López F, Gómez-Díez S, Sánchez J, et al. Dermoscopy of active lichen planus. Arch Dermatol 2007;143:1092.
49. Tan C, Min ZS, Xue Y, et al. Spectrum of dermoscopic patterns in lichen planus: a case series from China. J Cutan Med Surg 2014;18:28–32.
50. Michalek IM, Loring B, John SM. A systematic review of worldwide epidemiology of psoriasis. J Eur Acad Dermatol Venereol 2017;31:205–12.
51. Cather JC, Ryan C, Meeuwis K, et al. Patients' perspectives on the impact of genital psoriasis: a qualitative study. Dermatol Ther (Heidelb) 2017;7: 447–61.
52. Meeuwis KA, de Hullu JA, Massuger LF, et al. Genital psoriasis: a systematic literature review on this hidden skin disease. Acta Derm Venereol 2011;91: 5–11.
53. Ryan C, Sadlier M, De Vol E, et al. Genital psoriasis is associated with significant impairment in quality of life and sexual functioning. J Am Acad Dermatol 2015;72:978–83.
54. Meeuwis KA, de Hullu JA, van de Nieuwenhof HP, et al. Quality of life and sexual health in patients with genital psoriasis. Br J Dermatol 2011;164: 1247–55.
55. Lallas A, Kyrgidis A, Tzellos TG, et al. Accuracy of dermoscopic criteria for the diagnosis of psoriasis, dermatitis, lichen planus and pityriasis rosea. Br J Dermatol 2012;166:1198–205.

56. Lacarrubba F, Pellacani G, Gurgone S, et al. Advances in non-invasive techniques as aids to the diagnosis and monitoring of therapeutic response in plaque psoriasis: a review. Int J Dermatol 2015;54:626–34.
57. Lacarrubba F, Nasca MR, Micali G. Videodermatoscopy enhances diagnostic capability in psoriatic balanitis. J Am Acad Dermatol 2009;61:1084–6.
58. Lallas A, Apalla Z, Argenziano G, et al. Dermoscopic pattern of psoriatic lesions on specific body sites. Dermatology 2014;228:250–4.
59. Lynch PJ. Lichen simplex chronicus (atopic/neurodermatitis) of the anogenital region. Dermatol Ther 2004;17:8–19.
60. Virgili A, Levratti A, Marzola A, et al. Retrospective histopathologic reevaluation of 18 cases of plasma cell vulvitis. J Reprod Med 2005;50:3–7.
61. Zoon J. Balanoposthite chronique circonscrite benigne a plasmocytes (contra erythroplasie de Queyrat). Dermatologica 1952;105:1–7.
62. Garnier G. Vulvite erythemateuse circonscrite benigne a type erythroplasique. Bull Soc Fr Dermatol Syphiligr 1954;61:102.
63. Brix WK, Nassau SR, Patterson JW, et al. Idiopathic lymphoplasmacellular mucositis-dermatitis. J Cutan Pathol 2010;37:426–31.
64. Virgili A, Corazza M, Minghetti S, et al. Symptoms in plasma cell vulvitis: first observational cohort study on type, frequency and severity. Dermatology 2015;230:113–8.
65. Kyriakou A, Patsatsi A, Patsialas C, et al. Therapeutic efficacy of topical calcineurin inhibitors in plasma cell balanitis: case series and review of the literature. Dermatology 2014;228:18–23.
66. Corazza M, Virgili A, Minghetti S, et al. Dermoscopy in plasma cell balanitis: its usefulness in diagnosis and follow-up. J Eur Acad Dermatol Venereol 2016;30:182–4.
67. Errichetti E, Lacarrubba F, Micali G, et al. Dermoscopy of Zoon's plasma cell balanitis. J Eur Acad Dermatol Venereol 2016;30:e209–10.
68. Bornstein J, Bogliatto F, Haefner HK, et al. The 2015 International Society for the Study of Vulvovaginal Disease (ISSVD) terminology of vulvar squamous intraepithelial lesions. J Low Genit Tract Dis 2016;20:11–4.
69. Del Pino M, Rodriguez-Carunchio L, Ordi J. Pathways of vulvar intraepithelial neoplasia and squamous cell carcinoma. Histopathology 2013;62:161–75.
70. Oertell J, Caballero C, Iglesias M, et al. Differentiated precursor lesions and low-grade variants of squamous cell carcinomas are frequent findings in foreskins of patients from a region of high penile cancer incidence. Histopathology 2011;58:925–33.
71. Maione V, Errichetti E, Dehen L, et al. Usual-type vulvar intraepithelial neoplasia: report of a case and its dermoscopic features. Int J Dermatol 2016;55:e621–3.
72. Ferrari A, Zalaudek I, Argenziano G, et al. Dermoscopy of pigmented lesions of the vulva: a retrospective morphological study. Dermatology 2011;222:157–66.
73. Friedman BJ, Kohen LL. A case of pigmented penile intraepithelial neoplasia: dermoscopic and clinicohistopathologic analysis. J Am Acad Dermatol 2015;72:S71–2.
74. Kanitakis J. Mammary and extramammary Paget's disease. J Eur Acad Dermatol Venereol 2007;21:581–90.
75. Lentini M, Le Donne M. Asymmetrically pigmented patch on the vulvo-perineal area: a quiz. Pigmented extramammary Paget's disease. Acta Derm Venereol 2011;91:380–1.
76. Longo C, Fantini F, Cesinaro AM, et al. Pigmented mammary Paget disease: dermoscopic, in vivo reflectance-mode confocal microscopic, and immunohistochemical study of a case. Arch Dermatol 2007;143:752–4.
77. Coras-Stepanek B, von Portatius A, Dyall-Smith D, et al. Dermatoscopy of pigmented extramammary Paget disease simulating melanoma. J Am Acad Dermatol 2012;67:e144–6.
78. Brugués A, Iranzo P, Díaz A, et al. Pigmented mammary Paget disease mimicking cutaneous malignant melanoma. J Am Acad Dermatol 2015;201(72):e97–8.
79. Mun JH, Park SM, Kim GW, et al. Clinical and dermoscopic characteristics of extramammary Paget: a study of 35 cases. Br J Dermatol 2016;174:1104–7.

Dermatoscopy of Common Lesions in Pediatric Dermatology

Giuseppe Micali, MD[a,*], Anna Elisa Verzì, MD[a], Enrica Quattrocchi, MD[a], Chau Yee Ng, MD[b], Francesco Lacarrubba, MD[a]

KEYWORDS

• Dermatoscopy • Dermoscopy • Videodermatoscopy • Pediatric skin disorders

KEY POINTS

- Being non invasive, dermatoscopy is perfectly suitable for use in the pediatric population, and its applications are constantly increasing.
- Dermatoscopy has demonstrated usefulness in a variety of cutaneous growths and proliferative, infectious, parasitic, pigmentary, inflammatory, congenital, and genetic cutaneous and skin appendage disorders in children.
- This article focuses on the dermatoscopy features of juvenile xanthogranuloma, verrucous epidermal nevus, sebaceous naevus, Langerhans cell histiocytosis, vitiligo, cutaneous mastocytosis, median raphe cyst, aplasia cutis congenita of the scalp, and pseudoxanthoma elasticum.

INTRODUCTION

Being non invasive, dermatoscopy has demonstrated to be very useful in children to enhance the diagnosis of a variety of proliferative, infectious, pigmentary, inflammatory, malformative, and genetic cutaneous and skin appendage disorders (**Table 1**), and its use is constantly increasing.[1–3] This article focuses on those nonmelanocytic disorders typically encountered in pediatric age in which the diagnostic value of dermatoscopy has been reported and not otherwise described in this *Dermatologic Clinics* issue (see **Table 1**).

CUTANEOUS GROWTHS/PROLIFERATIVE DISORDERS

Juvenile Xanthogranuloma

Juvenile xanthogranuloma (JXG) is a benign non–Langerhans cell histiocytosis occurring in 40% to 70% of cases during the first year of life.[4,5] Adults are rarely affected.[6] Clinically, lesions appear as single or multiple yellow, orange, or reddish papules or nodules of different sizes (**Fig. 1**A). The head and the neck represent the most common involved sites, but trunk and extremities also may be affected.[7] Spontaneous regression may occur, sometimes leaving a residual atrophic or hyperpigmented scar. The diagnosis is generally clinical but, in some cases, histopathological examination is required.

Dermatoscopy of JXG shows a typical pattern consisting of diffuse, homogeneous orange-yellowish hue surrounded by a slight erythema, also known as "setting sun" appearance[7–13] (**Fig. 1**B). This finding is histopathologically related to the presence of aggregates of lipid-laden histiocytes ("foam cells") in the superficial dermis. The presence of linear and branched vessels may also be detected, especially when the

Disclosures: None.

[a] Dermatology Clinic, University of Catania, Via S. Sofia 78, Catania 95123, Italy; [b] Department of Dermatology, College of Medicine, Chang Gung Memorial Hospital, No. 199, Tun-Hwa North Road, Taipei 105, Taiwan
* Corresponding author. Dermatology Clinic, University of Catania, Via S. Sofia 78, Catania 95123, Italy.
E-mail address: cldermct@gmail.com

Dermatol Clin 36 (2018) 463–472
https://doi.org/10.1016/j.det.2018.05.012
0733-8635/18/

Table 1
Main indications of dermatoscopy in pediatric dermatology beyond melanocytic lesions

Cutaneous growths/proliferative disorders	
Juvenile xanthogranuloma[a]	Homogeneous orange-yellowish hue (setting sun appearance) Linear/branched vessels Yellow globules
Pyogenic granuloma	Reddish homogeneous area White collarette White rail lines Vascular structures Ulceration
Verrucous epidermal nevus[a]	Large brown circles Fissures, comedo-like openings, milia-like cysts, brown globules, brown-grayish dots, papillomatous surface, cerebriform and cobblestone appearance
Sebaceous naevus[a]	Roundish, yellowish/orange structures Bright yellow dots Telangiectasias Cerebriform patterns/verrucous proliferations
Langerhans cell histiocytosis[a]	Reddish-purple areas Whitish areas and brown dots
Infectious and parasitic skin disorders	
Anogenital warts	Whitish network circumscribing areas centered by dilated glomerular/dotted vessels (papular lesions) Multiple, irregular whitish projections arising from a common base containing elongated and dilated vessels (cauliflower-like lesions)
Cutaneous warts	Irregularly distributed, reddish to black dots on a whitish background (papular lesions) Multiple papillomatous projections containing elongated and dilated vessels (filiform lesions) Interrupted skin lines
Molluscum contagiosum	Yellowish-white, lobulated, amorphous central structures Crown of linear/fine/blurred vessels
Scabies	Low magnification: jet-shaped triangular structure (mite) and contrail-shaped segment (burrow) High magnification: mites, eggs, and feces
Pediculosis	Lice, full/empty nits fixed to the hair shaft
Cutaneous leishmaniasis	Diffuse erythema Yellow "tears," yellowish-orange areas Polymorphous vessels
Tinea capitis	Broken hairs Comma hairs, corkscrew hairs Interrupted hairs (Morse-code hairs) Zigzag hairs Erythema, scaling, pustules, and crusts
Disorders of pigmentation	
Vitiligo[a]	Pigmentary network reduced, reversed, or absent Perifollicular hyperpigmentation (progressive/active and repigmenting vitiligo) or depigmentation (stable disease) Leukotrichia
Inflammatory skin disorders	
Psoriasis	Low magnification: dotted/pinpoint capillaries, scaling High magnification: glomerular/bushy capillaries
Pityriasis lichenoides chronica	Orange-yellowish structureless areas Nondotted vessels (milky-red areas/globules, linear irregular and/or branching vessels)

Pityriasis lichenoides et varioliformis acuta	Amorphous, brownish crust/central whitish area Pinpoint/linear vessels
Pityriasis rosea	Peripheral whitish scaling (collarette sign) Dotted vessels in an irregular or focal pattern
Lichen aureus and Majocchi disease	Irregular, roundish, nonblanchable, purpuric, reddish dots/globules/patches Red-brownish/coppery background
Lichen nitidus	Smooth, roundish, homogeneous, whitish clouds
Lichen planus	Pinkish background Wickham striae Dotted/globular/linear vessels Pigmented structures
Lichen sclerosus	Whitish patches Linear branching/dotted vessels Erosions and hemorrhages Gray-blue dots Comedo-like openings
Morphea	Whitish fibrotic beams Linear branching vessels Pigment network-like structures
Cutaneous mastocytosis[a]	*Urticaria pigmentosa*: faint pigment network, light-brown blots, reticular telangiectasias, and erythematous background *Mastocytoma*: yellowish to orange discoloration
Congenital and genetic skin disorders	
Hemangiomas	Red round-oval structures (lacunae) Globular/circulated/comma-like/wavy/dilated/linear vessels Blue-whitish septa
Lymphatic malformations	Whitish or yellowish lacunae Scattered reddish areas or reddish lacunae
Vascular malformations	Red-dotted, globular vessels or red, dilated, linear vessels or round/sacular/glomerular structures Perifollicular pale halo Gray-whitish veil
Darier disease	Polygonal/star-like/roundish-shaped yellowish or brownish structures with a whitish halo
Median raphe cyst[a]	Homogeneous white/yellowish pattern Translucent tract (median raphe canal)
Aplasia cutis congenita of the scalp[a]	Scarring alopecia Telangiectatic vessels Horizontally and radially oriented hair follicles (starburst hair follicles pattern)
Pseudoxanthoma elasticum[a]	Multiple irregular yellowish areas Prominent linear vessels
Appendage disorders	
Alopecia areata	Dystrophic hair shafts (broken hairs, exclamation-mark hairs, black dots) Yellow dots Hypopigmented vellus hairs
Trichotillomania	Multiple hairs broken at different lengths Damaged hair shafts (flame hairs, coiled hairs, tulip hairs, V-sign) Hair powder
Congenital triangular alopecia	"Carpet" of short vellus hairs
Hair shaft disorders	Variable patterns
Nail disorders	Variable patterns

[a] Disorders described in this article.
Data from Refs.[1–3]

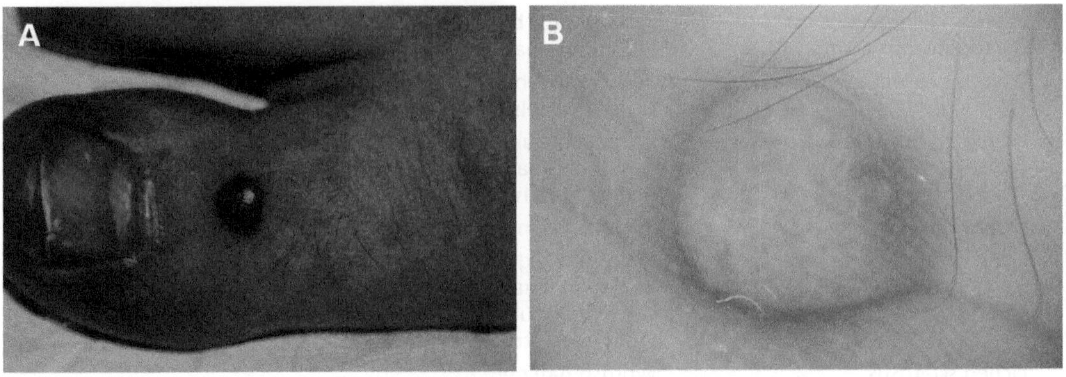

Fig. 1. Juvenile xanthogranuloma. (*A*) Reddish papule on the big toe of a 6-year-old boy. (*B*) Dermatoscopy shows diffuse, homogeneous yellowish hue and linear vessels (original magnification × 10).

dermatoscope is gently placed on the lesions, thus avoiding excessive pressure on the skin. Additional features include "clouds" of pale yellow globules, subtle pigment network, and whitish streaks, indicating foci of fibrosis.

The dermatoscopic features also have been related to the lesion stage[9,10,12,14]: in early and developed stages, the "setting sun" appearance is a constant finding; in the late regressive stage, surrounding erythema decreases, and the vacuolated cells transform to more xanthomatized cells, so that the yellow globules become more evident.

Verrucous Epidermal Nevus

Verrucous epidermal nevus (VEN) is a benign hamartoma mainly composed of keratinocytes that arise from pluripotential germ cells in the basal layer of the embryonic ectoderm.[15,16] It is thought that VEN is the result of mosaic post-zygotic mutations that have not yet been completely identified.[17] It clinically appears as well-demarcated, skin-colored to brown, velvet papules coalescing into plaques, which commonly have the appearance of being "stuck on" to the skin surface (**Fig. 2**A). Lesions display a linear arrangement according to either Blaschko lines or tension lines and usually tend to not cross the midline. They are usually present at birth or occur within the first years of life. Even though VEN is usually an isolated lesion, in some cases it may be associated with abnormalities affecting other systems (epidermal nevus syndrome).[15] Diagnosis of VEN is usually based on clinical presentation and, in selected cases, on histopathology examination.

At dermatoscopy, a characteristic presence of large brown circles (hyperchromic brown edge surrounding a hypochromic area) has recently been reported[18] (**Fig. 2**B). These structures, which histologically correspond to a peculiar disposition of pigmented keratinocytes surrounding the dermal papillae, appear adjacent each other and variable in size. Additional features, which are usually seen in other pigmented lesions, such as seborrheic keratosis, include fissures, comedo-like openings, milia-like cysts, brown globules,

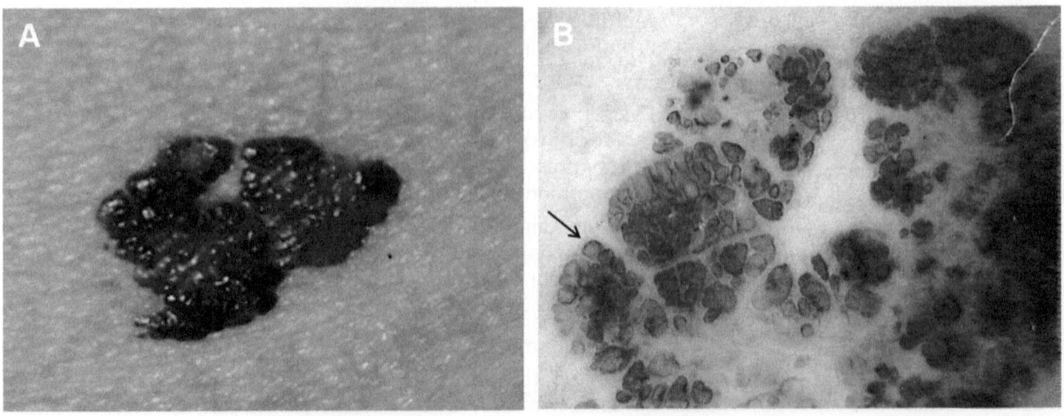

Fig. 2. Verrucous epidermal nevus. (*A*) Well-demarcated, light to dark-brown, velvet plaque on the trunk of a 10-year-old girl. (*B*) Dermatoscopy shows large brown circles (*arrow*) (original magnification × 10).

brown-grayish dots, papillomatous surface, and cerebriform and cobblestone appearance.

Sebaceous Naevus

Sebaceous naevus (SN), also known as naevus sebaceous of Jadassohn or organoid naevus, is a benign hamartoma that is mainly composed of sebaceous glands.[19] It occurs in approximately 0.3% of all neonates, although it may occasionally become apparent later in life. SN usually presents at birth, mainly involving the head, scalp, and neck, as a flat, hairless, pink/yellow/orange, waxy plaque (**Fig. 3**A). It generally develops a velvety and verrucous surface and becomes thickened at puberty. Most of the secondary neoplasms arising on SN are benign (syringocystadenoma papilliferum, trichoblastoma, and trichilemmoma) and, although it has the potential for malignant transformation (mainly into basal cell and squamous cell carcinoma),[20] this risk is less than 1% and unlikely in childhood.[21,22]

Dermatoscopy may assist the diagnosis of SN in doubtful cases. In early lesions it reveals the presence of roundish yellowish/orange structures of different sizes (**Fig. 3**B), bright yellow dots not associated with hair follicles, and thin telangiectasias.[23–27] In advanced lesions, dermatoscopy generally shows a cerebriform pattern as well as verrucous proliferations. Dermatoscopy also may be helpful for the identification of secondary arising tumors[24–27]: the detection of blue ovoid nests in the context of the lesion may indicate the presence of a basal cell carcinoma or trichoblastoma.

Langerhans Cell Histiocytosis

Langerhans cell histiocytosis is a rare condition characterized by abnormal proliferation and dissemination of clonal Langerhans cells in several organs, such as bone, lung, hypothalamus, posterior pituitary gland, lymph nodes, liver, mucous membranes, and skin. The clinical manifestations are variable, ranging from self-resolving single-organ disease to disseminated, aggressive condition, mimicking other childhood inflammatory, infectious, and neoplastic disorders. Cutaneous involvement is reported in approximately 50% of the cases and may be the presenting feature.[28] Lesions vary from purpuric macules to reddish papules, nodules, or blisters[29]; they may be single or multiple and are mainly located on the head, trunk, and skin folds (**Fig. 4**A). The diagnosis is based on the presence of characteristic S-100–positive Langerhans cells, along with histiocytes and eosinophils, on histopathological examination.

Few reports described the dermatoscopic findings of cutaneous Langerhans cell histiocytosis.[30–32] Dermatoscopy of maculo-papular lesions reveals the presence of reddish-purple areas, corresponding to dermal hemorrhage, and peripheral telangiectasias (**Fig. 4**B). Whitish areas, related to the proliferation of Langerhans cells in the dermis, and brown dots, linked to the infiltration and necrosis of the epidermis by Langerhans cells, have also been reported.[30–32]

DISORDERS OF PIGMENTATION

Vitiligo

Vitiligo is an acquired disorder of pigmentation that results from a progressive loss of functional melanocytes. It has an estimated prevalence of 0.5% of the general population and 30% to 40% of patients have a positive family history.[33] Although various theories have been suggested for the pathogenesis, the contribution of both genetic and environmental factors remains to be elucidated. Lesions appear as single or multiple, variable sized, milk-white patches surrounded by normal skin. The pigment loss may be partial or complete, also in the same areas (trichrome vitiligo). There is a

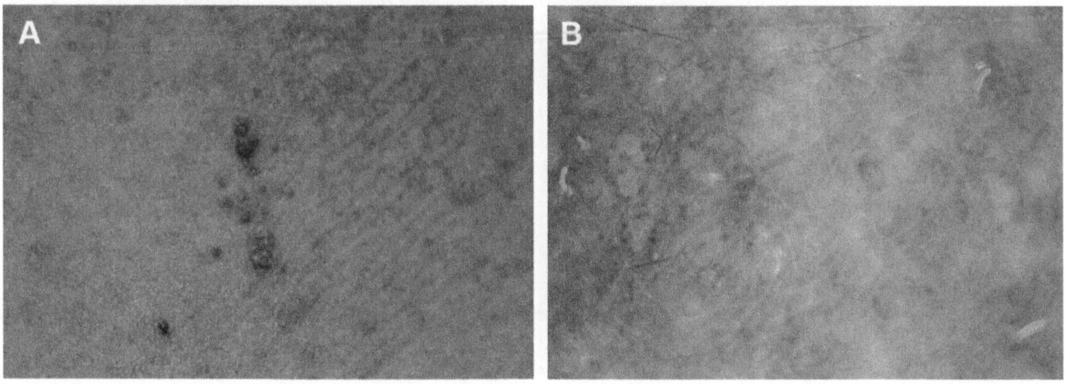

Fig. 3. Sebaceous nevus. (*A*) Flat, yellowish plaque on the chest of a 3-year-old girl. (*B*) Dermatoscopy shows roundish, yellowish structures of different sizes (original magnification × 10).

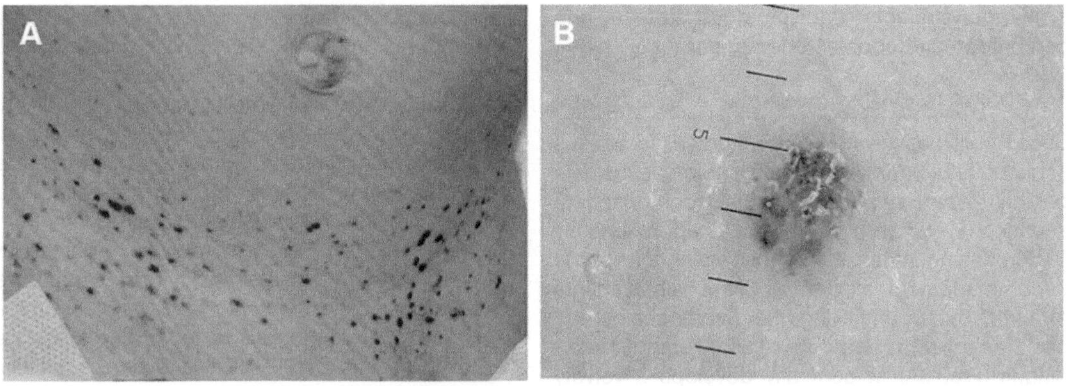

Fig. 4. Langerhans cell histiocytosis. (*A*) Multiple erythematous maculo-papules on the abdomen of a 10-month-old boy. (*B*) Dermatoscopy of a lesion shows reddish-purple areas and brown dots (original magnification × 10).

predilection for sites that are normally hyperpigmented, including the face, axillae, groins, areolae, and genitalia, as well as areas subjected to repeated trauma and friction, as dorsal aspect of the hands, feet, elbows, knees, and ankles.[34] In segmental vitiligo, which is more frequent in children, the progressive loss of melanocytes results in a unilateral patch of depigmentation that may be arranged in a linear or block-like pattern.[35]

Diagnosis of vitiligo is straightforward, and Wood lamp examination may accentuate lesions in lightly pigmented patients, revealing a striking contrast between vitiliginous areas and the surrounding skin.

Few studies have reported the dermatoscopic features of vitiligo, consisting of a different degree of pigmentary network and perifollicular changes along with leukotrichia.[36,37] In the lesional areas, the pigmentary network may be reduced, reversed, or absent. Perifollicular hyperpigmentation has been found more frequently in both progressive/active and repigmenting vitiligo, whereas depigmentation is associated to stable disease. The detection of leukotrichia seems to be a negative prognostic factor for repigmentation.[38] Finally, perilesional changes or marginal hyperpigmentation are usually seen in repigmenting vitiligo.[37]

INFLAMMATORY SKIN DISORDERS

Cutaneous Mastocytosis

Mastocytosis is a disorder characterized by mast cell proliferation and accumulation in several organs.[39] Cutaneous lesions, reported in 95% of patients, may develop during childhood, usually without evident involvement of other organs, or adulthood, often associated with extracutaneous manifestations (including bone marrow, gastrointestinal tract, liver, spleen, and lymphatic tissues).[40–44] The main forms of cutaneous mastocytosis are represented by urticaria pigmentosa, clinically characterized by red, tan, or brown macules and papules that vary in size and number and preferentially involve the trunk (**Fig. 5**A), and localized mastocytoma, which typically appears as a single red, pink, or yellowish nodule or plaque measuring up to 3 to 4 cm in diameter. In both varieties, the lesions may become erythematous

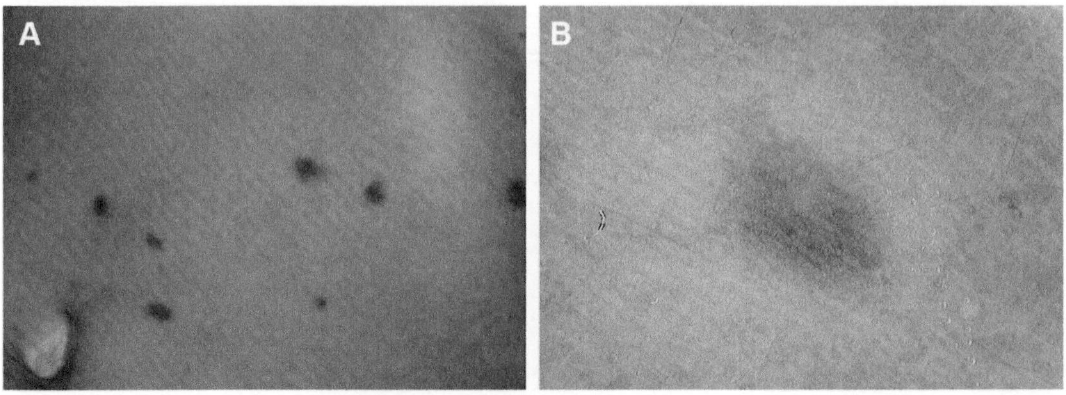

Fig. 5. Urticaria pigmentosa. (*A*) Multiple brown macules on the trunk of a 3-year-old boy. (*B*) Dermatoscopy of a lesion shows a faint pigment network (original magnification × 10).

and/or urticated after gentle scratching or rubbing (Darier sign).[45] The diagnosis of cutaneous mastocytosis is based on the presence of a typical skin lesion (major criterion) and 1 or 2 of the following minor criteria: a histologically confirmed infiltrate of mast cells in the dermis and a detection of a KIT mutation at codon 816 in lesional skin.[46,47]

Some studies have reported the usefulness of dermatoscopy in cutaneous mastocytosis. In urticaria pigmentosa, it shows a combination of light-brown blots and pigment network[48–52] (**Fig. 5**B), likely related to hyperpigmentation of basal keratinocytes induced by high concentration of mast cell growth factor that stimulates melanocyte proliferation and melanogenesis.[45] In addition, thin reticular telangiectasias on a mild erythematous background can be appreciated. Mastocytomas are characterized by yellowish to orange discoloration with an ill-defined margin (more prominent after Darier sign) that histopathologically correlates with a dense infiltration of mast cells along the papillary and reticular dermis.[50] However, a similar yellowish pattern also can be detected in xanthogranulomatous dermal infiltrate-associated disorders.[8]

CONGENITAL AND GENETIC SKIN DISORDERS

Median Raphe Cyst

Median raphe cyst is an uncommon developmental defect involving any site along the midline of the ventral side of the male genital area, from the meatus to the scrotum and perineum.[53,54] Although the underlying etiopathogenetic mechanisms are not well understood, it might occur for incomplete ventral fusion of the urethral or genital folds, ectopic periurethral glands of Littre, or separated outgrowths of urethral endoderm. Median raphe cyst usually appears as an asymptomatic, translucent, yellowish solitary cyst.[55] When multiple, linearly arranged lesions are interconnected, the term of median raphe canal may be used. Lesions are usually unrecognized during childhood and diagnosed in adulthood because they enlarge and become symptomatic following traumas and/or bacterial infections.

Dermatoscopy has been reported to support the clinical diagnosis by showing the presence of a homogeneous, white/yellowish pattern. Moreover, it may highlight the presence of a clinically undetected connection by revealing a translucent tract between multiple cysts, so to address to the final diagnosis of median raphe canal and, consequently, to plan the correct therapeutic approach.[56,57]

Aplasia Cutis Congenita of the Scalp

Aplasia cutis congenita is a rare malformation with an incidence of approximately 1.0 to 2.8 per 10,000 births, characterized by a failure of skin development.[58] It is usually located on the scalp (85% of cases) but can occur anywhere, including the face, trunk, and extremities.[59,60] The pathogenetic mechanisms are still unclear, although many abnormalities have been suggested, including neural tube defects (encephalocele/meningocele), focal pressure, necrosis, paucity or impaired vascular development in the cranial vertex, incomplete healing and fusion of the mesoderm, ischemic or thrombotic episodes, teratogen drugs (methimazole and carbimazole), and congenital infections.[61] The clinical aspect at birth is variable, varying from a single ulcerated/eroded lesion to a well-demarcated, alopecic patch covered with a thin, fragile, transparent membrane, usually involving the midline vertex. Moreover, lesions may be surrounded by a ring of dark, coarse, thick hairs ("hair collar sign").[62] Diagnosis is usually based on clinical presentation and on anamnestic data.

At dermatoscopy, aplasia cutis congenita of the scalp is characterized by a central area of scarring alopecia with no evidence of follicular openings, along with the presence of some telangiectatic vessels. At the hair-bearing margin, hair bulbs can be easily identified through a semi-translucent epidermis.[63–67] The hair follicles appear horizontally and radially oriented, configuring a starburst hair follicle pattern,[63] probably due to aberrant shearing forces occurring early at some point of follicle development, forcing them to bend.[62]

Pseudoxanthoma Elasticum

Pseudoxanthoma elasticum (PXE) is a rare genetic syndrome due to a mutation of the ABCC6 gene codifying an ATP-transmembrane transporter protein and characterized by progressive mineralization and fragmentation of elastic fibers, called elastorrhexia, affecting several tissues (skin, retina, blood vessels).[68,69] Its incidence is estimated to be from 1 per 25,000 to 1 per 100,000.[70] This wide range is correlated with the difficult diagnosis of PXE, with many cases going unrecognized. The first symptoms usually occur in childhood, with a female sex predilection (M:F = 1:2).[68] Cutaneous lesions of PXE are often the first manifestations of the disease, and in childhood may be the unique signs anticipating the onset of ocular (visual impairment) and cardiovascular (myocardial infarction, angina pectoris) symptoms.[71,72] They appear as soft, small, yellowish asymptomatic papules confluent in plaques with cobblestone aspect, leading to the "Moroccan leather" or "chicken skin" appearance.

Neck, axillae, antecubital and popliteal fossae, inguinal, and periumbilical areas are the main involved sites. The diagnosis of PXE is based on major and minor criteria, including skin, eye, and genetic findings, codified in 1994 and revised in 2000 by Plomp and colleagues.[70]

Recently, dermatoscopy has been reported to reveal a typical aspect consisting of multiple irregular yellowish areas, related both to the elastolysis of elastic fibers and/or to the presence of calcium deposits, alternating with prominent linear vessels.[73–75] In some fields, these yellowish areas coalesce to form parallel strands. Dermatoscopy may be useful for a noninvasive prompt diagnosis of PXE, so to address the appropriate diagnostic work-up.[74]

SUMMARY

The use of semi-invasive and/or invasive dermatologic diagnostic procedures may be often difficult to carry out in the pediatric population. In these subjects, dermatoscopy, being noninvasive and quick to perform, is a helpful imaging technique in daily clinical practice to assist the diagnosis and the follow-up in a variety of skin diseases.[76–78]

REFERENCES

1. Micali G, Lacarrubba F. Possible applications of videodermatoscopy beyond pigmented lesions. Int J Dermatol 2003;42(6):430–3.
2. Lacarrubba F, D'Amico V, Nasca MR, et al. Use of dermatoscopy and videodermatoscopy in therapeutic follow-up: a review. Int J Dermatol 2010;49(8): 866–73.
3. Micali G, Lacarrubba F, Massimino D, et al. Dermatoscopy: alternative uses in daily clinical practice. J Am Acad Dermatol 2011;64(6):1135–46.
4. Janssen D, Harms D. Juvenile xanthogranuloma in childhood and adolescence: a clinicopathologic study of 129 patients from the Kiel pediatric tumor registry. Am J Surg Pathol 2005;29:21.
5. Cypel TK, Zuker RM. Juvenile xanthogranuloma: case report and review of the literature. Can J Plast Surg 2008;16:175–7.
6. Chang SE, Cho S, Choi JC, et al. Clinicohistopathologic comparison of adult type and juvenile type xanthogranulomas in Korea. J Dermatol 2001;28: 413–8.
7. Palmer A, Bowling J. Dermoscopic appearance of juvenile xanthogranuloma. Dermatology 2007;215: 256–9.
8. Hussain SH, Kozic H, Lee JB. The utility of dermatoscopy in the evaluation of xanthogranulomas. Pediatr Dermatol 2008;25:505–6.
9. Kim JH, Lee SE, Kim SC. Juvenile xanthogranuloma on the sole: dermoscopic findings as a diagnostic clue. J Dermatol 2011;38:84–6.
10. Song M, Kim SH, Jung DS, et al. Structural correlations between dermoscopic and histopathological features of juvenile xanthogranuloma. J Eur Acad Dermatol Venereol 2011;25:259–63.
11. Pajaziti L, Hapçiu SR, Pajaziti A. Juvenile xanthogranuloma: a case report and review of the literature. BMC Res Notes 2014;7:174.
12. Pretel M, Irarrazaval I, Lera M, et al. Dermoscopic "setting sun" pattern of juvenile xanthogranuloma. J Am Acad Dermatol 2015;72:S73–5.
13. Mun JH, Ohn J, Kim KH. Dermoscopy of giant juvenile xanthogranuloma. J Am Acad Dermatol 2017; 76(2S1):S76–8.
14. Unno T, Minagawa A, Koga H, et al. Alteration of dermoscopic features in a juvenile xanthogranuloma during follow-up of 43 months. Int J Dermatol 2014;53:e590–1.
15. Rogers M. Epidermal nevi and the epidermal nevus syndromes: a review of 233 cases. Pediatr Dermatol 1992;9(4):342–4.
16. Kim R, Marmon S, Kaplan J, et al. Verrucous epidermal nevus. Dermatol Online J 2013;19(12): 20707.
17. Paller AS, Syder AJ, Chan YM, et al. Genetic and clinical mosaicism in a type of epidermal nevus. N Engl J Med 1994;331(21):1408–15.
18. Carbotti M, Coppola R, Graziano A, et al. Dermoscopy of verrucous epidermal nevus: large brown circles as a novel feature for diagnosis. Int J Dermatol 2016;55:653–6.
19. Moody MN, Landau JM, Goldberg LH. Nevus sebaceous revisited. Pediatr Dermatol 2012;29(1):15–23.
20. Taher M, Feibleman C, Bennett R. Squamous cell carcinoma arising in a nevus sebaceous of Jadassohn in a 9-year-old girl: treatment using Mohs micrographic surgery with literature review. Dermatol Surg 2010;36:1203–8.
21. Idriss MH, Elston DM. Secondary neoplasms associated with nevus sebaceus of Jadassohn: a study of 707 cases. J Am Acad Dermatol 2014;70:332–7.
22. Wali GN, Felton SJ, McPherson T. Management of naevus sebaceous: a national survey of UK dermatologists and plastic surgeons. Clin Exp Dermatol 2018;43(5):589–91. [Epub ahead of print].
23. Neri I, Savoia F, Giacomini F, et al. Usefulness of dermatoscopy for the early diagnosis of sebaceous naevus and differentiation from aplasia cutis congenita. Clin Exp Dermatol 2009;34(5):e50–2.
24. Bruno CB, Cordeiro FN, Soares Fdo E, et al. Dermoscopic aspects of syringocystadenoma papilliferum associated with nevus sebaceus. An Bras Dermatol 2011;86(6):1213–6.
25. Enei ML, Paschoal FM, Valdés G, et al. Basal cell carcinoma appearing in a facial nevus sebaceous

of Jadassohn: dermoscopic features. An Bras Dermatol 2012;87(4):640–2.
26. Zaballos P, Serrano P, Flores G, et al. Dermoscopy of tumours arising in naevus sebaceous: a morphological study of 58 cases. J Eur Acad Dermatol Venereol 2015;29:2231–7.
27. Duman N, Ersoy-Evans S. Erkin Özaygen G, et al. Syringocystadenoma papilliferum arising on naevus sebaceus: a 6-year-old child case described with dermoscopic features. Australas J Dermatol 2015; 56(2):e53–4.
28. Howarth DM, Gilchrist GS, Mullan BP, et al. Langerhans cell histiocytosis: diagnosis, natural history, management and outcome. Cancer 1999;85:2278–90.
29. Morren MA, Vanden Broecke K, Vangeebergen L, et al. Diverse cutaneous presentations of Langerhans cell histiocytosis in children: a retrospective cohort study. Pediatr Blood Cancer 2016;63(3): 486–92.
30. Behera B, Malathi M, Prabhakaran N, et al. Dermoscopy of Langerhans cell histiocytosis. J Am Acad Dermatol 2017;76(2S1):S79–81.
31. Murata S, Yoshida Y, Adachi K, et al. Solitary, late-onset, self-healing Langerhans cell histiocytosis. Acta Derm Venereol 2011;91(1):103–4.
32. Rubio-González B, García-Bracamonte B, Ortiz-Romero PL, et al. Multisystemic Langerhans cell histiocytosis mimicking diffuse neonatal hemangiomatosis. Pediatr Dermatol 2014;31(3):e87–9.
33. Boniface K, Seneschal J, Picardo M, et al. Vitiligo: focus on clinical aspects, immunopathogenesis, and therapy. Clin Rev Allergy Immunol 2018;54(1): 52–67.
34. Anstey AV. Disorders of skin colour. In: Griffiths CEM, Barker J, Bleiker T, et al, editors. Rook's textbook of dermatology, 58, 9th edition. Oxford (England): Wiley-Blackwell; 2016. p. 46–58.
35. Rodrigues M, Ezzedine K, Hamzavi I, et al. New discoveries in the pathogenesis and classification of vitiligo. J Am Acad Dermatol 2017;77(1):1–13.
36. Thatte SS, Khopkar US. The utility of dermoscopy in the diagnosis of evolving lesions of vitiligo. Indian J Dermatol Venereol Leprol 2014;80(6):505–8.
37. Kumar Jha A, Sonthalia S, Lallas A, et al. Dermoscopy in vitiligo: diagnosis and beyond. Int J Dermatol 2018;57(1):50–4.
38. Kim MS, Cho EB, Park EJ, et al. Effect of excimer laser treatment on vitiliginous areas with leukotrichia after confirmation by dermoscopy. Int J Dermatol 2016;55(8):886–92.
39. Grattan CEH, Radia DH. Mastocytosis. In: Griffiths CEM, Barker J, Bleiker T, et al, editors. Rook's textbook of dermatology, 46, 9th edition. Oxford (England): Wiley-Blackwell; 2016. p. 1–10.
40. Azaña JM, Torrelo A, Matito A. Update on mastocytosis (part 1): pathophysiology, clinical features, and diagnosis. Actas Dermosifiliogr 2016;107(1):5–14.
41. Azaña JM, Torrelo A, Matito A. Update on mastocytosis (part 2): categories, prognosis, and treatment. Actas Dermosifiliogr 2016;107:15–22.
42. Brockow K. Epidemiology, prognosis, and risk factors in mastocytosis. Immunol Allergy Clin North Am 2014;34(2):283–95.
43. Hartmann K, Escribano L, Grattan C, et al. Cutaneous manifestations in patients with mastocytosis: Consensus report of the European Competence Network on Mastocytosis; the American Academy of Allergy, Asthma & Immunology; and the European Academy of Allergology and Clinical Immunology. J Allergy Clin Immunol 2016;137(1):35–45.
44. Horny HP, Akin C, Arber D, et al. Mastocytosis. In: Swerdlow SH, Campo E, Harris NL, et al, editors. World Health Organization (WHO) classification of tumours. Pathology & genetics. Tumours of haematopoietic and lymphoid tissues. Lyon (France): IARC Press; 2017. p. 61–9.
45. Maluf LC, Barros JA, Machado Filho CD. Mastocytosis. An Bras Dermatol 2009;84:213–25.
46. Valent P, Akin C, Escribano L, et al. Standards and standardization in mastocytosis: consensus statements on diagnostics, treatment recommendations and response criteria. Eur J Clin Invest 2007;37(6): 435–53.
47. Valent P, Akin C, Hartmann K, et al. Advances in the classification and treatment of mastocytosis: current status and outlook toward the future. Cancer Res 2017;77(6):1261–70.
48. Arpaia N, Cassano N, Vena GA. Lessons on dermoscopy: pigment network in nonmelanocytic lesions. Dermatol Surg 2004;30(6):929–30.
49. Akay BN, Kittler H, Sanli H, et al. Dermatoscopic findings of cutaneous mastocytosis. Dermatology 2009;218:226–30.
50. Vano-Galvan S, Alvarez-Twose I, De las Heras E, et al. Dermoscopic features of skin lesions in patients with mastocytosis. Arch Dermatol 2011;147: 932–40.
51. Miller MD, Nery NS, Gripp AC, et al. Dermatoscopic findings of urticaria pigmentosa. An Bras Dermatol 2013;88(6):986–8.
52. Gutiérrez-González E, Ginarte M, Toribio J. Letter: cutaneous mastocytosis with systemic involvement mimicking clinical and dermatoscopically multiple melanocytic nevi. Dermatol Online J 2011;17(11):15.
53. Shao IH, Chen TD, Shao HT, et al. Male median raphe cysts: serial retrospective analysis and histopathological classification. Diagn Pathol 2012;7:121.
54. Navalón-Monllor V, Ordoño-Saiz MV, Ordoño-Domínguez F, et al. Median raphe cysts in men. Presentation of our experience and literature review. Actas Urol Esp 2017;41(3):205–9.
55. Nishida H, Kashima K, Daa T, et al. Pigmented median raphe cyst of the penis. J Cutan Pathol 2012; 39:808–10.

56. Lacarrubba F, Tedeschi A, Francesconi L, et al. Canal versus cysts of the penile median raphe: advancing diagnostic methods using videodermatoscopy. Pediatr Dermatol 2010;27:667–9.
57. Micali G, Lacarrubba F. Augmented diagnostic capability using videodermatoscopy on selected infectious and non-infectious penile growths. Int J Dermatol 2011;50:1501–5.
58. Silberstein E, Pagkalos VA, Landau D, et al. Aplasia cutis congenita: clinical management and a new classification system. Plast Reconstr Surg 2014; 134:766e–74e.
59. Kruk-Jeromin J, Janik J, Rykała J. Aplasia cutis congenita of the scalp. Report of 16 cases. Dermatol Surg 1998;24:549–53.
60. Frieden IJ. Aplasia cutis congenita: a clinical review and proposal for classification. J Am Acad Dermatol 1986;14:646–60.
61. Mesrati H, Amouri M, Chaaben H, et al. Aplasia cutis congenita: report of 22 cases. Int J Dermatol 2015; 54:1370–5.
62. Drolet BA, Clowry L Jr, McTigue MK, et al. The hair collar sign: marker for cranial dysraphism. Pediatrics 1995;96:309–13.
63. Verzì AE, Lacarrubba F, Micali G. Starburst hair follicles: a dermoscopic clue for aplasia cutis congenita. J Am Acad Dermatol 2016;75(4):e141–2.
64. Rakowska A, Maj M, Zadurska M, et al. Trichoscopy of focal alopecia in children - new trichoscopic findings: hair bulbs arranged radially along hair-bearing margins in aplasia cutis congenita. Skin Appendage Disord 2016;2(1–2):1–6.
65. Pinheiro AMC, Mauad EBS, Fernandes LFA, et al. Aplasia cutis congenita: trichoscopy findings. Int J Trichology 2016;8(4):184–5.
66. Damiani L, Aguiar FM, da Silva MV, et al. Dermoscopic findings of scalp aplasia cutis congenita. Skin Appendage Disord 2017;2(3–4):177–9.
67. Lozano-Masdemont B. A case of membranous aplasia cutis congenita and dermoscopic features. Int J Trichology 2017;9(1):33–4.
68. Chassaing N, Martin L, Calvas P, et al. Pseudoxanthoma elasticum: a clinical, pathophysiological and genetic update including 11 novel ABCC6 mutations. J Med Genet 2005;42:881–92.
69. Hosen M, Lamoen A, De Paepe A, et al. Histopathology of pseudoxanthoma elasticum and related disorders: histological hallmarks and diagnostic clues, 2012. Cairo (Egypt): Scientifica; 2012. p. 598262.
70. Plomp AS, Toonstra J, Bergen AA, et al. Proposal for updating the pseudoxanthoma elasticum classification system a review of the clinical findings. Am J Med Genet A 2010;152:1049–58.
71. Marconi B, Bobyr I, Campanati A, et al. Pseudoxanthoma elasticum and skin: clinical manifestations, histopathology, pathomechanism, perspectives of treatment. Intractable Rare Dis Res 2015;4:113–22.
72. Nouri M, Boisseau C, Bonicel P, et al. Manifestations of pseudoxanthoma elastic in childhood. Br J Dermatol 2009;161:635–9.
73. Nasca MR, Lacarrubba F, Caltabiano R, et al. Perforating pseudoxanthoma elasticum with secondary elastosis perforans serpiginosa-like changes: dermoscopy, confocal microscopy and histopathological correlation. J Cutan Pathol 2016;43(11):1021–4.
74. Lacarrubba F, Verzì AE, Caltabiano R, et al. Dermoscopy of pseudoxanthoma elasticum. J Am Acad Dermatol 2017;76:69–70.
75. Singh A, Bhari N, Bhari A. Dermoscopy of pseudoxanthoma elasticum. BMJ Case Rep 2017;2017 [pii: bcr-2017-221365].
76. Lacarrubba F. The role of imaging in dermatology. G Ital Dermatol Venereol 2015;150(5):505–6.
77. Lacarrubba F, Verzì AE, Dinotta F, et al. Dermatoscopy in inflammatory and infectious skin disorders. G Ital Dermatol Venereol 2015;150(5):521–31.
78. Micali G, Verzì AE, Lacarrubba F. Alternative uses of dermatoscopy in daily clinical practice: an update. J Am Acad Dermatol 2018 [pii:S0190-9622(18) 32143-1]. [Epub ahead of print].

Dermoscopy of Pigmentary Disorders in Brown Skin

Manas Chatterjee, MD, DNB[a], Shekhar Neema, MD[b,*]

KEYWORDS

• Dermoscopy • Pigmentary disorders • Melasma • Lichen planus

KEY POINTS

- Dermoscopy is an invaluable tool in the diagnosis of pigmentary disorders in brown skin.
- Dermoscopy can reliably differentiate epidermal from dermal pigmentation and helps in planning treatment.
- Dermoscopy is also helpful in the diagnosis of vitiligo and examining its differentiation from other hypopigmentary disorders.

INTRODUCTION

Disorders of pigmentation are quite common in brown skin. Almost 11% of patients attending the dermatology outpatient department in Western India present with pigmentary disorders.[1] Disorders of hypopigmentation bring patients to physicians early, as they appear as a contrast to brown skin and evoke fear of leprosy and vitiligo in the minds of patients. Hyperpigmentation is also quite common, as individuals with darker skin tend to develop postinflammatory hyperpigmentation (PIH) in response to skin trauma more commonly.

Dermoscopy was introduced and is most commonly used as a tool to differentiate benign nevi from malignant melanoma in Caucasian skin. Malignant melanoma is uncommon in darker skin, with the exception of acral lentiginous melanoma. Over the years, dermoscopy has been used for the diagnosis of various other dermatoses like papulosquamous disorders, infections, and infestations. It has also become an invaluable tool in the assessment of pigmentary disorders other than melanomas in brown skin. Dermoscopy can be used for diagnosis, prognosis, and treatment monitoring in pigmentary disorders.

PATTERN IDENTIFICATION IN PIGMENTARY DISORDERS

Dermoscopic diagnosis of pigmentary disorders in brown skin requires a basic understanding of the normal pattern. It is important to imagine skin as a 3-dimensional structure while performing dermoscopy. The third dimension or depth can be assessed by observing the color of pigment on dermoscopy. Melanin is the main chromophore in the skin, and anatomic location of melanin determines the color perceived on dermoscopy. The presence of pigment in superficial epidermis, epidermis, papillary dermis, and reticular dermis results in the observed color being black, brown, gray, and blue, respectively. Dermoscopy of normal skin on the trunk shows a reticular pattern of pigmentation (**Fig. 1**), whereas normal facial skin shows a pseudoreticular pattern in which the reticular pattern is interrupted by the presence of the pilosebaceous apparatus (**Fig. 2**).

DISORDERS OF HYPERPIGMENTATION

Facial Melanoses

Melasma

It is a commonly acquired hypermelanosis of multifactorial cause. It is characterized by

Disclosure statement: No conflict of interest.

[a] Department of Dermatology, INHS Asvini, Colaba, Mumbai 400005, India; [b] Department of Dermatology, Command Hospital, 17/1E, Alipore Road, Alipore Police Line, Alipore, Kolkata, West Bengal 700027, India
* Corresponding author.
E-mail address: shekharadvait@gmail.com

Dermatol Clin 36 (2018) 473–485
https://doi.org/10.1016/j.det.2018.05.014

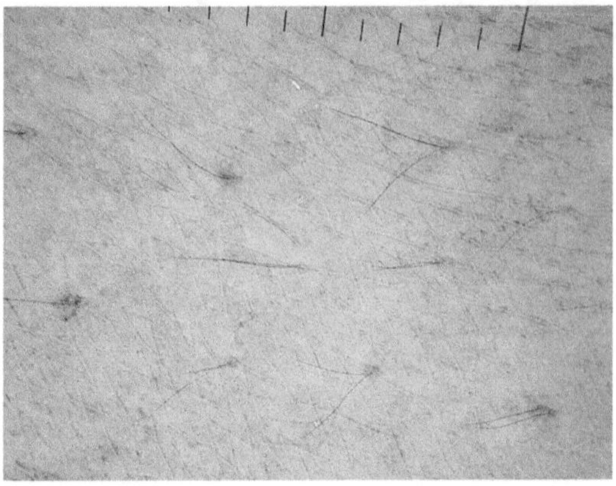

Fig. 1. Reticular pigment network seen in trunk on brown skin.

symmetric brown macules on sun-exposed areas, particularly over the forehead and malar areas; but it can also occur on extrafacial sites like the forearms and trunk (Fig. 3A). It is classified as epidermal, dermal, and mixed variants by clinical features and the Wood lamp examination.[2] However, this classification has its fallacies in brown skin.

Dermoscopy in melasma is used for

- Diagnosis and differentiation form other facial pigmentary disorders
- Monitoring of treatment
- Treatment-associated adverse effect monitoring: steroid-damaged face and hydroquinone-induced exogenous ochronosis

Dermoscopic features of melasma[3]

- Light brown to dark brown pigment
- Pseudoreticular pigment network (Fig. 3B)
- Annular and arcuate structures, brown dots and globules (Fig. 4)
- Sparing of perifollicular and peri-appendageal regions (see Fig. 3B)

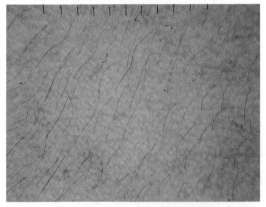

Fig. 2. Pseudoreticular pigment network seen on face; reticular pigment network obliterated by presence of sebaceous gland openings.

The presence of gray dots suggests a dermal component of melasma. Telangiectasia on dermoscopy can be an indicator of vascular component of melasma or prolonged steroid use (Fig. 5).

Exogenous ochronosis on dermoscopy appears as the presence of blue-gray amorphous areas obliterating follicular openings and irregular, brown-gray globular, annular, or arciform structures[4] (Fig. 6).

Lichen planus pigmentosus

It is an uncommon variant of lichen planus, occurring most commonly in darker skin. It is characterized by symmetrically distributed, brown to gray-brown macules on sun-exposed areas of the head and neck and flexural areas (Fig. 7A). Pigmentation observed in lichen planus pigmentosus (LPP) is generally diffuse; but reticular, follicular, and linear variants may be seen.[5,6] Histopathologic examination of affected skin reveals atrophic epidermis, lichenoid interface dermatitis, and melanophages in the upper dermis.

Dermoscopic features of LPP[7,8]:

- Absence of Wickham striae
- Diffuse brown color and pseudoreticular pigment network (Fig. 7B)
- Slate-gray to blue dots and globules
- Perifollicular and peri-eccrine gray to brown/gray blue pigment deposition (Fig. 8)
- Hemlike pigment pattern

Riehl melanosis or pigmented contact dermatitis

It was first described by Riehl in Vienna. It is characterized by diffuse or patchy brown pigmentation on forehead and cheeks (Fig. 9A). The exact pathomechanism of the development of pigmented contact dermatitis (PCD) is unknown. Most of the cases occur in individuals with brown skin due to direct contact with allergens like fragrances. It has been hypothesized that a low concentration of allergen does not produce spongiotic dermatitis but damages the basal layer of the epidermis and results in pigmentary incontinence. Patch testing can identify the offending allergen. Histopathology reveals normal epidermis, mild perivascular infiltrate, and melanophages in the upper dermis.[9,10]

Dermoscopic features of PCD

- There is a diffuse brown-colored, pseudoreticular pigment network.

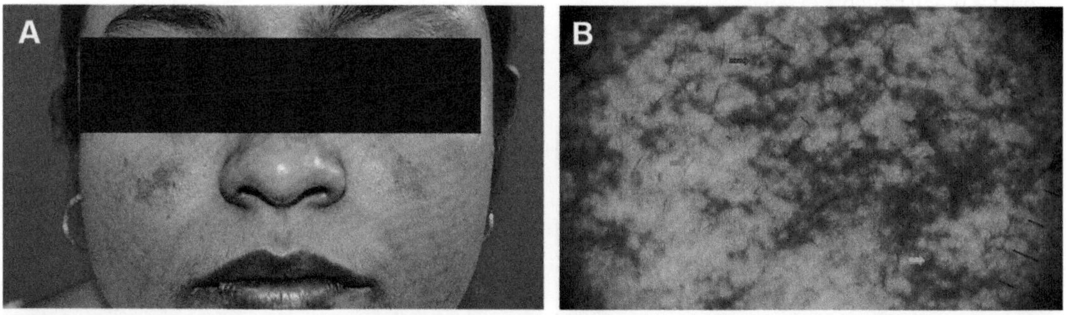

Fig. 3. (*A*) Clinical image of melasma involving nose and malar areas. (*B*) Dermoscopy shows pseudoreticular network of pigmentation, light-brown pigment (*blue arrow*), sparing of peri-follicular and peri-appendageal areas (*orange arrow*), and arcuate structure (*green arrow*).

- There is a regular distribution of brown to gray dots. Dots in PCD are smaller, uniformly distributed, and gray to blue as compared with LPP whereby they appear larger, irregularly distributed, and brown to gray. Also, the dots in PCD are unpatterned, representing melanophages in the deeper dermis, whereas those in LPP roughly follow a reticulo-globular pattern due to the more superficial location of the melanophages being nearer the dermal papillae and epidermal rete-ridges (Fig. 9B).
- There is no predilection of pigment dots for perifollicular and peri-appendageal areas, unlike what is seen in LPP.

Pigmentary demarcation lines

They are areas of transition between normal skin color and darker skin color that are seen on the face, extremities, and trunk and are more commonly seen in individuals with darker skin because of the different melanocyte distribution. There are 8 groups of pigmentary demarcation lines (PDLs) (A–H), out of which PDL F to H occur on the face. PDL F has been described as an inverted-cone–shaped hyperpigmented area on the lateral aspect of the face, extending from the orbital rim inferiorly. PDL G has been described in a similar location as PDL F; however, it appears as a W-shaped area of hyperpigmentation. PDL H occurs on the lower face as a hyperpigmented band, extending from the angle of the mouth to the chin (Fig. 10). PDLs appear around puberty or pregnancy and remain constant thereafter. Because of the site and timing of appearance, they can be confused clinically with melasma or they can coexist with melasma (Fig. 11A). They also need to be differentiated from PIH.

Dermoscopy of PDL shows an exaggerated or prominent pseudoreticular pattern normally seen on the face and is described as unpatterned (Fig. 11B). It can be of help in differentiating PDLs from other differential diagnoses.[11]

Nevus of Ota

It is a dermal melanocytosis observed along the distribution of ophthalmic and maxillary branches of trigeminal nerves. It is generally unilateral, more commonly occurs in females, and is mostly present at birth. However, it can be bilateral and can occur later in life. The nevus of Ota (NOO) is

Fig. 4. Presence of brown granules at dermoscopy suggests dermal component of melasma (*orange arrows*).

Fig. 5. Dermoscopy of partially treated melasma showing areas of clearing (*green arrow*) and telangiectasia (*blue arrow*) due to steroid application.

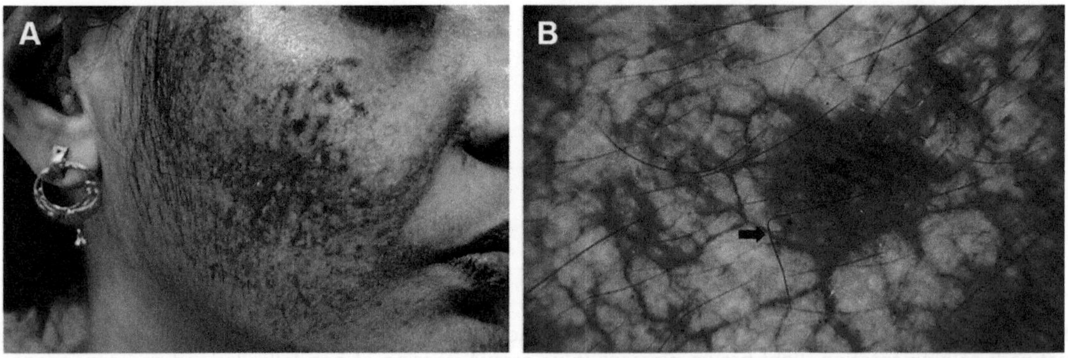

Fig. 6. (*A*) Clinical image of hydroquinone-induced exogenous ochronosis. (*B*) Dermoscopy shows amorphous gray-brown area obliterating follicular opening (*blue arrow*) and telangiectasia (*black arrow*).

characterized by mottled blue-gray macules over zygomatic and temporal area; scleral pigmentation can also be seen in two-thirds of cases[12] (**Fig. 12**A).

Dermoscopy of NOO reveals gray to blue color; pigmented lines are thick and broad, and the hypopigmented area appears as distinct globular structures (**Fig. 12**B).

Postinflammatory hyperpigmentation

It is an acquired hypermelanosis, which may occur after any form of injury to the skin. Injuries may be thermal, chemical, or inflammatory due to some skin disorders, such as acne or psoriasis. PIH is much more common in darker skin because of the higher amount of epidermal melanin and propensity of darker skin to produce more melanin in response to trauma. In darker skin types, PIH can results from several forms of trivial injuries and may aggravate on sun exposure. These entities are ill defined and cannot be distinguished histopathologically, always requiring a clinical correlation.[13]

Dermoscopy can help guide treatment in these cases, suggesting whether pigmentation is predominantly epidermal or mixed. The epidermal component appears as brown, whereas the dermal component appears as gray dots and/or blotches. There is no consistent pattern of pigmentation seen on dermoscopy (**Fig. 13**).

Primary Cutaneous Amyloidosis

It is a disorder characterized by the deposition of amyloid in previously healthy skin, without any evidence of amyloid deposition in internal organs. It can be classified as macular amyloidosis, lichen amyloidosis, and biphasic amyloidosis. Macular amyloidosis is characterized by the presence of rippled hyperpigmentation on the extensor aspect of the arm, forearm, and upper back. Lichen amyloidosis shows dome-shaped brown papules predominantly on the legs but can be generalized (**Fig. 14**A). Biphasic amyloidosis can have features of both macular and lichen amyloidosis. Macular amyloidosis needs to be differentiated from extrafacial melasma, PIH, and frictional melanosis.

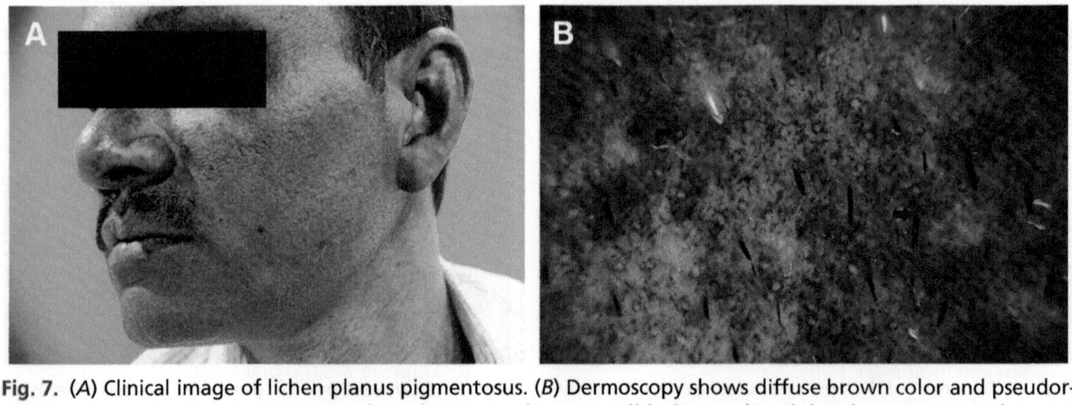

Fig. 7. (*A*) Clinical image of lichen planus pigmentosus. (*B*) Dermoscopy shows diffuse brown color and pseudoreticular pigment network, peri-appendageal pigment deposition (*black arrow*) and slate brown to gray dots and globules (*blue arrow*).

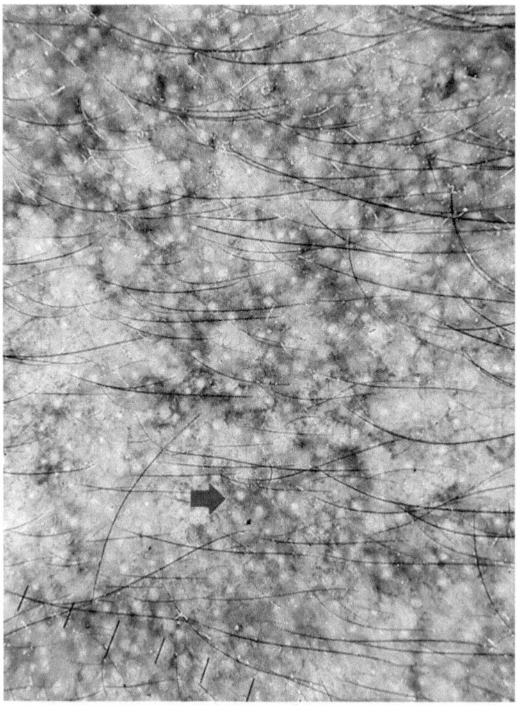

Fig. 8. Dermoscopy of lichen planus pigmentosus showing brown to gray pigment network, hem like pattern of pigment network and peri-appendageal pigment deposition (*red arrow*).

Histopathological examination and demonstration of amyloid is diagnostic; however, dermoscopy can help in the diagnosis of cutaneous amyloidosis.[14]

Dermoscopy of cutaneous amyloidosis reveals a brown or white central hub and radiating fine streaks, called a hub-and-spoke pattern. Frictional melanosis is a close differential diagnosis of macular amyloidosis and can result from friction resulting from a loofah while bathing. Dermoscopy of frictional melanosis shows a reticular network of pigmentation without a central hub[15] (**Figs. 14**B and **15**).

Acanthosis Nigricans

It is characterized by hyperpigmented, velvety plaques over the neck and flexures. It can be generalized, acral, or facial (**Fig. 16**A). The most common cause of acanthosis nigricans (AN) is obesity associated, other rare causes being hereditary, drugs, and internal malignancy. Classic AN is a clinical diagnosis; however, acral AN and facial AN can sometimes pose a diagnostic dilemma and require histopathology for confirmation of diagnosis. Histopathology reveals papillomatosis, hyperkeratosis, and hyperpigmentation of the basal layer.[16]

Dermoscopy can also help in the diagnosis of AN by showing hyperpigmented dots in addition to linear crista cutis along with the presence of sulcus cutis[17] (**Fig. 16**B).

Seborrheic Melanosis

It is an ill-defined entity described mainly in the Indian subcontinent and characterized by darkening of seborrheic areas of the face, especially alar groves, labiomental crease, and angles of the mouth (**Fig. 17**A). The exact cause of this condition is unknown; however, it has been linked with seborrheic dermatitis and responds to topical steroids and calcineurin inhibitors.

Dermoscopy of seborrheic melanosis shows a vascular, pigmented, or mixed pattern[18] (**Fig. 17**B).

DISORDERS OF HYPOPIGMENTATION

Vitiligo

It is a depigmenting disorder of unknown cause, affecting approximately 0.5% of the world's population. It is characterized by depigmented macules (**Fig. 18**). It is classified as segmental vitiligo or

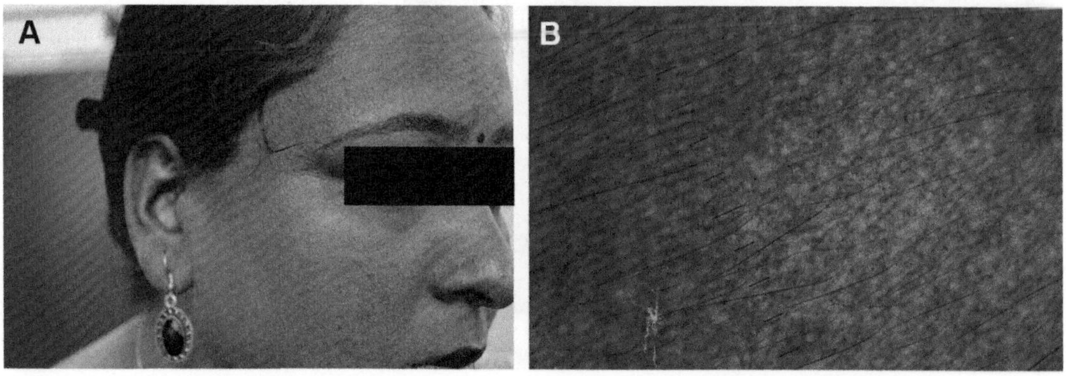

Fig. 9. (*A*). Clinical image of pigmented contact dermatitis. (*B*). Dermoscopy shows diffuse brown color and pseudoreticular network; dots are brown to gray, smaller, and more uniformly distributed (*blue arrow*).

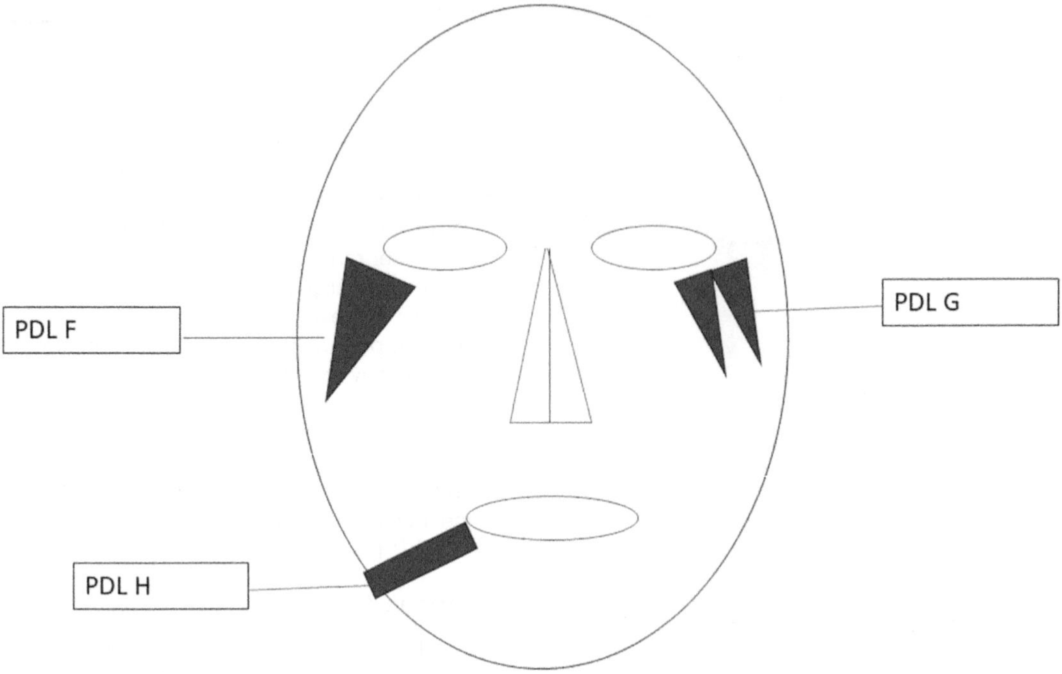

Fig. 10. PDL of the face.

nonsegmental vitiligo/vitiligo vulgaris. Vitiligo severely impacts the quality of life of affected individuals, more so in skin of color, as it results in a striking contrast with skin color. It is associated with social stigma, so much so that patients cannot function effectively in society and have psychiatric morbidities. Treatment options of vitiligo include medical treatments, in the form of immunosuppressive therapy and phototherapy, or surgical therapy, such as punch grafting, once the disease gets stabilized on medical therapy.

Diagnosis of fully evolved vitiligo is straightforward and does not require any special investigations. Dermoscopy has an important role to play in differentiating evolving vitiligo from other hypopigmentary disorders, response to therapy, and determining the stability of vitiligo lesions before surgery.

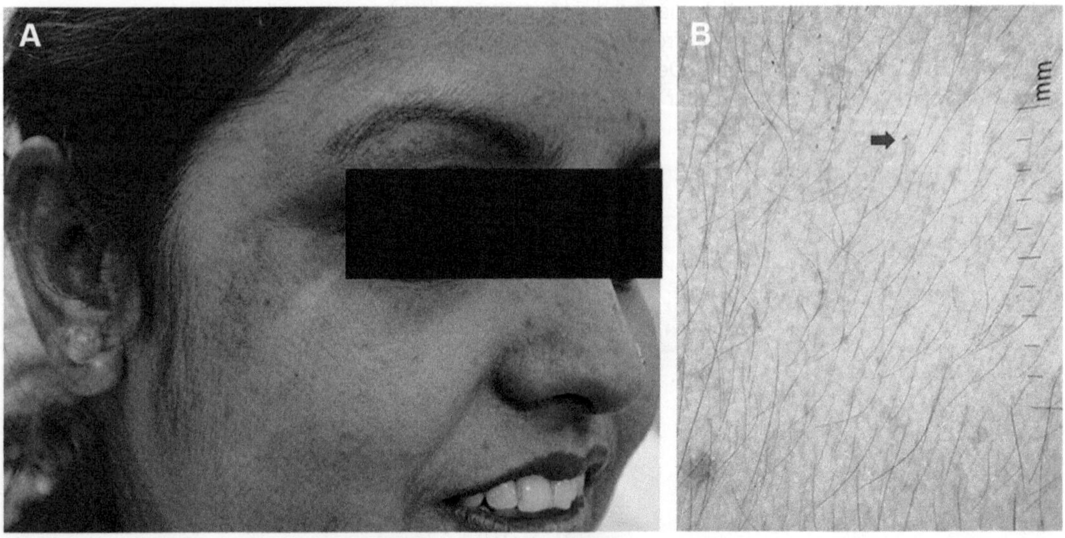

Fig. 11. (*A*). Clinical image of PDL F. (*B*). Dermoscopy shows exaggerated pseudoreticular pattern of pigmentation (*blue arrow*).

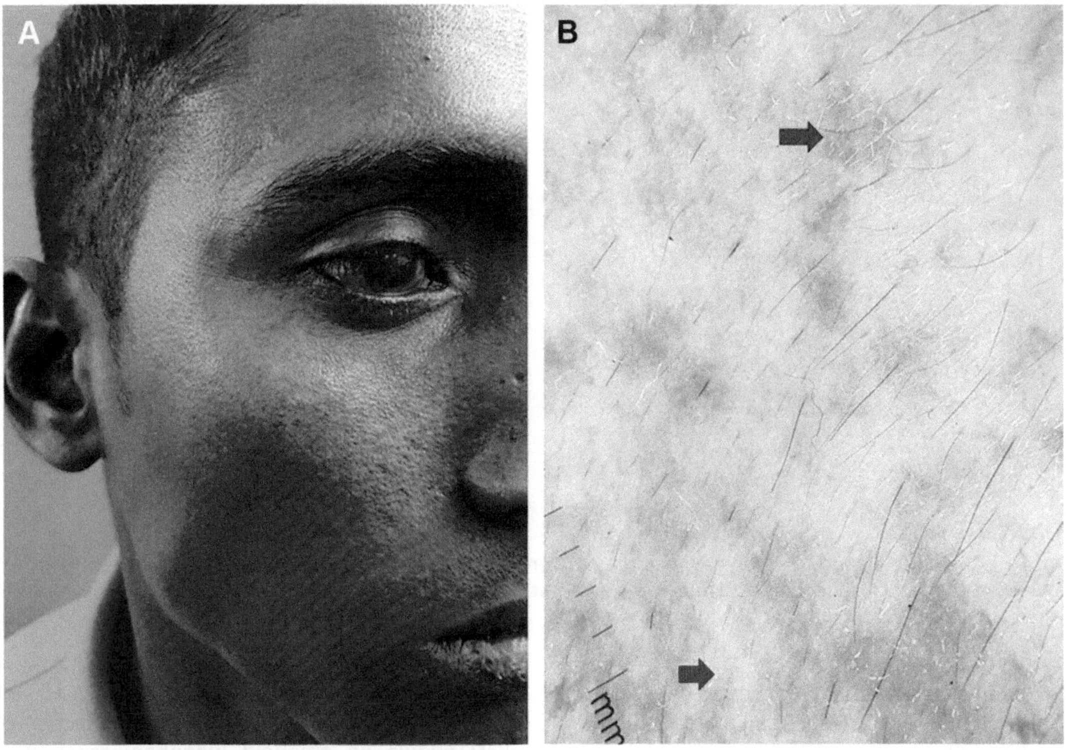

Fig. 12. (*A*). Clinical image of nevus of Ota. (*B*). Dermoscopy shows thick broad blue pigmentary lines (*blue arrow*) and globular hypopigmented areas (*red arrow*).

Dermoscopy has been used to diagnose various stages of vitiligo; various dermoscopic features have been described for evolving vitiligo, a fully evolved vitiligo patch, and repigmenting vitiligo. Dermoscopic features of stable and unstable vitiligo have also been described.

- The evolving lesions of vitiligo can be confused with other disorders of hypopigmentation. Dermoscopic features of evolving vitiligo are reduced or absent pigmentary network, reversed pigmentary network, perilesional hypopigmentation, and diffuse white glow[19] (**Fig. 19**).
- Dermoscopy of fully evolved lesions of vitiligo shows complete absence of a pigmentary network and leukotrichia in addition to diffuse white glow. Repigmenting lesions of vitiligo shows perifollicular pigmentation[20] (**Fig. 20**).
- Dermoscopy of progressive or unstable vitiligo shows a polka dot or confettilike pattern, trichrome pattern, comet-tail pattern, and star burst/feathery pattern. A tapioca or sago grain pattern in normal skin adjacent to a vitiligo lesion has also been recently described in progressive vitiligo.[21] Perifollicular depigmentation with evolving leukotrichia in areas of clinically unaltered pigmentation has also been described as early predictive features of impending vitiligo. Dermoscopy has become an essential tool to determine the stability of a lesion before performing vitiligo surgery. Stable vitiligo is associated with ameboid or petaloid patterns. These two patterns are also seen in idiopathic guttate hypomelanosis, as mentioned later (**Figs. 21** and **22**). Repigmenting or stable vitiligo shows

Fig. 13. Dermoscopy showing unpatterned brown pigment (*blue arrow*) in predominantly epidermal PIH.

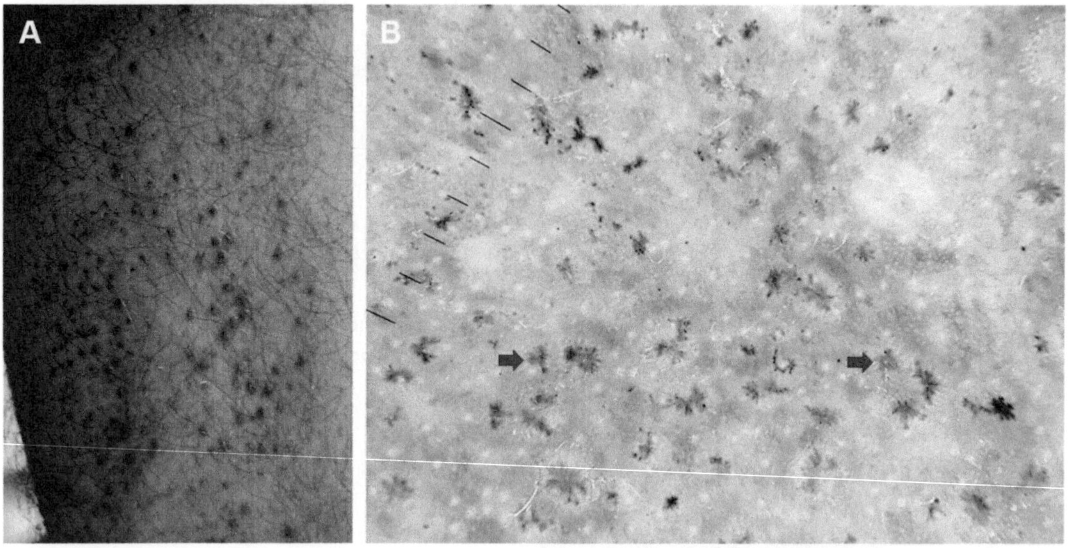

Fig. 14. (*A*). Clinical image of lichen amyloidosis. (*B*). Dermoscopy shows brown central hub and radiating brown lines from the center, described as a hub-and-spoke pattern. (*blue arrows*). This pattern is more conspicuous in lichen amyloidosis than macular amyloidosis.

perifollicular pigmentation, marginal hyperpigmentation, and reticular pigmentation[22,23] (**Fig. 23**).

The presence of any white patch causes so much concern in the mind of affected individuals that it is imperative to appropriately diagnose the condition. Most of the times, patients visit physicians out of fear of vitiligo or leprosy, which should be ruled out by clinical examination. Dermoscopy is of great help in the diagnosis of various conditions that can mimic vitiligo:

Idiopathic guttate hypomelanosis

It is a disorder of unknown cause, characterized by porcelain white macules on the extremities (more commonly) and trunk (**Fig. 24**A). The prevalence of idiopathic guttate hypomelanosis (IGH) increases with an increase in age. Dermoscopy of IGH shows an ameboid (periphery resembling pseudopods of ameba) (**Fig. 24**B) or petaloid pattern (**Fig. 25**). Most IGH lesions shows distinct margins from surrounding skin, whereas in vitiligo margins may merge into surrounding skin.[24] Other dermoscopic features include multiple small areas coalescing into irregular/polycyclic macules, with several white shades and both well- and ill-defined edges, surrounded by a patchy hyperpigmented network (cloudy skylike pattern) and cloudy pattern (well or ill-defined roundish homogeneous whitish areas surrounded by patchy hyperpigmented network).

Fig. 15. Dermoscopy of macular amyloidosis showing hub-and-spoke pattern, which is not as well defined as in lichen amyloidosis (*blue arrows*).

Nevus depigmentosus

Also known as achromic nevus, it is characterized by hypopigmented macules of varying size (**Fig. 26**A). It is present at birth in most cases; however, it may also be noticed later in life. It can create diagnostic confusion from childhood vitiligo and dermoscopy can help in differentiating it. Dermoscopy of nevus depigmentosus shows the presence of a reticular pigment pattern within the lesion; however, the intensity of pigment is less than normal skin[25] (**Fig. 26**B).

Ash-leaf macules

They are a sign of tuberous sclerosis and are one of the earliest cutaneous manifestations of tuberous sclerosis. They present as ovoid or ash-leaf–shaped hypopigmented macules. Dermoscopy can help in differentiating these lesions from other

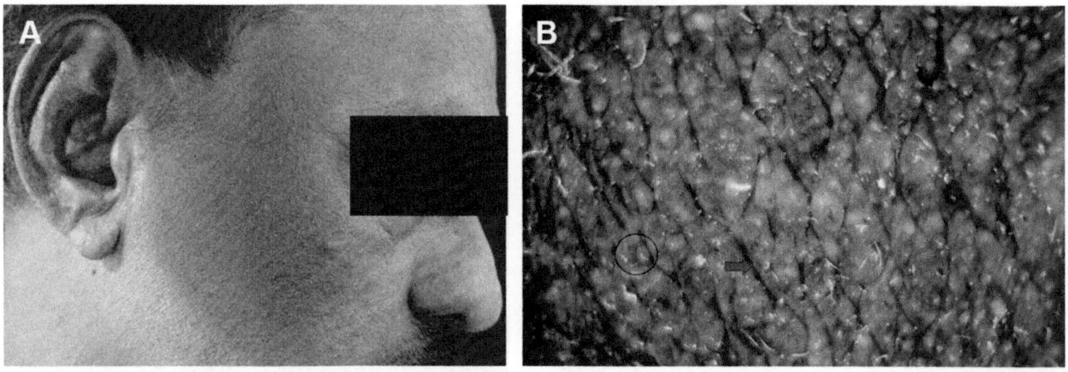

Fig. 16. (*A*). Clinical image of facial AN. (*B*). Dermoscopy shows sulcus cutis (*blue arrow*) and hyperpigmented dots (*black circle*).

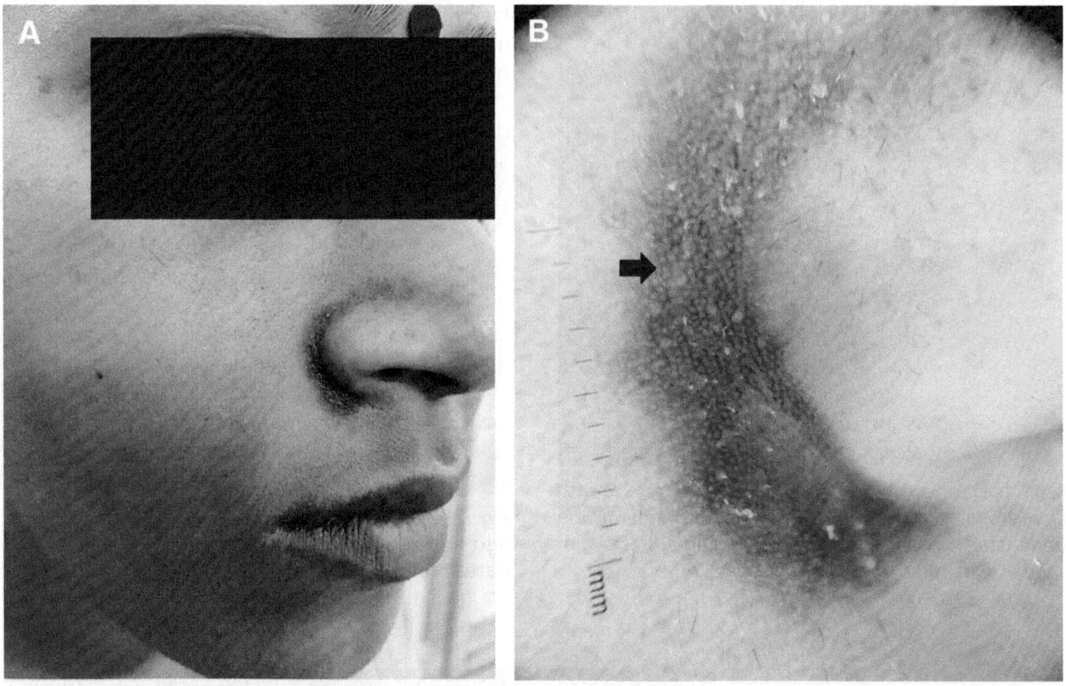

Fig. 17. (*A*). Clinical image of seborrheic melanosis. (*B*). Dermoscopy shows hyperpigmented pseudonetwork (*black arrow*).

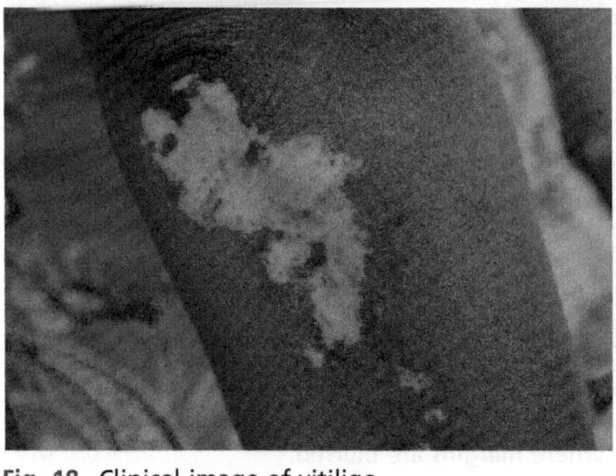

Fig. 18. Clinical image of vitiligo.

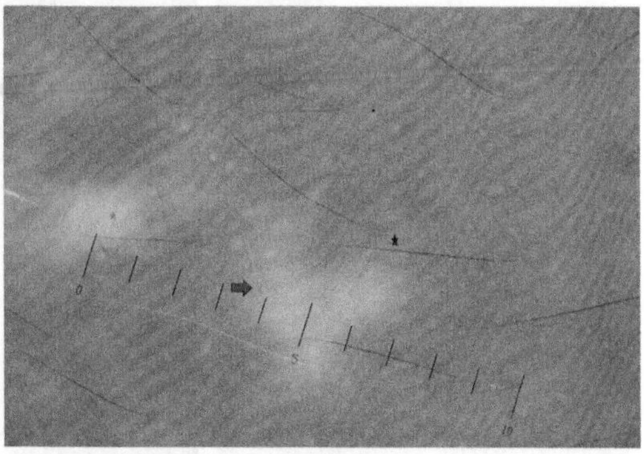

Fig. 19. Dermoscopy of evolving vitiligo showing reversed pigmentary network (*blue arrow*), diffuse white glow (*orange star*), and perilesional hypopigmentation (*black star*). Leukotrichia can also be visualized on dermoscopic field.

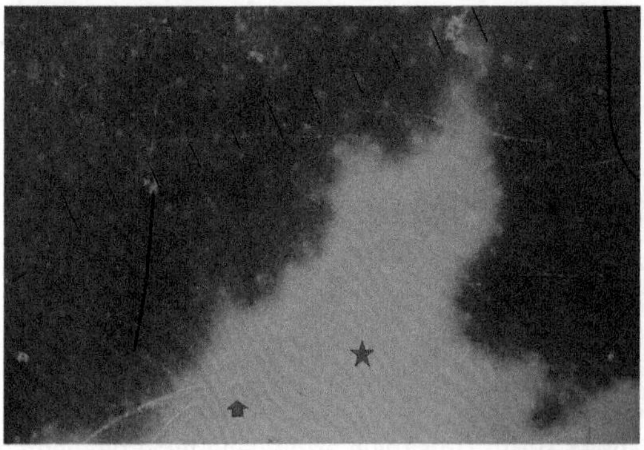

Fig. 20. Dermoscopy of fully evolved vitiligo showing absence of pigment network (*blue star*), leukotrichia (*blue arrow*), and diffuse white glow.

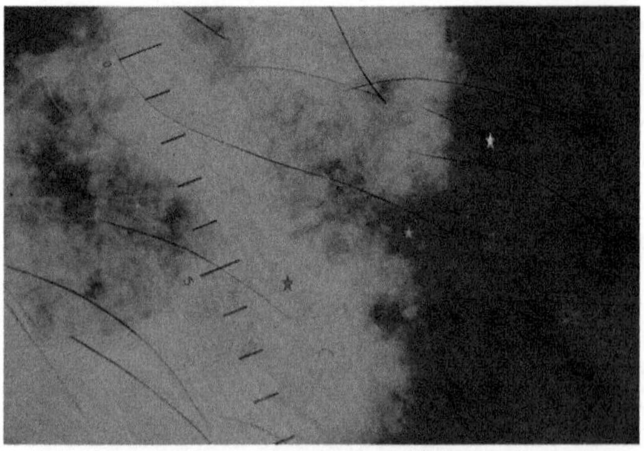

Fig. 21. Dermoscopy of unstable or progressive vitiligo showing a trichrome pattern. Depigmentation (*blue star*), hypopigmentation (*orange star*), and normal skin color (*green star*).

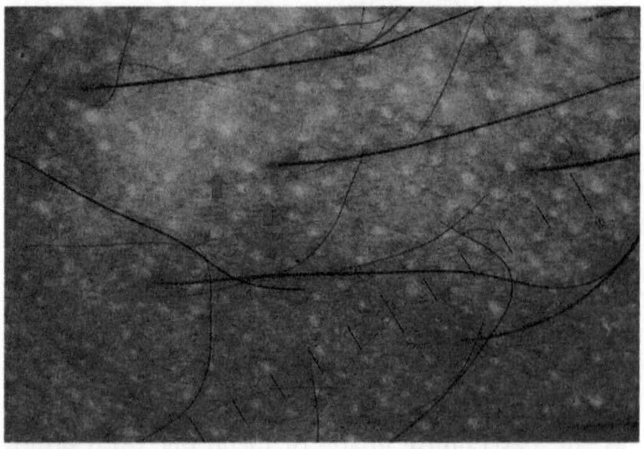

Fig. 22. Dermoscopy of perilesional skin in unstable vitiligo showing tapioca or sago grain pattern (*blue arrows*).

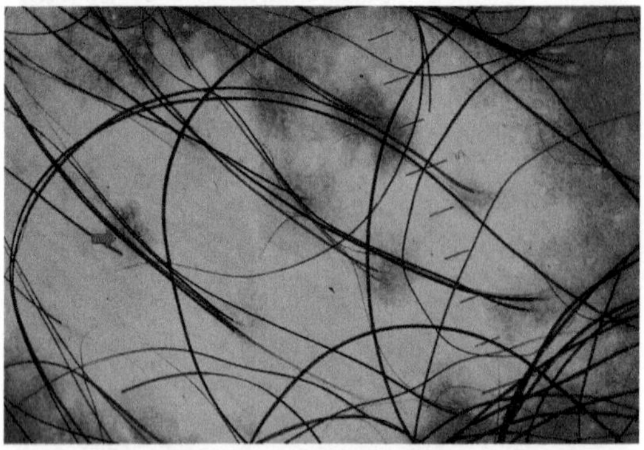

Fig. 23. Dermoscopy of repigmenting or stable vitiligo showing perifollicular pigmentation and reticular pattern of pigmentation (*blue arrow*).

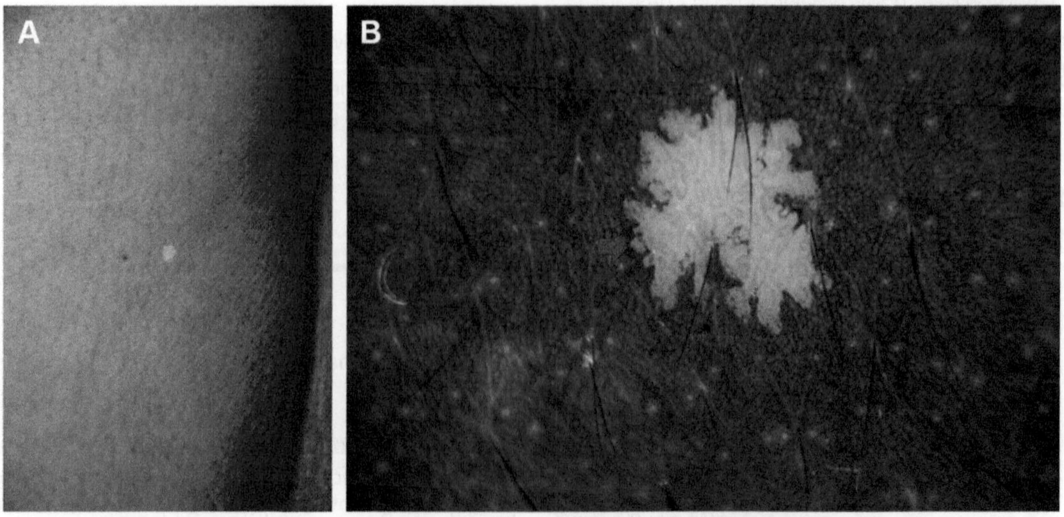

Fig. 24. (*A*). Clinical image of idiopathic guttate hypomelanosis. (*B*). Dermoscopy shows ameboid pattern (*blue arrow*). Lesional margins are distinct in contrast to vitiligo where margins are blurred.

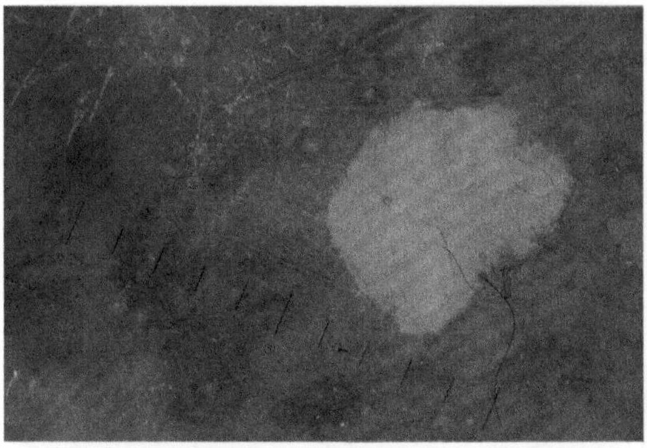

Fig. 25. Dermoscopy of IGH showing petaloid pattern (*blue arrow*) and distinct margins.

hypopigmentary conditions. The presence within the lesion of a reticular pigment pattern in some areas and a total absence of pigmentary pattern in other areas is suggestive of ash-leaf macules, whereas nevus depigmentosus shows the presence of a reticular pigment pattern throughout the lesion (unpublished observations).

Leprosy

It is a chronic granulomatous disorder caused by *Mycobacterium leprae*, characterized by a hypopigmented, hypoaesthetic patch (**Fig. 27**A). Histopathology of the skin is the gold standard for the diagnosis. Dermoscopy is increasingly used as a noninvasive modality to help in the early diagnosis where clinical features are not characteristic and biopsy may not be feasible, like hypopigmented lesions on the face of children. Dermoscopy of borderline tuberculoid leprosy shows white areas, decreased hair, and white dots, suggestive of a decreased density of pilosebaceous openings and sweat duct. Yellow globules with a distorted pigment network can also be seen in infiltrated plaques, which are histopathologically correlated with the presence of dermal granulomas. However, it is difficult to differentiate indeterminate leprosy from other hypopigmentary disorders on dermoscopy; more detailed studies are needed before dermoscopy can be used as a screening tool for the diagnosis of early leprosy[26] (**Fig. 27**B).

Discoid lupus erythematosus

It is a chronic autoimmune disorder that generally involves the head and neck and is characterized by discoid plaques. End-stage or burnt-out DLE can be confused with vitiligo and can be difficult to differentiate clinically (**Fig. 28**A). Dermoscopy of DLE shows follicular keratotic plugs, a perifollicular whitish halo, and telangiectatic vessels. However, burnt-out lesions may not show any keratotic plugs and only perifollicular white dots may be seen. These areas indicate the end stage of the disease process and suggest scarring (**Fig. 28**B).

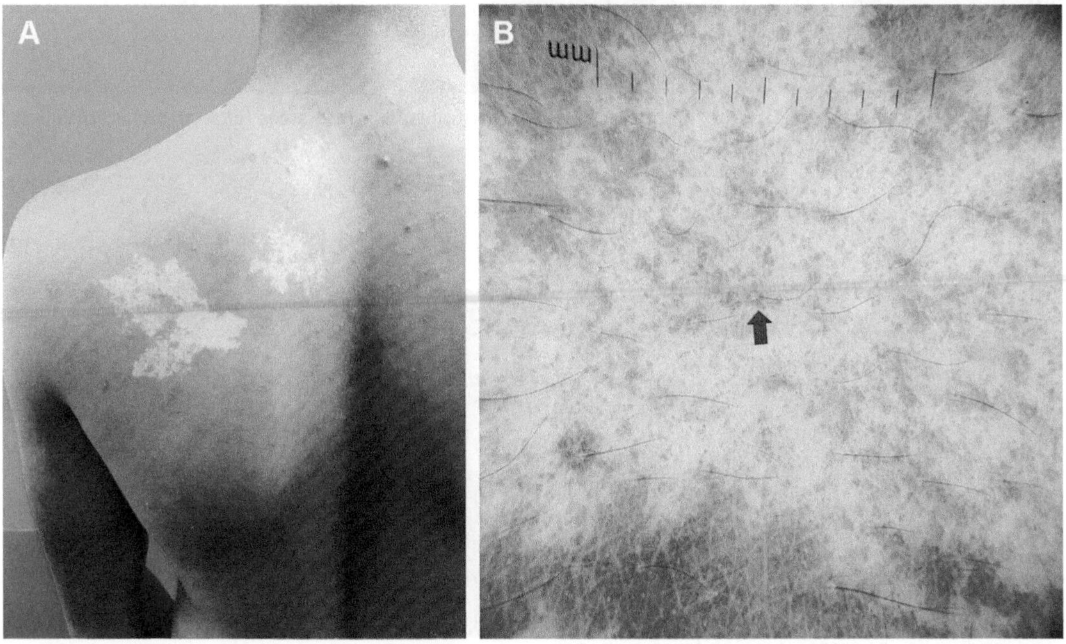

Fig. 26. (*A*). Clinical image of nevus depigmentosus. (*B*). Dermoscopy shows presence of reticular pigment network within the lesion (*blue arrow*).

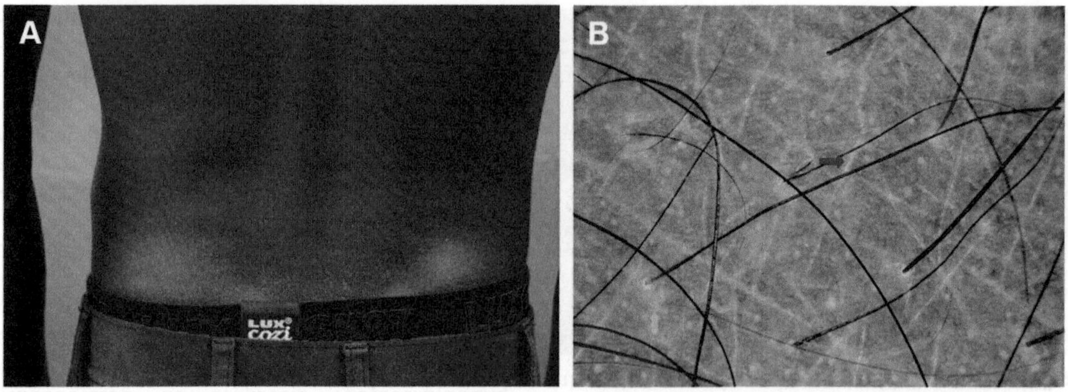

Fig. 27. (*A*). Clinical image of borderline tuberculoid leprosy. (*B*). Dermoscopy shows white areas (*green arrow*) and white scales (*blue arrow*). Yellow areas suggesting granulomas are not very evident. (*Courtesy of* B.S. Ankad, MBBS, Bagalkot, India.)

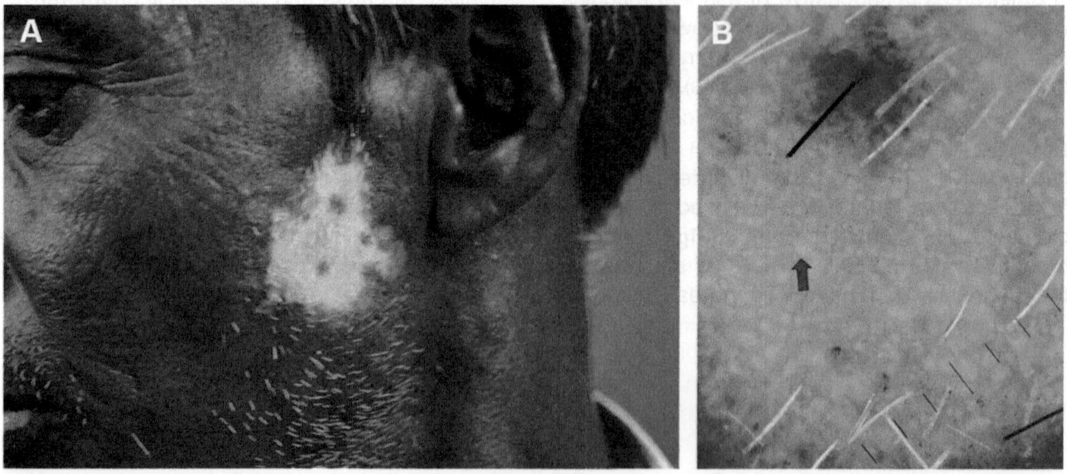

Fig. 28. (*A*). Clinical image of DLE. (*B*). Dermoscopy shows perifollicular white areas (*blue arrow*). Clinically it is difficult to differentiate this lesion from vitiligo lesion.

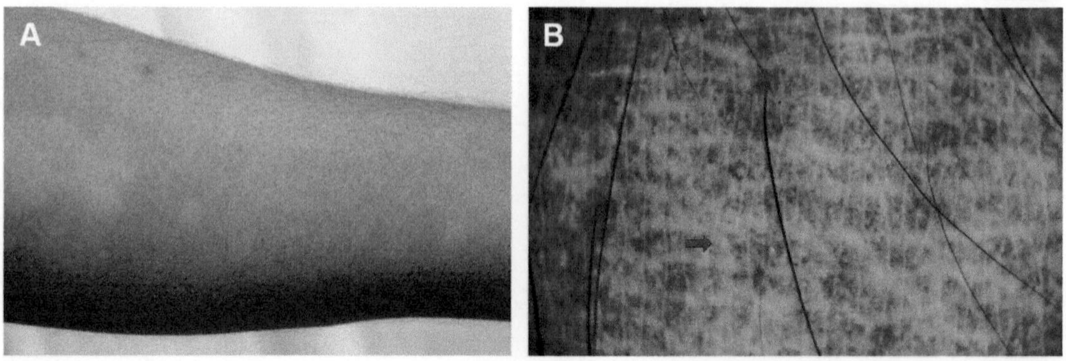

Fig. 29. (*A*). Clinical image of progressive macular hypomelanosis. (*B*). Dermoscopy shows ill-defined white areas without scaling (*blue arrow*).

Progressive macular hypomelanosis

This hypopigmentation disorder is caused by *Propionibacterium acnes*. It is characterized by asymptomatic, ill-defined to discoid, nonscaly, symmetric, hypopigmented macules that sometimes coalesce into patches (**Fig. 29**A). The eruptions are often seen on the trunk, face, and a satellite extension to the extremities, neck, and buttocks. Dermoscopy reveals ill-defined whitish areas without scaling[27] (**Fig. 29**B).

SUMMARY

Dermoscopy is evolving as an important tool for diagnosis, prognosis, and monitoring of inflammatory disorders. In these parts of the world where cutaneous malignancies are relatively uncommon, these so-called alternative uses of dermoscopy are actually its most common uses. A handheld dermoscope is cheap, noninvasive, and does not require much infrastructure for its use; it can be connected to widely available smart phones, and images can be captured easily making it a popular instrument to be used in developing countries.

REFERENCES

1. Sayal SK, Das AL, Gupta CM. Pattern of skin diseases among civil population and armed forces personnel at Pune. Indian J Dermatol Venereol Leprol 1997;63:29–32.
2. Sarkar R, Ailawadi P. Treatment of melasma: the journey ahead. Indian J Dermatol 2017;62:555–7.
3. Sonthalia S, Jha AK, Langar S. Dermoscopy of melasma. Indian Dermatol Online J 2017;8(6):525.
4. Khunger N, Kandhari R. Dermoscopic criteria for differentiating exogenous ochronosis from melasma. Indian J Dermatol Venereol Leprol 2013;79:819–21.
5. Bhutani LK, Bedi TR, Pandhi RK, et al. Lichen planus pigmentosus. Dermatology 1974;149(1):43–50.
6. Rieder E, Kaplan J, Kamino H, et al. Lichen planus pigmentosus. Dermatol Online J 2013;19(12).
7. Neema S, Jha A. Lichen planus pigmentosus. Pigment International 2017;4(1):48–9.
8. Pirmez R, Duque-Estrada B, Donati A, et al. Clinical and dermoscopic features of lichen planus pigmentosus in 37 patients with frontal fibrosing alopecia. Br J Dermatol 2016;175(6):1387–90.
9. Nakayama H. Pigmented contact dermatitis and chemical depigmentation. Springer (Berlin): Heidelberg; 2011. p. 377–93. InContact Dermatitis.
10. Shenoi SD, Rao R. Pigmented contact dermatitis. Indian J Dermatol Venereol Leprol 2007;73(5):285.
11. Singh N, Thappa DM. Pigmentary demarcation lines. Pigment International 2014;1(1):13.
12. Redkar NN, Rawat KJ, Warrier S, et al. Nevus of ota. J Assoc Physicians India 2016;64:70.
13. Sofen B, Prado G, Emer J. Melasma and post inflammatory hyperpigmentation: management update and expert opinion. Skin Therapy Lett 2016;21(1):1–7.
14. Vijaya B, Dalal BS, Manjunath GV. Primary cutaneous amyloidosis: a clinico-pathological study with emphasis on polarized microscopy. Indian J Pathol Microbiol 2012;55(2):170.
15. Chuang YY, Lee DD, Lin CS, et al. Characteristic dermoscopic features of primary cutaneous amyloidosis: a study of 35 cases. Br J Dermatol 2012;167(3):548–54.
16. Phiske MM. An approach to acanthosis nigricans. Indian Dermatol Online J 2014;5(3):239.
17. Uchida S, Oiso N, Suzuki T, et al. Dermoscopic features of hyperpigmented dots in crista cutis in two siblings in a japanese family with inherited acanthosis nigricans. J Chem Dermatol Sci Appl 2012; 2(04):252.
18. Verma SB, Vasani RJ, Chandrashekar L, et al. Seborrheic melanosis: an entity worthy of mention in dermatological literature. Indian J Dermatol Venereol Leprol 2017;83:285–9.
19. Thatte SS, Khopkar US. The utility of dermoscopy in the diagnosis of evolving lesions of vitiligo. Indian J Dermatol Venereol Leprol 2014;80(6):505.
20. Chuh AA, Zawar V. Demonstration of residual perifollicular pigmentation in localized vitiligo—a reverse and novel application of digital epiluminescence dermoscopy. Comput Med Imaging Graph 2004; 28(4):213–7.
21. Jha AK, Sonthalia S, Lallas A. Dermoscopy as an evolving tool to assess vitiligo activity. J Am Acad Dermatol 2017. https://doi.org/10.1016/j.jaad.2017.12.009.
22. Kumar Jha A, Sonthalia S, Lallas A, et al. Dermoscopy in vitiligo: diagnosis and beyond. Int J Dermatol 2017. https://doi.org/10.1111/ijd.13795.
23. Thappa DM, Chandrashekar L, Malathi M. Dermoscopy in vitiligo. In: Handog EB, Enriquez-Macarayo MJ, editors. Melasma and vitiligo in brown skin. Springer India; 2017. p. 207–16.
24. Ankad BS, Beergouder SL. Dermoscopic evaluation of idiopathic guttate hypomelanosis: a preliminary observation. Indian Dermatol Online J 2015; 6(3):164.
25. Naoki OI, Kawada A. The diagnostic usefulness of dermoscopy for nevus depigmentosus. Eur J Dermatol 2011;21(4):639–40.
26. Ankad BS, Sakhare PS. Dermoscopy of borderline tuberculoid leprosy. Int J Dermatol 2017. https://doi.org/10.1111/ijd.13731.
27. Desai SR, Owen JL. Progressive macular hypomelanosis: an update. Pigment Int 2014;1:52–5.

Dermatoscopy and Reflectance Confocal Microscopy Correlations in Nonmelanocytic Disorders

Check for updates

Francesco Lacarrubba, MD[a,*], Marco Ardigò, MD[b],
Alessandro Di Stefani, MD[c], Anna Elisa Verzì, MD[a], Giuseppe Micali, MD[a]

KEYWORDS

• Reflectance confocal microscopy • Dermatoscopy • Histopathology • Nonmelanocytic disorders

KEY POINTS

- Dermatoscopy and in vivo reflectance confocal microscopy are noninvasive techniques that are increasingly used in different fields of dermatology for diagnosis and treatment monitoring.
- Some studies have reported interesting correlations between dermatoscopic and confocal reflectance features in selected cutaneous disorders.
- The combined use of both techniques represents a promising option to reach a definitive diagnosis without the need of invasive procedures.

INTRODUCTION

Dermatoscopy and in vivo reflectance confocal microscopy (RCM) are noninvasive techniques mainly used for pigmented skin lesion evaluation that however may assist the clinical diagnosis in a variety of inflammatory and infectious cutaneous disorders.[1–12] Both techniques provide a horizontal approach, with an en face view of the skin structures. Dermatoscopy allows the magnified observation from the top, of the skin structures from the surface to the mid-dermis. RCM provides real-time virtual skin biopsies offering microscopic details of the different skin layers up to the papillary dermis. The aim of this article, based on the existing literature and on the authors' personal experience, is to correlate the features obtained with these techniques along with the histopathologic findings in a series of skin disorders (**Table 1**).

PSORIASIS

Psoriasis is an inflammatory, chronic-relapsing, erythematous-desquamative dermatosis affecting about 3% of the overall population of the world. Plaque-type psoriasis is the most common presentation and is characterized by reddish plaques covered by silver/white scales.

Dermatoscopy at ×10 of psoriatic lesions (**Fig. 1**A) shows the presence of diffuse white scales and uniformly distributed pinpoint red capillaries or red dots over a light-red background.[8,13–15] At high magnification (≥×100), the red dots appear as dilated and twisted capillaries, with a typical bushy or basket-like appearance (**Fig. 1**B); each bush measures about 70 to 90 μm in diameter vs 15–25 μm of the normal capillary loops of healthy skin.[16–24]

The whitish scales seen at dermatoscopy correspond at RCM and histopathology to a thickened

Disclosures: None.

[a] Dermatology Clinic, University of Catania, Via Santa Sofia 78, Catania 95123, Italy; [b] Department of Clinical Dermatology, San Gallicano Dermatological Institute, Rome, Italy; [c] Institute of Dermatology, Catholic University of the Sacred Heart, Rome, Italy
* Corresponding author. Dermatology Clinic, University of Catania, Via Santa Sofia 78, Catania 95123, Italy.
E-mail address: francesco.lacarrubba@unict.it

Dermatol Clin 36 (2018) 487–501
https://doi.org/10.1016/j.det.2018.05.015

Table 1
Main dermatoscopy and reflectance confocal microscopy findings and their histopathologic correlation in some cutaneous disorders

	Dermatoscopy	RCM	Histopathology
Inflammatory Disorders			
Psoriasis	Whitish scales	Thickened stratum corneum with parakeratosis	Thickened stratum corneum with parakeratosis
	Red dots (×10)/bushy capillaries (>×100)	Uplocated, enlarged dermal papillae (roundish dark areas) filled with prominent round or linear dark, canalicular structures	Tortuous, ectatic capillaries within elongated dermal papillae
Eczematous dermatitis	Yellowish scales	Disrupted stratum corneum	Exudates within the stratum corneum
	—	Broadband intercellular spaces, intraepidermal dark areas, and small, mildly refractive cells	Spongiosis, vesicles, and epidermal and dermal inflammatory cells
	Irregularly distributed dotted vessels on an erythematous background	Dilated vessels in the upper dermis	Dilated dermal vessels
Seborrheic dermatitis	Whitish/yellowish scales	Thickened stratum corneum	Thickened stratum corneum
	—	Broadband intercellular spaces and small, mildly refractive cells	Spongiosis and inflammatory cells in the upper dermis
	Pinpoint and linear vessels	Focal areas of dilated and crowded dermal papillae and horizontally distributed vessels	Dilated vessels in the dermis
Cutaneous discoid lupus erythematous (active lesions)	Follicular yellowish plugs with a perifollicular whitish halo	Large, roundish hyper-reflective, amorphous areas	Follicular hyperkeratosis
	Disappearance of the normal capillary loops	Dermoepidermal junction obscuration (multiple, small, bright cells at the level of the interface between the epidermis and the upper dermis with focal disappearance of the normal edged papillae)	Inflammatory cells infiltrate modifying the normal aspect of the dermoepidermal junction (interface dermatitis)
Cutaneous discoid lupus erythematous (late-stage lesions)	Whitish structureless areas, telangiectatic vessels	Epidermal atrophy and hyper-reflecting thickened fibers in the upper dermis	Epidermal atrophy and diffuse dermal fibrosis
	Hyperpigmentation	Polygonal, plump, bright cells located in the upper dermis	Melanophages in the upper dermis

Lichen planus	Network of pearly, whitish lines that may display a reticular, arboriform, annular, globular, or homogeneous configuration	Hypergranulosis	Hypergranulosis
	—	Diffuse dermoepidermal junction obscuration (sheets of inflammatory cells at the level of the interface between the epidermis and the upper dermis)	Massive lymphocytic infiltrate modifying the normal aspect of the dermoepidermal junction (interface dermatitis)
	Prominent linear vessels with a characteristic radial distribution at the periphery of the whitish lines	Dilated dermal vessels	Dilated dermal vessels
Lichen sclerosus (anogenital and extragenital)	Patchy, whitish, homogenous areas	Epidermal atrophy and hyper-reflecting thickened fibers in the upper dermis	Epidermal atrophy and dermal fibrosis
	Yellow circles (extragenital lesions)	Round dark structures containing bright amorphous material	Follicular keratotic plugs
Pityriasis rubra pilaris	Whitish hyperkeratotic perifollicular areas on a yellowish background	Stratum granulosum and corneum in confluent arrangement especially around follicles, with alternating orthokeratosis and parakeratosis	Checkerboard pattern, with alternating orthokeratosis and parakeratosis and follicular parakeratotic "lipping"
	Pinpoint/linear vessels	Irregularly shaped papillae with enlarged blood vessels	Irregularly shaped papillae with enlarged blood vessels
Zoon balanitis	Fairly focused curved vessels	Tortuous vessels running parallel to the surface (vermicular vessels) at the epithelium-lamina propria junction	Vascular dilatation/proliferation
	Red to orange, structureless, homogeneous areas	—	Hemosiderin deposition
	—	Small bright cells in the upper dermis	Band-like infiltrate of predominantly plasma cells
Darier disease	Polygonal, star-like, or roundish-oval yellowish/brownish structures surrounded by a thin whitish halo	Low-reflectant areas of variable shape extending through the whole epidermis and containing structureless, high-reflectant material	Hyperparakeratotic areas
	—	Epidermal, large, roundish, bright cells	Corps ronds and grains

(*continued on next page*)

Table 1
(continued)

	Dermatoscopy	RCM	Histopathology
Darier-like Grover disease	Polygonal, star-like, or roundish-oval yellowish/brownish structures surrounded by a thin whitish halo	Low-reflectant areas of variable shape extending through the whole epidermis and containing structureless, high-reflectant material	Hyperparakeratotic areas
	—	Intraepidermal bright cells and dark spaces	Acantholytic keratinocytes and intraepidermal clefts
	—	Intraepidermal target-like cells with a dark center and a highly reflectant halo	Dyskeratotic cells
Acne	Dilated, roundish, central pore filled with a brown-yellow plug (comedo)	Enlarged follicular ostium filled with hyper-reflecting amorphous material (comedo)	Dilated follicular infundibulum filled with keratin and debris
	Erythematous roundish area (inflammatory papule) that can be centered by a white-yellowish structure (pustule)	Dark roundish structure containing amorphous material and/or organized hyper-reflecting inflammatory infiltrate (papule); accumulation of hyper-reflecting material surrounded by inflammatory cells and dilated vessels (pustule)	Folliculitis and suppurative folliculitis
Infectious Disorders			
Molluscum contagiosum	Central yellowish-white, roundish or poly-lobular amorphous structure	Hyporefractive roundish lobules containing hyper-refractive cells	Lobulated, endophytic hyperplasia and enlarged keratinocytes containing characteristic intracytoplasmic viral inclusions
	Crown of fine, linear, and blurred vessels	Dilated dermal vessels	Dilated dermal vessels
Cutaneous and anogenital warts	Whitish network, regularly distributed dotted vessels, hemorrhagic black dots or streaks (papular lesions) Multiple irregular, whitish projections filled with elongated and dilated vessels (papillomatous lesions)	Elongated and enlarged dermal papillae containing dilated capillary vessels	Elongated and enlarged dermal papillae containing dilated capillary vessels
	—	Large cells at the level of the spinous-granulous layer (anogenital warts)	Koilocytes
Scabies	Mites in migration within the burrow, eggs, and feces (high magnification)	Mites in migration within the burrow, eggs, and feces	Burrow containing mites, eggs, and feces

Demodicosis	Dilated follicular openings containing either the *Demodex* tails protruding from the follicular orifice or grayish to brown plugs surrounded by an erythematous halo	Dilated follicular openings and *Demodex* tails appearing as elongated, cone-shaped structures superficially located in the follicle	Dilated follicular openings and *Demodex folliculorum*
Tinea nigra	Brown dots and pigmented spicules with a filamentous arrangement, over a homogeneous brownish pigmentation	Multiple bright, roundish and elongated, filamentous structures at the level of the stratum corneum	Arthroconidia and filamentous, septate hyphae
Miscellanea			
Juvenile xanthogranuloma	Homogeneous yellow hue	Multiple large atypical cells of different sizes with a highly refractive periphery	Foamy histiocytes
Argyria	Gray dots	Small, hyper-reflective particles in the papillary dermis arranged in clusters or forming a network	Dermal deposition of brown-black granules
Aquagenic palmar wrinkling	Hypertrophic stratum corneum with deepening of normal dermatoglyphics and dilatation of eccrine ostia	Increased size of keratinocytes and hyper-reflective intercellular spaces in the stratum granulosum and abnormally dilated eccrine ostia and ducts	Edematous changes of the stratum corneum and dilated eccrine ducts

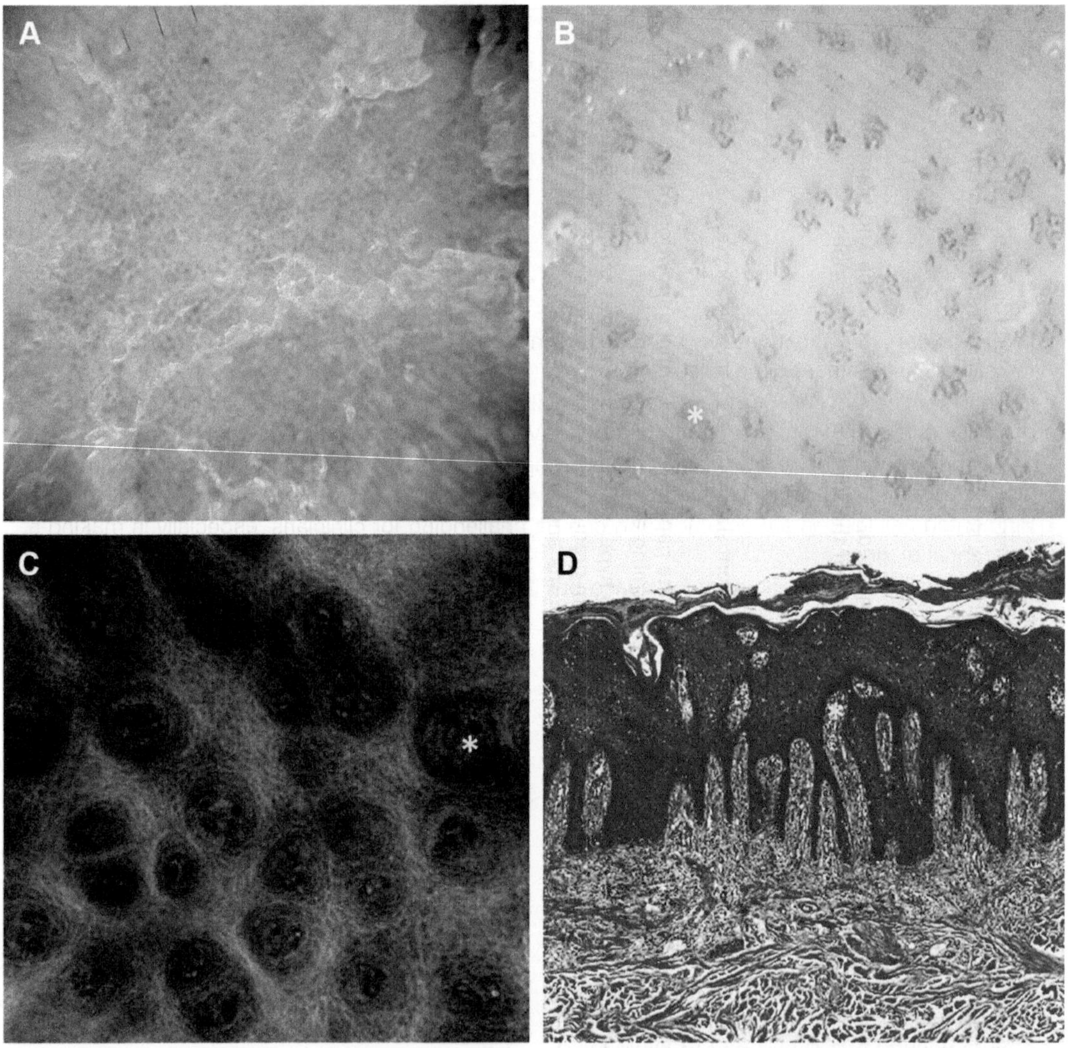

Fig. 1. Plaque psoriasis. (*A*) Dermatoscopy showing white scales and regularly distributed dotted vessels (original magnification ×10); (*B*) high-magnification videodermatoscopy showing a uniform pattern of bushy dilated capillaries (*asterisk*) (original magnification ×200); (*C*) RCM (1 × 1 mm) of the papillary dermis showing nonrimmed, enlarged dermal papillae (*asterisk*) fulfilled by dilated blood vessels; (*D*) histopathology showing hyperparakeratosis and elongated dermal papillae (*asterisk*) containing ectatic capillaries (H&E, original magnification ×50).

stratum corneum showing parakeratosis. The red dots/bushy capillaries match with RCM for the presence of diffuse superficial, enlarged dermal papillae (**Fig. 1**C), which appear as dark areas (>80 μm in diameter), typically filled with prominent round or linear dark canalicular structures, each representing a capillary loop containing circulating blood cells.[10,11,15,25] These structures represent the horizontal view of the tortuous, ectatic capillaries within the elongated dermal papillae (papillomatosis) seen at histopathologic examination (**Fig. 1**D). Another characteristic RCM feature of psoriasis is represented by the absence of the normal rim of variable bright basal keratinocytes surrounding the dermal papillae; this is probably related to the hypopigmentation of basal keratinocytes secondary to the release of tumor necrosis factor-α in psoriasis inhibiting melanocyte activity.[10,11]

ECZEMATOUS DERMATITIS

The term *eczematous dermatitis* includes a variety of inflammatory skin diseases histopathologically characterized by spongiosis and vesicles. The most common clinical presentation is represented by contact dermatitis (allergic and irritant) and atopic dermatitis.

Dermatoscopy of eczematous lesions shows a low-specific pattern characterized by the presence of yellowish scales with a patchy distribution and irregularly distributed dotted vessels on an erythematous background.[5,7,8]

The yellowish scales seen at dermatoscopy correspond at RCM to a disrupted stratum corneum characterized by highly refractile, polygonal, detached corneocytes and, histopathologically, to the presence of exudates within the stratum corneum. In the upper dermis, dilated vessels are generally detectable as round to canalicular structures.[10,11] RCM also reveals the characteristic histopathologic epidermal features of eczematous dermatitis, that is, spongiosis, presenting as areas with broadband intercellular spaces in comparison with the surrounding epithelium; vesicles, detectable as intraepidermal dark areas; and small, mildly refractive cells corresponding to intraepidermal and dermal inflammatory cells. The dermoepidermal junction is typically preserved.[10,11]

SEBORRHEIC DERMATITIS

Seborrheic dermatitis (SD) is a common chronic inflammatory skin disorder, mainly localized on seborrheic areas of the body (scalp, face, trunk) and characterized by erythema, scaling, and itch.

On dermatoscopy, SD is characterized by the presence of whitish/yellowish scaling and both pinpoint and linear vessels.[8] Both features are well visible at RCM, which shows a thickened stratum corneum, focal areas of dilated and crowded dermal papillae, and horizontally distributed vessels that are generally detected around adnexal structures.[25] Moreover, RCM shows the presence of spongiosis in the epidermis and inflammatory cells in the upper dermis, with a good histopathology correlation.[25]

CUTANEOUS DISCOID LUPUS ERYTHEMATOSUS

Cutaneous discoid lupus erythematosus is an autoimmune disease triggered by ultraviolet light exposure but whose exact cause is not well understood. It is clinically characterized by erythematous to violaceous scaly plaques with prominent follicular plugging that mainly arise in sun-exposed areas and may result in atrophy, hyperpigmentation, and scarring. It may occur in association with systemic lupus erythematosus.

In active lesions, dermatoscopy shows a diffuse homogeneous erythema, irregular vessels (the normal capillary loops are no more detectable), and follicular yellowish plugs with a perifollicular whitish halo (**Fig. 2**A). Late, scarring lesions display whitish structureless areas, telangiectatic vessels, and hyperpigmentation.[5]

At RCM, the yellowish plugs observed at dermatoscopy appear as large, roundish, hyperreflective, amorphous areas (**Fig. 2**B) histopathologically related to follicular hyperkeratosis (**Fig. 2**D). The dermatoscopic disappearance of the normal capillary loops could be related to the typical RCM feature of cutaneous discoid lupus erythematosus that is represented by the so-called dermoepidermal junction obscuration at the level of the interface between the epidermis and the upper dermis; it consists of the presence of multiple small, bright cells and the focal disappearance of the normal edged papillae (**Fig. 2**C), defined as roundish dark structures surrounded by a well-demarcated rim of bright basal cells.[10,11] Histopathologically, this aspect corresponds to the inflammatory cells infiltrate that modifies the normal aspect of the dermoepidermal junction (interface dermatitis) (see **Fig. 2**D).

In late-stage lesions, the whitish structureless areas observed at dermatoscopy correspond at RCM to diffuse dermal fibrosis, whereas the hyperpigmentary changes correlate to the presence of polygonal, plump, bright cells located in the upper dermis; they represent melanophages that can be observed in all types of interface dermatitis as an expression of the basal layer damage with diffusion of melanin in the upper dermis.[10,11]

LICHEN PLANUS

Lichen planus is a chronic-relapsing inflammatory disorder of unknown origin (probably autoimmune) that may involve the skin, mucosal membranes, hair, and nails. The classic cutaneous lesions are represented by multiple, symmetric, pruritic, pinkish, polygonal papules mainly involving the flexural aspects of arms and legs. On the lesion surface, a whitish network (known as Wickham striae) may be often observed. Postinflammatory hyperpigmentation is common.

Cutaneous lichen planus at $\times 10$ dermatoscopy shows a pinkish to light red background color and a network of pearly, whitish lines (clinically corresponding to the Wickham striae)[3] that may display a reticular, arboriform, annular, globular, or homogeneous configuration (**Fig. 3**A). Moreover, prominent linear vessels with a characteristic radial distribution may be observed at the periphery of the whitish lines.[5,26,27]

The Wickham striae observed at dermatoscopy likely correspond to areas of wedge-shaped hypergranulosis (**Fig. 3**C), a characteristic histopathology feature of lichen planus that is also well visible at RCM.[10,11,28] Another typical RCM feature of lichen planus is the dermoepidermal junction obscuration (**Fig. 3**B) that seems to be more diffuse in lichen

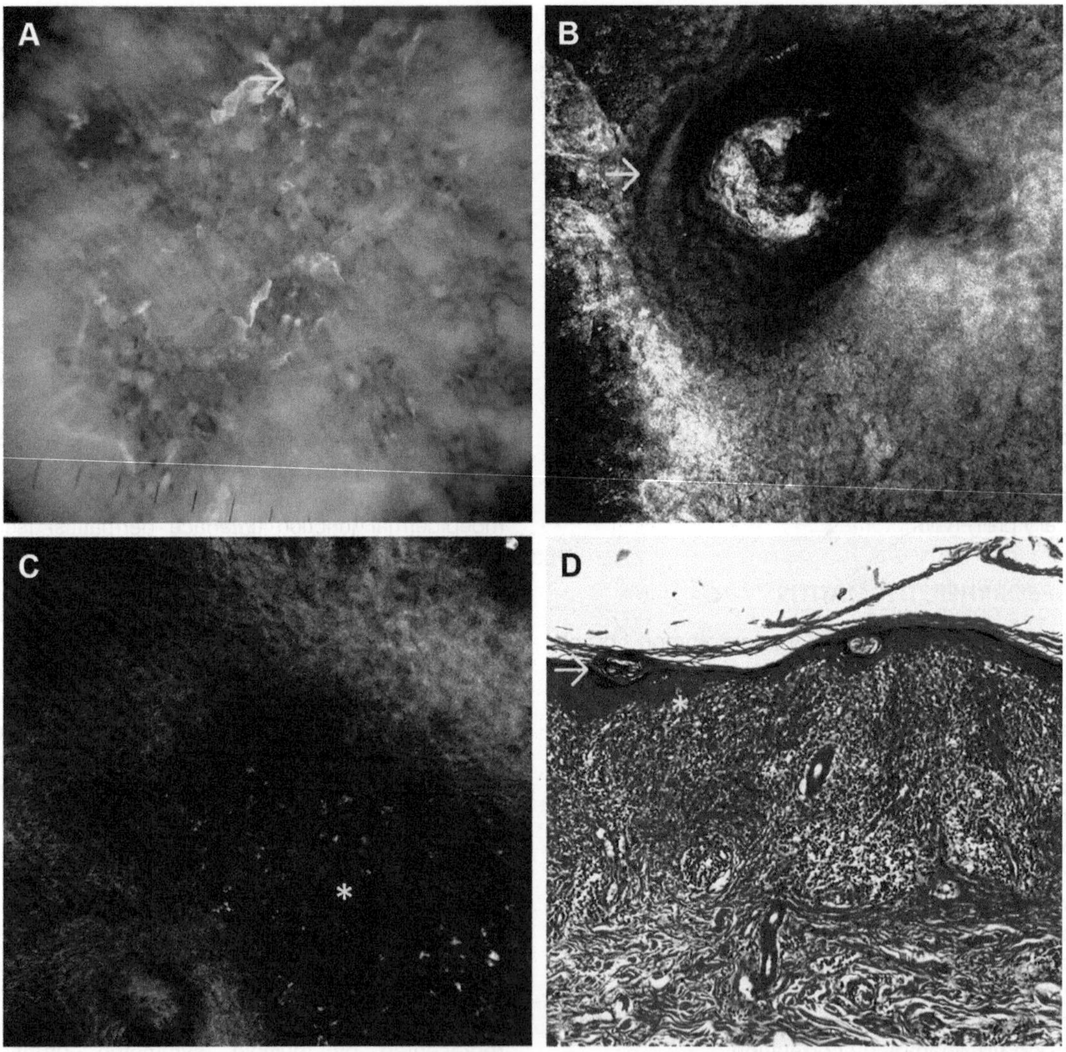

Fig. 2. Cutaneous discoid lupus erythematous. (*A*) Dermatoscopy showing a reddish background, irregular vessels, whitish scales, and yellowish plugs (*arrow*) (original magnification ×10); (*B*) RCM (1 × 1 mm) of the epidermis showing a large, roundish hyper-reflective, amorphous area (*arrow*); (*C*) RCM (1 × 1 mm) of the dermoepidermal junction showing multipl small, bright cells and absence of normal edged papillae (*asterisk*); (*D*) histopathology showing follicular hyperkeratotic plugs (*arrow*) and diffuse inflammatory cells infiltrate with disarrangement of the dermoepidermal junction (*asterisk*) (H×E, original magnification ×50).

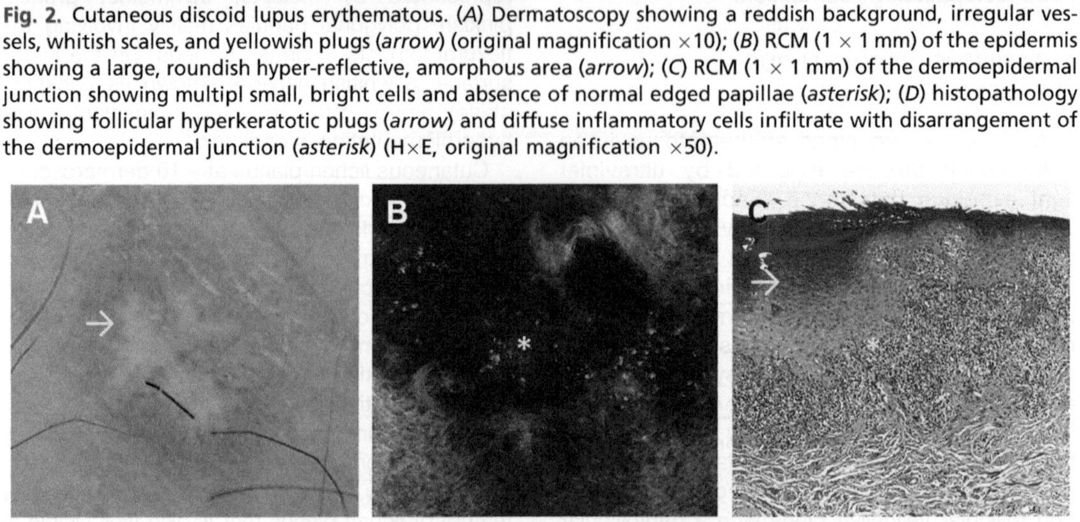

Fig. 3. Lichen planus. (*A*) Dermatoscopy showing a network of whitish lines (*arrow*) over a light-red background (original magnification ×10); (*B*) RCM (1 × 1 mm) of the dermoepidermal junction showing multiple small, bright cells obscuring the junction (*asterisk*); (*C*) histopathology showing hyperkeratosis, wedge-shaped hypergranulosis (*arrow*) and a dense lymphocytic lichenoid infiltrate (*asterisk*) (H&E, original magnification ×50).

planus compared with cutaneous lupus erythematous. In lichen planus, sheets of inflammatory cells distributed along the front of the lesion are often observable and histopathologically correspond to the lymphocytic lichenoid infiltrate (see **Fig. 3**C). Melanophages are also visible on RCM, especially in late stages of the disease.[10,11,28]

LICHEN SCLEROSUS

Lichen sclerosus is a chronic inflammatory disease of unknown cause that may involve both anogenital and extragenital areas. It is clinically characterized by whitish, atrophic plaques that may show hemorrhagic spots. In anogenital areas, these lesions may result in scarring and adhesion, with pain and sexual and/or urinary dysfunction. Extragenital lesions are usually asymptomatic.

At dermatoscopy, anogenital lichen sclerosus shows patchy, whitish areas associated with linear and/or dotted vessels; erosions and hemorrhages may also be detected.[29–31] The whitish areas correspond at RCM to a disarray of the normal papillary architecture (obscuration of the epithelium-lamina propria junction) and to hyper-reflecting thickened fibers in the upper dermis (reflecting dermal fibrosis at histopathology). Small bright cells are generally observed, whereas the normal honeycomb pattern of the epidermis is preserved.

Dermatoscopy of extragenital lichen sclerosus shows the presence of whitish, homogenous bright areas associated with follicular yellow circles (comedo-like openings).[5,32–35] At RCM, the whitish areas correlate to the presence of coarse collagen structures in bundles in the upper dermis, histopathologically corresponding to dermal fibrosis, whereas the yellow circles correspond to round dark structures containing bright amorphous material, histopathologically correlated to follicular keratotic plugs.[34,36,37] RCM also reveals the presence of bright inflammatory cells in the upper dermis.

PITYRIASIS RUBRA PILARIS

Pityriasis rubra pilaris is a rare chronic inflammatory papulosquamous skin disease clinically characterized by coalescing papules that may progress to erythroderma showing small areas of spared normal skin.

The dermatoscopic pattern consists of whitish keratotic follicular plugs on a yellowish background, surrounded by vessels of mixed morphology, mostly pinpoint and linear.[38–40]

The whitish keratotic plugs correlate at RCM with stratum granulosum and corneum in a confluent arrangement, especially around follicles; histologically these aspects correspond to the typical checkerboard pattern, with alternating orthokeratosis and parakeratosis and follicular parakeratotic “lipping.”[41] Moreover, the presence at RCM of irregularly shaped and elongated papillae with enlarged blood vessels matches with histopathology and to the mixed vascular appearance at dermatoscopy.[41]

ZOON BALANITIS

Zoon plasma cell balanitis is an idiopathic, chronic, benign inflammatory disease of the glans and the inner foreskin usually affecting middle-aged to elderly men and clinically characterized by shiny, well-defined erythematous plaques.

At dermatoscopy it shows the presence of fairly focused curved vessels having different widths (including serpentine, convoluted, chalice-shaped, and spermatozoa-like vessels); red to orange, structureless, homogeneous areas, corresponding to hemosiderin deposition, are also common.[42–44]

At RCM, the curved vessels appear as tortuous vessels running parallel to the surface (vermicular vessels) at the epithelium-lamina propria junction that histopathologically correspond to vascular dilatation/proliferation. Moreover, RCM examination of the affected areas reveals a normal nucleated honeycomb pattern in the superficial layers (able to differentiate Zoon balanitis from carcinoma in situ, the latter showing a disarranged epidermal pattern)[44,45] and small bright cells in the upper dermis histologically corresponding to the band-like infiltrate of predominantly plasma cells.

DARIER DISEASE AND DARIER-LIKE GROVER DISEASE

Darier disease is an autosomal dominantly inherited genodermatosis due to mutations in the gene ATP2A2 and clinically characterized by hyperkeratotic, skin-colored, yellowish and/or reddish papules mainly located in seborrheic areas and skin folds. Grover disease, also known as transient acantholytic dermatosis, is a benign condition of unknown origin characterized by erythematous, papulovesicular lesions of the trunk; among the different histopathological subtypes, the Darier-like is the most frequent.

The main dermatoscopic feature of Darier disease is represented by polygonal, star-like, or roundish-oval, yellowish/brownish structures surrounded by a thin whitish halo. A pinkish, homogeneous, structureless background, whitish scales, and dotted/linear vessels may also be observed.[46] The same findings have been described in the Darier-like subtype of Grover disease.[47–50]

In both Darier disease and the Darier-like Grover disease, the polygonal areas observed at dermatoscopy appear at RCM as low-reflectant areas of variable shape extending through the epidermis and containing structureless, high-reflectant material.[48,50] Histopathologically, they correspond to hyperparakeratotic areas of a different shape and size in the epidermis. Moreover, RCM allows the recognition of additional findings closely correlated to histopathologic features. In Darier disease, the presence in the epidermis of large, roundish, bright cells likely corresponds to the corps ronds.[50] In Darier-like Grover disease, RCM shows the presence of intraepidermal dark spaces corresponding to intraepidermal clefts, roundish, bright cells correlating to acantholytic keratinocytes, and target-like cells with a dark center and a highly reflectant halo corresponding to dyskeratotic cells.[48]

ACNE

Acne is a polymorphic chronic inflammatory disorder that clinically may present with open and/or closed comedones and inflammatory lesions, including papules, pustules, and nodules. Lesions typically affect body areas with a high density of sebaceous glands, such as the face, back, and chest. The clinical picture embraces a spectrum of signs, ranging from mild comedonal acne, with or without inflammatory lesions, to acne conglobata or aggressive fulminate disease with deep-seated inflammation, nodules, and associated systemic symptoms.

On dermatoscopy, acne lesions can be easily visualized. Comedones reveal a dilated, roundish, central pore filled with a brown-yellow plug (more evident in open comedones) corresponding to oxidic/melanized keratin. Inflammatory lesions appear as erythematous roundish areas that can be centered by a white-yellowish structure, a consequence of suppuration.[51,52] On RCM, the central pore observed at dermatoscopy in comedones appears as an enlarged follicular ostium filled with hyper-reflecting amorphous material (keratin).[53–55] Closed comedones reveal a smaller infundibular diameter and a better outlined roundish contour than open comedones.[54] Inflammatory papules appear at RCM as dark roundish structures containing amorphous material and/or organized hyper-reflecting inflammatory infiltrate.[54] Pustules show a central accumulation of hyper-reflecting material surrounded by inflammatory cells and dilated vessels.[54,55]

MOLLUSCUM CONTAGIOSUM

Molluscum contagiosum is a common cutaneous infection due to a poxvirus of the Molluscipox virus genus and characterized by single or multiple umbilicated, smooth, skin-colored papules.

A typical lesion shows at dermatoscopy the presence of a central yellowish-white, roundish or polylobular amorphous structure (corresponding to clinical umbilication) surrounded by a crown of fine, linear, and blurred vessels.[56] At RCM examination, the central structure observed at dermatoscopy corresponds to a well-circumscribed area consisting of hyporefractive roundish lobules containing hyper-refractive cells; these structures correlate to the typical histopathologic features of well-defined, lobulated, endophytic hyperplasia and of enlarged keratinocytes containing characteristic intracytoplasmic viral inclusions displacing the nucleus peripherally (Henderson-Paterson bodies).[57]

CUTANEOUS AND ANOGENITAL WARTS

Cutaneous and anogenital warts are very common infections from human papillomaviruses (HPVs). Clinically, they appear either as papular or papillomatous lesions with a hyperkeratotic (common warts) or smooth (anogenital warts) surface.

The dermatoscopic aspect of both cutaneous and anogenital warts depends on the clinical presentation. Papular lesions show a whitish network associated with regularly distributed dotted vessels (mosaic pattern) with hemorrhagic black dots or streaks sometimes being present.[5,58–60] Papillomatous lesions display multiple, irregular, whitish projections filled with elongated and dilated vessels (finger-like pattern).

The mosaic and the finger-like patterns observed at dermatoscopy correlate to the observation at RCM of elongated dermal papillae containing enlarged capillary vessels, a typical aspect seen also at histopathology. Moreover, in anogenital lesions RCM may show the presence of koilocytes, appearing as large cells at the level of the spinous-granulous layer.[61]

SCABIES

Scabies is a highly contagious, intensely pruritic skin infestation caused by *Sarcoptes scabiei hominis*. Clinically, it presents with typical serpiginous grayish tracts (burrows), erythematous papules and vesicles, and scratching marks with a symmetric distribution.

At low-magnification dermatoscopy (×10), the burrow is well recognizable and appears as a jet with contrail, whereby a jet-shaped, dark triangular structure corresponds to the pigmented mouth and anterior legs of the mite. High-magnification (>×100) dermatoscopy allows the detection of details, such as the mite in migration within the burrow, eggs and feces, usually not appreciable at a lower magnification.[62–67]

Similarly to high-magnification dermatoscopy, the RCM examination allows the identification of the burrow, visible as a tortuous large empty space at the level of the stratum granulosum/spinosum surrounded by the characteristic honeycomb pattern of the epidermis, and of the mite. RCM allows the in vivo visualization of the anatomic details of *Sarcoptes scabiei* (length 30 μm, width 25 μm), for example, the head, the legs, and the parasite's peristalsis. Moreover, the eggs (15 × 8 μm) containing mite embryos and high-refractive fecal material can also be observed within the burrow.[67,68]

DEMODICOSIS

The term *demodicosis* refers to a group of disorders caused by *Demodex folliculorum* and characterized by variable degree of spinulosis, erythema, and papules of the face, generally accompanied by a burning or pruritic sensation.[69]

Dermatoscopy at ×10 shows the presence of dilated follicular openings containing either the *Demodex* tails, appearing as a whitish creamy thread, 1 to 3 mm in length, protruding from the follicular orifice or grayish to brown plugs surrounded by an erythematous halo.[69–71]

At RCM examination, both dilated follicular openings and the *Demodex* tails are better visualized. The latter appear as elongated, cone-shaped structures superficially located in the follicle, which, when the RCM device is positioned completely perpendicular to the follicle, present as clusters of bright, round structures approximately 4 to 9 μm in diameter.[71]

TINEA NIGRA

Tinea nigra is a superficial mycosis due to *Hortaea werneckii* and typically observed in the palmoplantar regions as ill-defined brown macules.

Dermatoscopy shows the presence of brown dots and pigmented spicules with a filamentous arrangement, which do not follow any furrow or ridge pattern, over a homogeneous brownish pigmentation.[72,73]

The dots and spicules observed at dermatoscopy correspond at RCM to multiple bright, roundish and elongated, filamentous structures in the stratum corneum[74,75] likely representing arthroconidia and filamentous, septate hyphae, respectively[75]; their hyper-reflectance is probably due to the melanin presence in the cell wall.[74] Interestingly, the speckled aspect observed in some cases is morphologically similar to the hyphae identified on direct mycological examination.[74,75]

JUVENILE XANTHOGRANULOMA

Juvenile xanthogranuloma is a benign non-Langerhans cell histiocytosis that is more frequent in childhood. It is clinically characterized by single or multiple yellow to orange papulonodular lesions.

At dermatoscopy, juvenile xanthogranuloma displays a homogeneous orange-yellowish hue (**Fig. 4**A), which has been described as a setting-sun appearance, with or without linear and branched vessels. Other features include clouds of pale-yellow globules, subtle pigment network, and whitish streaks.[76–78]

The yellow hue correlates at RCM with the observation in the superficial dermis of multiple large atypical cells of different sizes with a highly refractive periphery (**Fig. 4**B), which likely reflect the foamy histiocytes at histopathology (**Fig. 4**C).[79,80]

ARGYRIA

Argyria is a cutaneous or mucosal deposition of silver salts often resulting in a permanent diffuse or

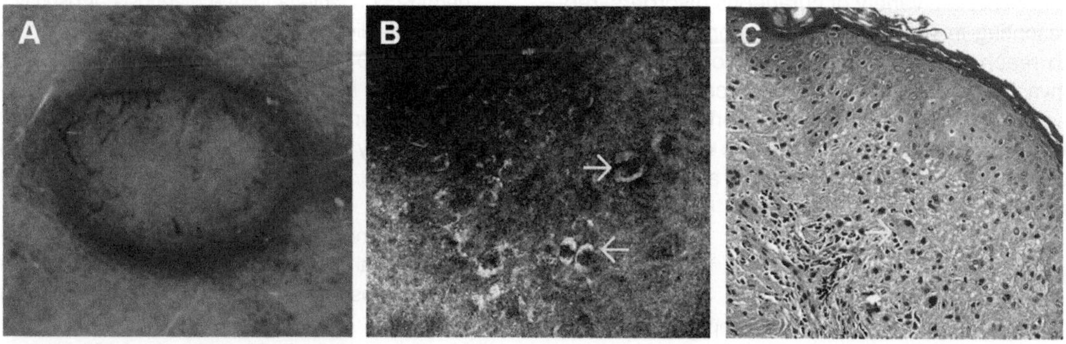

Fig. 4. Juvenile xanthogranuloma. (*A*) Dermatoscopy showing a homogeneous orange-yellowish hue and linear and branched vessels (original magnification ×10); (*B*) RCM (1 × 1 mm) of the superficial dermis showing large atypical cells with a highly refractile periphery (*arrows*); (*C*) histopathology showing foamy histiocytes (*arrow*) and Touton cells (H×E, original magnification ×50).

localized blue-gray pigmentation that may be caused by intake or a prolonged topical application of compounds containing silver.[81,82]

Dermatoscopic evaluation at ×10 reveals the presence of gray dots that at RCM correspond to small hyper-reflective particles in the papillary dermis arranged in clusters or forming a network. Both structures are related to the histopathologic presence of brown-black granules in the dermis.[81,82]

AQUAGENIC PALMAR WRINKLING

Aquagenic palmar wrinkling (or aquagenic syringeal acrokeratoderma) is characterized by the presence of whitish papules and plaques on the palms and excessive wrinkling after a few minutes of contact with water. This phenomenon is related to cystic fibrosis (40%–80% of patients and 25% of carriers).

Dermatoscopy shows the presence of a hypertrophic stratum corneum with deepening of normal dermatoglyphics and a marked dilatation of eccrine ostia.[83–85] At incident light high-magnification dermatoscopy, this pattern has been defined “gruyere-like.”[85–86]

RCM examination of the lesions is similar, showing a hypertrophic stratum corneum and abnormally dilated eccrine ostia and ducts (acrosyringium),[85,87] along with increased size of keratinocytes and hyper-reflective intercellular spaces in the stratum granulosum. As palmar wrinkling is a transient phenomenon, histopathology generally does not reveal significant alterations; however, some studies reported edematous changes of the stratum corneum with increased thickness and dilated eccrine ducts.[88]

SUMMARY

In conclusion, the combined use of dermatoscopy and RCM may be useful to enhance the clinical diagnosis in a variety of cutaneous disorders, representing in several instances a promising option to reach the final diagnosis without the need of invasive procedures. In many cases dermatoscopy and RCM have shown concordance, and further studies on large series are desirable in order to define precise correlation also with histopathologic findings.

REFERENCES

1. Micali G, Lacarrubba F. Possible applications of videodermatoscopy beyond pigmented lesions. Int J Dermatol 2003;42:430–3.
2. Lacarrubba F, D’Amico V, Nasca MR, et al. Use of dermatoscopy and videodermatoscopy in therapeutic follow up: a review. Int J Dermatol 2010;49:866–73.
3. Micali G, Lacarrubba F, Massimino D, et al. Dermatoscopy: alternative uses in daily clinical practice. J Am Acad Dermatol 2011;64:1135–46.
4. Lacarrubba F. The role of imaging in dermatology. G Ital Dermatol Venereol 2015;150(5):505–6.
5. Lacarrubba F, Verzì AE, Dinotta F, et al. Dermatoscopy in inflammatory and infectious skin disorders. G Ital Dermatol Venereol 2015;150(5): 521–31.
6. Zalaudek I, Giacomel J, Cabo H, et al. Entodermoscopy: a new tool for diagnosing skin infections and infestations. Dermatology 2008;216:14–23.
7. Lallas A, Zalaudek I, Argenziano G, et al. Dermoscopy in general dermatology. Dermatol Clin 2013; 31:679–94.
8. Errichetti E, Stinco G. The practical usefulness of dermoscopy in general dermatology. G Ital Dermatol Venereol 2015;150(5):533–46.
9. Lacarrubba F, de Pasquale R, Micali G. Videodermatoscopy improves the clinical diagnostic accuracy of multiple clear cell acanthoma. Eur J Dermatol 2003;13(6):596–8.
10. Ardigò M, Agozzino M, Franceschini C, et al. Reflectance confocal microscopy algorithms for inflammatory and hair diseases. Dermatol Clin 2016;34(4): 487–96.
11. Ardigo M, Longo C, Gonzalez S, International Confocal Working Group Inflammatory Skin Diseases Project. Multicentre study on inflammatory skin diseases from The International Confocal Working Group: specific confocal microscopy features and an algorithmic method of diagnosis. Br J Dermatol 2016;175(2):364–74.
12. Lacarrubba F, Verzì AE, Pippione M, et al. Reflectance confocal microscopy in the diagnosis of vesicobullous disorders: case series with pathologic and cytologic correlation and literature review. Skin Res Technol 2016;22(4):479–86.
13. Lallas A, Kyrgidis A, Tzellos TG, et al. Accuracy of dermoscopic criteria for the diagnosis of psoriasis, dermatitis, lichen planus and pityriasis rosea. Br J Dermatol 2012;166:1198–205.
14. Errichetti E, Lacarrubba F, Micali G, et al. Differentiation of pityriasis lichenoides chronica from guttate psoriasis by dermoscopy. Clin Exp Dermatol 2015; 40(7):804–6.
15. Lacarrubba F, Pellacani G, Gurgone S, et al. Advances in non-invasive techniques as aids to the diagnosis and monitoring of therapeutic response in plaque psoriasis: a review. Int J Dermatol 2015; 54:626–34.
16. Micali G, Nardone B, Scuderi A, et al. Videodermatoscopy enhances the diagnostic capability of palmar and/or plantar psoriasis. Am J Clin Dermatol 2008;9:119–22.

17. Lacarrubba F, Nasca MR, Micali G. Videodermatoscopy enhances diagnostic capability in psoriatic balanitis. J Am Acad Dermatol 2009;61:1084–6.
18. Micali G, Lacarrubba F, Musumeci ML, et al. Cutaneous vascular patterns in psoriasis. Int J Dermatol 2010;49:249–56.
19. Lacarrubba F, Potenza MC, Micali G. Enhanced videodermoscopic visualization of superficial vascular patterns on skin using a 390- to 410-nm light. Arch Dermatol 2012;148(2):276.
20. Lacarrubba F, Musumeci ML, Ferraro S, et al. A three-cohort comparison with videodermatoscopic evidence of the distinct homogeneous bushy capillary microvascular pattern in psoriasis vs atopic dermatitis and contact dermatitis. J Eur Acad Dermatol Venereol 2016;30(4):701–3.
21. Musumeci ML, Lacarrubba F, Verzì AE, et al. Evaluation of the vascular pattern in psoriatic plaques in children using videodermatoscopy: an open comparative study. Pediatr Dermatol 2014;31:570–4.
22. Musumeci ML, Lacarrubba F, Catalfo P, et al. Videodermatoscopy evaluation of the distinct vascular pattern of psoriasis improves diagnostic capability for inverse psoriasis. G Ital Dermatol Venereol 2017;152(1):88–90.
23. Musumeci ML, Lacarrubba F, Fusto CM, et al. Combined clinical, capillaroscopic and ultrasound evaluation during treatment of plaque psoriasis with oral cyclosporine. Int J Immunopathol Pharmacol 2013;26:1027–33.
24. Micali G, Lacarrubba F, Santagati C, et al. Clinical, ultrasound, and videodermatoscopy monitoring of psoriatic patients following biological treatment. Skin Res Technol 2016;22(3):341–8.
25. Agozzino M, Berardesca E, Donadio C, et al. Reflectance confocal microscopy features of seborrheic dermatitis for plaque psoriasis differentiation. Dermatology 2014;229(3):215–21.
26. Vázquez-López F, Alvarez-Cuesta C, Hidalgo-García Y, et al. The handheld dermatoscope improves the recognition of Wickham striae and capillaries in lichen planus lesions. Arch Dermatol 2001;137:1376.
27. Vázquez-López F, Gómez-Díez S, Sánchez J, et al. Dermoscopy of active lichen planus. Arch Dermatol 2007;143:1092.
28. Pezzini C, Piana S, Longo C, et al. A solitary pink lesion: dermoscopy and RCM features of lichen planus. Dermatol Pract Concept 2017;7(4):43–5.
29. Larre Borges A, Tiodorovic-Zivkovic D, Lallas A, et al. Clinical, dermoscopic and histopathologic features of genital and extragenital lichen sclerosus. J Eur Acad Dermatol Venereol 2013;27:1433–9.
30. Lacarrubba F, Dinotta F, Nasca MR, et al. Localized vascular lesions of the glans in patients with lichen sclerosus diagnosed by dermatoscopy. G Ital Dermatol Venereol 2012;147:510–1.
31. Borghi A, Corazza M, Minghetti S, et al. Dermoscopic features of vulvar lichen sclerosus in the setting of a prospective cohort of patients: new observations. Dermatology 2016;232(1):71–7.
32. Garrido-Ríos AA, Alvarez-Garrido H, Sanz-Muñoz C, et al. Dermoscopy of extragenital lichen sclerosus. Arch Dermatol 2009;145:1468.
33. Shim WH, Jwa SW, Song M, et al. Diagnostic usefulness of dermatoscopy in differentiating lichen sclerous et atrophicus from morphea. J Am Acad Dermatol 2012;66:690–1.
34. Lacarrubba F, Pellacani G, Verzì AE, et al. Extragenital lichen sclerosus: clinical, dermoscopic, confocal microscopy and histologic correlations. J Am Acad Dermatol 2015;72:S50–2.
35. Errichetti E, Lallas A, Apalla Z, et al. Dermoscopy of morphea and cutaneous lichen sclerosus: clinicopathological correlation study and comparative analysis. Dermatology 2017;233(6):462–70.
36. Kreuter A, Gambichler T, Sauermann K, et al. Extragenital lichen sclerosus successfully treated with topical calcipotriol: evaluation by in vivo confocal laser scanning microscopy. Br J Dermatol 2002;146(2):332–3.
37. Jacquemus J, Debarbieux S, Depaepe L, et al. Reflectance confocal microscopy of extra-genital lichen sclerosus atrophicus. Skin Res Technol 2016;22(2):255–8.
38. Lallas A, Apalla Z, Karteridou A, et al. Photoletter to the editor: dermoscopy for discriminating between pityriasis rubra pilaris and psoriasis. J Dermatol Case Rep 2013;7(1):20–2.
39. López-Gómez A, Vera-Casaño Á, Gómez-Moyano E, et al. Dermoscopy of circumscribed juvenile pityriasis rubra pilaris. J Am Acad Dermatol 2015;72(1 Suppl):S58–9.
40. Abdel-Azim NE, Ismail SA, Fathy E. Differentiation of pityriasis rubra pilaris from plaque psoriasis by dermoscopy. Arch Dermatol Res 2017;309(4):311–4.
41. Pietroleonardo L, Di Stefani A, Campione E, et al. Confocal reflectance microscopy in pityriasis rubra pilaris. J Am Acad Dermatol 2013;68(4):689–91.
42. Errichetti E, Lacarrubba F, Micali G, et al. Dermoscopy of Zoon's plasma cell balanitis. J Eur Acad Dermatol Venereol 2016;30(12):e209–10.
43. Corazza M, Virgili A, Minghetti S, et al. Dermoscopy in plasma cell balanitis: its usefulness in diagnosis and follow-up. J Eur Acad Dermatol Venereol 2016;30(1):182–4.
44. Lacarrubba F, Verzì AE, Ardigò M, et al. Handheld reflectance confocal microscopy, dermatoscopy and histopathological correlation of common inflammatory balanitis. Skin Res Technol 2018. https://doi.org/10.1111/srt.12460.
45. Arzberger E, Komericki P, Ahlgrimm-Siess V, et al. Differentiation between balanitis and carcinoma in

situ using reflectance confocal microscopy. JAMA Dermatol 2013;149(4):440–5.
46. Errichetti E, Stinco G, Lacarrubba F, et al. Dermoscopy of Darier's disease. J Eur Acad Dermatol Venereol 2016;30(8):1392–4.
47. Errichetti E, De Francesco V, Pegolo E, et al. Dermoscopy of Grover's disease: variability according to histological subtype. J Dermatol 2016;43(8):937–9.
48. Lacarrubba F, Boscaglia S, Nasca MR, et al. Grover's disease: dermoscopy, reflectance confocal microscopy and histopathological correlation. Dermatol Pract Concept 2017;7(3):51–4.
49. Sadayasu A, Maumi Y, Hayashi Y, et al. Dermoscopic features of a case of transient acantholytic dermatosis. Australas J Dermatol 2017;58(1):50–2.
50. Lacarrubba F, Verzì AE, Errichetti E, et al. Darier's disease: dermoscopy, confocal microscopy and histological correlations. J Am Acad Dermatol 2015; 73(3):e97–9.
51. Alfaro-Castellón P, Mejía-Rodríguez SA, Valencia-Herrera A, et al. Dermoscopy distinction of eruptive vellus hair cysts with molluscum contagiosum and acne lesions. Pediatr Dermatol 2012;29(6):772–3.
52. Lacarrubba F, Dall'Oglio F, Musumeci ML, et al. Secondary comedones in a case of acne conglobata correlate with double-ended pseudocomedones in hidradenitis suppurativa. Acta Derm Venereol 2017;97(8):969–70.
53. Lora V, Capitanio B, Ardigò M. Noninvasive, in vivo assessment of comedone re-formation. Skin Res Technol 2015;21(3):384–6.
54. Manfredini M, Mazzaglia G, Ciardo S, et al. Acne: in vivo morphologic study of lesions and surrounding skin by means of reflectance confocal microscopy. J Eur Acad Dermatol Venereol 2015;29(5): 933–9.
55. Manfredini M, Greco M, Farnetani F, et al. In vivo monitoring of topical therapy for acne with reflectance confocal microscopy. Skin Res Technol 2017;23(1):36–40.
56. Morales A, Puig S, Malvehy J, et al. Dermoscopy of molluscum contagiosum. Arch Dermatol 2005;141:1644.
57. Lacarrubba F, Verzì AE, Ardigò M, et al. Handheld reflectance confocal microscopy for the diagnosis of molluscum contagiosum: histopathology and dermoscopy correlation. Australas J Dermatol 2017; 58(3):e123–5.
58. Dong H, Shu D, Campbell TM, et al. Dermatoscopy of genital warts. J Am Acad Dermatol 2011;64:859–64.
59. Micali G, Lacarrubba F. Augmented diagnostic capability using videodermatoscopy on selected infectious and non-infectious penile growths. Int J Dermatol 2011;50:1501–5.
60. Lacarrubba F, Dinotta F, Nasca MR, et al. Enhanced diagnosis of genital warts with videodermatoscopy: histopatologic correlation. G Ital Dermatol Venereol 2012;147:215–6.
61. Veasey JV, Framil VM, Nadal SR, et al. Genital warts: comparing clinical findings to dermatoscopic aspects, in vivo reflectance confocal features and histopathologic exam. An Bras Dermatol 2014;89(1):137–40.
62. Micali G, Lacarrubba F, Lo Guzzo G. Scraping versus videodermatoscopy for the diagnosis of scabies: a comparative study. Acta Derm Venereol 1999;79(5):396.
63. Lacarrubba F, Musumeci ML, Caltabiano R, et al. High-magnification videodermatoscopy: a new noninvasive diagnostic tool for scabies in children. Pediatr Dermatol 2001;18(5):439–41.
64. Micali G, Tedeschi A, West DP, et al. The use of videodermatoscopy to monitor treatment of scabies and pediculosis. J Dermatolog Treat 2011;22(3): 133–7.
65. Micali G, Lacarrubba F, Verzì AE, et al. Low-cost equipment for diagnosis and management of endemic scabies outbreaks in underserved populations. Clin Infect Dis 2015;60(2):327–9.
66. Lacarrubba F, Micali G. Videodermatoscopy and scabies. J Pediatr 2013;163(4):1227–1227.e1.
67. Micali G, Lacarrubba F, Verzì AE, et al. Scabies: advances in noninvasive diagnosis. PLoS Negl Trop Dis 2016;10(6):e0004691.
68. Lacarrubba F, Verzì AE, Micali G. Detailed Analysis of in vivo reflectance confocal microscopy for Sarcoptes scabiei hominis. Am J Med Sci 2015;350(5):414.
69. Segal R, Mimouni D, Feuerman H, et al. Dermoscopy as a diagnostic tool in demodicidosis. Int J Dermatol 2010;49(9):1018–23.
70. Friedman P, Sabban EC, Cabo H. Usefulness of dermoscopy in the diagnosis and monitoring treatment of demodicidosis. Dermatol Pract Concept 2017; 7(1):35–8.
71. Turgut Erdemir A, Gurel MS, Koku Aksu AE, et al. Reflectance confocal microscopy vs. standardized skin surface biopsy for measuring the density of Demodex mites. Skin Res Technol 2014;20(4):435–9.
72. Piliouras P, Allison S, Rosendahl S, et al. Dermoscopy improves diagnosis of tinea nigra: a study of 50 cases. Australas J Dermatol 2011;52:191–4.
73. Lacarrubba F, Dall'oglio F, Dinotta F, et al. Photoletter to the editor: Exogenous pigmentation of the sole mimicking in situ acral melanoma on dermoscopy. J Dermatol Case Rep 2012;6(3):100–1.
74. Veasey JV, Avila RB, Ferreira MAMO, et al. Reflectance confocal microscopy of tinea nigra: comparing images with dermoscopy and mycological examination results. An Bras Dermatol 2017; 92(4):568–9.
75. Uva L, Leal-Filipe P, Soares-de-Almeida L, et al. Reflectance confocal microscopy for the diagnosis of tinea nigra. Clin Exp Dermatol 2018;43(3):332–4.
76. Palmer A, Bowling J. Dermoscopic appearance of juvenile xanthogranuloma. Dermatology 2007;215: 256–9.

77. Pretel M, Irarrazaval I, Lera M, et al. Dermoscopic "setting sun" pattern of juvenile xanthogranuloma. J Am Acad Dermatol 2015;72:S73–5.
78. Song M, Kim SH, Jung DS, et al. Structural correlations between dermoscopic and histopathological features of juvenile xanthogranuloma. J Eur Acad Dermatol Venereol 2011;25:259–63.
79. Lovato L, Salerni G, Puig S, et al. Adult xanthogranuloma mimicking basal cell carcinoma: dermoscopy, reflectance confocal microscopy and pathological correlation. Dermatology 2010;220(1):66–70.
80. Koku Aksu AE, Turgut Erdemir AV, Gurel MS, et al. In vivo evaluation of juvenile xanthogranuloma with high-resolution optical coherence tomography and reflectance confocal microscopy and histopathological correlation. Skin Res Technol 2015;21(4): 508–10.
81. García-Martínez P, López Aventín D, Segura S, et al. In vivo reflectance confocal microscopy characterization of silver deposits in localized cutaneous argyria. Br J Dermatol 2016;175(5):1052–5.
82. Cinotti E, Labeille B, Douchet C, et al. Dermoscopy, reflectance confocal microscopy, and high-definition optical coherence tomography in the diagnosis of generalized argyria. J Am Acad Dermatol 2017; 76(2S1):S66–8.
83. Ghosh SK, Agarwal M, Ghosh S, et al. Aquagenic palmar wrinkling in two Indian patients with special reference to its dermoscopic pattern. Dermatol Online J 2015;21(6) [pii:13030/qt0hr3d0bn].
84. Gualdi G, Pavoni L, Monari P, et al. Dermoscopy of drug-induced aquagenic wrinkling phenomenon. J Eur Acad Dermatol Venereol 2016;30(7): 1211–2.
85. Lacarrubba F, Verzì AE, Leonardi S, et al. Palmar wrinkling: identification of a peculiar pattern at incident light dermoscopy with confocal microscopy correlation. J Am Acad Dermatol 2016; 75(4):e143–5.
86. Micali G, Verzì AE, Lacarrubba F. Alternative uses of dermatoscopy in daily clinical practice: an update. J Am Acad Dermatol 2018 Jun 16. pii: S0190-9622(18)32143-1. [Epub ahead of print].
87. Okuhira H, Matsunaka H, Iwahashi Y, et al. Case report of aquagenic wrinkling of the palms associated with impaired stratum corneum function. J Dermatol 2015;42(9):913–4.
88. Bielicky L, Braun-Falco M, Ruzicka T, et al. Aquagenic wrinkling of the palms: morphological changes in reflectance confocal microscopy and high-definition optical coherence tomography. Dermatology 2015;230:208–12.

Printed and bound by CPI Group (UK) Ltd, Croydon, CR0 4YY
03/10/2024
01040299-0003